Predicting Heart Failure

Predicting Heart Failure

Invasive, Non-Invasive, Machine Learning, and Artificial Intelligence Based Methods

Edited by

Kishor Kumar Sadasivuni
Qatar University
Doha, Qatar

Hassen M. Ouakad
Sultan Qaboos University
Muscat, Oman

Somaya Al-Maadeed
Qatar University
Doha, Qatar

Huseyin C. Yalcin
Qatar University
Doha, Qatar

Issam Bait Bahadur
Sultan Qaboos University
Muscat, Oman

WILEY

This edition first published 2022

Registered Offices
John Wiley & Sons, Inc., 111 River Street, Hoboken, NJ 07030, USA
John Wiley & Sons Ltd, The Atrium, Southern Gate, Chichester, West Sussex, PO19 8SQ, UK

Editorial Office
9600 Garsington Road, Oxford, OX4 2DQ, UK

For details of our global editorial offices, customer services, and more information about Wiley products visit us at www.wiley.com.

Wiley also publishes its books in a variety of electronic formats and by print-on-demand. Some content that appears in standard print versions of this book may not be available in other formats.

Library of Congress Cataloging-in-Publication Data
Names: Kumar Sadasivuni, Kishor, 1986- author.
Title: Predicting heart failure : invasive, non-invasive,machine learning
and artificial intelligence based methods / edited by Kishor Kumar Sadasivuni, Qatar University, Doha, Qatar, Hassen M. Ouakad, Sultan Qaboos University, Muscat, Oman, Somaya Al-Maadeed, Qatar University, Doha, Qatar, Huseyin C. Yalcin, Qatar University, Doha, Qatar, Issam Bait Bahadur, Sultan Qaboos University, Muscat, Oman.
Description: Hoboken, NJ : John Wiley & Sons, 2022. | Includes bibliographical references and index.
Identifiers: LCCN 2021043721 (print) | LCCN 2021043722 (ebook) | ISBN 9781119813019 (hardback) | ISBN 9781119813026 (pdf) | ISBN 9781119813033 (epub) | ISBN 9781119813040 (obook)
Subjects: LCSH: Heart failure--Risk factors. | Heart failure--Treatment. | Heart--Diseases--Patients.
Classification: LCC RC685.C53 P74 2023 (print) | LCC RC685.C53 (ebook) | DDC 616.1/29--dc23/eng/20211028
LC record available at https://lccn.loc.gov/2021043721
LC ebook record available at https://lccn.loc.gov/2021043722

Cover image: Courtesy of Kishor Kumar Sadasivuni
Cover design by Wiley

Set in 9.5/12.5pt STIXTwoText by Integra Software Services Pvt. Ltd, Pondicherry, India

Contents

Preface

Our knowledge of human biology, especially related to the heart, increases every day. This makes it nearly impossible for physicians to stay current on the latest research in their fields, let alone in all of the others that directly affect their ability to treat their patients properly. This book will help in learning the mechanics and symptoms of heart failure and the various approaches, including conventional and modern techniques for diagnosing it. Moreover, the book provides a detailed presentation of the latest research data for preventing and treating heart failure.

In this book, 13 chapters address different conditions related to the heart, with detailed descriptions of each. The first chapter discusses invasive, non-invasive, machine learning, and artificial intelligence-based methods for predicting heart failure. In addition, it discusses heart failure causes, symptoms, and treatment, as well as research related to heart failure. In the second chapter, we examine the traditional methods of predicting heart diseases and the implementation of artificial intelligence technology to predict heart diseases accurately. A discussion of the main characteristics of cardiovascular biosensors is presented in Chapter 3, along with their open issues for development and application. We summarize the difficulties of wireless sensor communication and power transfer in Chapters 4, 5, and 6, which outline the utility of artificial intelligence in cardiology. Chapter 7 discusses how to predict heart diseases using data mining classification techniques. Applied machine learning is discussed in Chapters 8 and 9 as are advanced methods for estimating heart failure severity and for diagnosing and predicting heart failure. In Chapter 10, the present state of artificial intelligence and biosensors based on materials is briefly discussed. The underlying technologies of various invasive and non-invasive devices, and their benefits, are discussed and analyzed in Chapter 11. A discussion of the risks and issues associated with remote monitoring systems is also included in this chapter. An overview of these heart failure prediction devices is presented in Chapter 12 along with their invasive and non-invasive alternatives. The chapter also highlights the potential of artificial intelligence in mobile monitoring technologies to provide clinicians with improved treatment options, ultimately easing access to healthcare by all patient populations. Chapter 13 assesses the potential applications of implantable and wearable devices in heart failure detection, summarizes the available data for wearables and machine learning for improving patients' cardiac health, and discusses the future of wearables for early prediction of heart failure.

Finally we strongly believe this book will provides a comprehensive but concise guide to all modern cardiological practice, emphasizing practical clinical management in many different contexts. The book provides readers with trustworthy insights into all aspects of heart failure, including essential background information on clinical practice guidelines, in-depth, peer-reviewed articles, and broad coverage of this fast-moving field. It provides the latest research data needed for the diagnosis and treatment of heart failure. Moreover, this book is an excellent resource for nurses, nurse practitioners, physician assistants, medical students, and general practitioners to gain a better understanding of bedside cardiology.

Abbreviations

Chapter 1

3-D	Three-dimensional, 10
BNP	Brain Natriuretic Peptide, 9
CAD	Coronary Artery Disease, 2
CHF	Congestive Heart Failure, 3
CRP	C-reactive Protein, 8
HF	Heart Failure, 3
HRV	Heart Rate Variability, 24
IoT	Internet of Things, 11
LS-SVM	Least Squares SVM, 24
LV	Left Ventricular, 23
SVM	Support Vector Machine, 18

Chapter 2

ACS	Acute Coronary Syndrome, 8
AI	Artificial Intelligence, 18 bp Blood Pressure, 12
CAC	Coronary Artery Calcium, 21
CCA	Common Carotid Artery, 19
CHF	Congestive Heart Failure, 20
CNN	Convolutional Neural Network, 20
CQ-NSGT	Constant-Q Non-Stationary Gabor Transform, 20
CT	Computed Tomography, 19
CVDs	Cardiovascular Diseases, 19
DNN	Deep Neural Network, 20
DOE	Dyspnea on Exertion, 10
ECG	Electrocardiogram, 5
ELM	Extreme Learning Machines, 20
FCN	Fully Convolutional Network, 20
GERD	Gastroesophageal Reflux Disease, 9
HDL	High-density Lipoprotein, 12
ICA	Internal Carotid Artery, 19
IMT	Intima-Media Thickness, 19
LDL	Low-density Lipoprotein, 12

LI	Lumen-intima, 19
LII	Lumen-Intima Interface, 20
MA	Media Adventitia, 19
MAI	Media-Adventitia Interface, 20
MLP	Multilayer Perceptron, 21
MPI	Myocardial Perfusion Imaging, 22
NSR	Normal Sinus Rhythm, 20
PND	Paroxysmal Nocturnal Dyspnea, 11

Chapter 3

BNP	Brain Natriuretic Peptide, 5
CRP	C-Reactive Protein, 3
CSGMs	Comb Structured Gold Microelectrode Arrays, 28
cTnI	Cardiac Troponin I, 5
CV	Cyclic Voltammetry, 28
CVDs	Cardiovascular Diseases, 1
DPV	Differential Pulse Voltammetry, 28
EIS	Electrochemical Impedance Spectroscopy, 28
ELISA	Enzyme-Linked Immunosorbent Assay, 29
ENPs	Enzyme Nanoparticles, 29
GDF	Growth Differentiation Factor, 7
GK	Glycerol Kinase, 29
GO	Graphene Oxide, 28
GPO	Glycerol-3- Phosphate Oxidase, 29
HDL	High-density Lipoprotein, 8
hour-FABP	Heart Fatty Acid-Binding Protein, 7
IL-6	Interleukin-6, 7
LDL	Low-density Lipoprotein, 8
LOD	Limit of Detection, 10
LSPR	Localized Surface Plasmon Resonance, 12
miRNAs	Micro RNAs, 6
MPO	Myeloperoxidase, 6
NPs	Nanoparticles, 29
NSE	Neuron-specific Enolase, 6
PCT	Procalcitonin, 5
PEC	Photoelectrochemical, 28
PG	Pencil Graphite, 29
QDs	Quantum Dots, 28
SEM	Scanning Electron Microscopy, 28
SERS	Surface-Enhanced Raman Scattering, 12
SPEs	Screen-Printed Electrodes, 28
SPGEs	Screen-Printed Gold Electrodes, 28
SPR	Surface Plasmon Resonance, 12
SPRi	Surface Plasmon Resonance Imaging, 12
sST2	Soluble Suppressor of Tumorgenicity 2, 8

TG	Triglycerides, 9
TNF-α,	Tumor Necrosis Factor-alpha, 7

Chapter 4

AC	Alternative Current, 9
BSN	Body Sensor Network, 2 CE Counter Electrode, 5
CMT	Coupled-Mode Theory, 12
EDAS	European Aeronautic Defense and Space Company, 10
EM	Electromagnetic Interference, 11
EMF	Electromagnetic Field, 9
HPF	High-Pass Filter, 17
IoT	Internet of Things, 2
LPF	Low Pass Filter, 17
MEMS	Micro-Electromechanical Systems, 4
MPT	Microwave Power Transmission, 8
RE	Reference Electrode, 5
RF	Radio Frequency, 3
SHM	Structural Health Supervising, 2
SoC	System on a Chip, 5
VSWR	Voltage Standing Wave Ratio, 24
WBAN	Wireless Body Area Network, 2
WE	Working Electrode, 5

Chapter 5

BCG	Ballistocardiography, 13
BLUE	Bedside Lung Ultrasound, 10
BNP	B-type Natriuretic Peptide, 14
C.A.USE	Cardiac Arrest Ultrasound Exam, 10
CHF	Chronic Heart Failure, 2
DNN	Deep Neural Network, 12
ECG	Electrocardiography, 3
EVLW	Extravascular Lung Water, 8
FALLS	Fluid Administration Limited by Lung Sonography, 10
GPS	Global Positioning System, 6
HF	Heart failure, 2
ICD	Implantable Cardioverter Defibrillator, 12
LuCUS	Lung and Cardiac Ultrasound, 10
LUS	Lung Ultrasound, 8
LV	Left Ventricular, 7
MEMS	Microelectromechanical System, 6
MFCCs	Mel-frequency Cepstral Coefficients, 12
NT-proBNP	Amino-terminal Pro-B-type Natriuretic Peptide, 14
PA	Pulmonary Arterial, 7
PCG	Phonocardiogram, 12

PPG	Photoplethysmogram, 14
RCTs	Randomized Control Trials, 15
ReDS	Remote Dielectric Sensing Technology, 5
RPM	Remote Patient Monitoring, 15
RV	Right Ventricular, 7
SCG	Seismocardiography, 12

Chapter 6

ACM	All-cause Mortality, 8
AI	Artificial Intelligence, 3, 8
ANN	Artificial Neural Networks, 3,12
AUC	Area Under the Curve, 9
CAD	Coronary Artery Disease, 8
CCTA	Cardiac Computed Tomographic Angiography, 8
CMR	Cardiac Magnetic Resonance, 12
CNN	Convolutional Neural Networks, 12
DL	Deep learning, 12
ECG	Electrocardiogram, 9
FDA	Food and Drug Administration, 17
FFR	Fractional Flow Reserve, 9
FRS	Framingham Risk Score, 8
GAN	Generative Adversarial Networks, 11
GAN	Generative Adversarial Networks, 3
HFpEF	Heart Failure with Preserved Ejection Fraction, 10
HMM	Hidden Markov Model, 15
LASSO	Least Absolute Shrinkage and Selection Operator, 3
LV	Left Ventricle, 9
LVEF	Left Ventricular Ejection Fraction, 12
MDI	Modified Duke Index, 8
MFR	Myocardial Flow Reserve, 9
ML	Machine Learning, 3
MPI	Myocardial Perfusion Imaging, 15
MPS	Myocardial Perfusion Scan, 9
NER	Names Entity Recognition, 15
NLP	Natural Language Processing, 15
POS	Part of Speech, 15
PSA	Parsing or Syntactic Analysis, 15
RNN	Recurrent Neural Networks, 12
SIS	Segment Involvement Score, 8
SSS	Segment Stenosis Score, 8
STE	Speckle-tracking Echocardiography, 11
SVMs	Support Vector Machines, 8
TPD	Total Perfusion Deficit, 15
TTE	Transthoracic Echocardiogram, 12

Chapter 7

DT	Decision Tree, 2
K-NN	K-Nearest Neighbor, 5
LDA	Linear Discriminant Analysis, 2
MAFIA	Maximal Frequent Itemset Algorithm, 4
NB	Naïve Bayes, 2
NN	Neural Networks, 4
RF	Random Forest, 2
SVM	Support Vector Machine, 2

Chapter 8

AUPRC	Area Under Precision Recall curve, 10
AUROC	Area Under ROC Curve, 10
BNP	Brain Natriuretic Peptide, 4
CNN	Convolutional Neural Networks, 7
DAE	Denoising Autoencoder, 7
DBNs	Deep Belief Networks, 7
DT	Decision Tree, 7
ECG	Electrocardiogram, 3
EHR	Electronic Health Records, 5
EMB	Endomyocardial Biopsy, 7
ESC	European Society of Cardiology, 4
GBM	Gradient-boosted Model, 11
GRU RNNs	Gated Recurrent Unit Recurrent Neural Networks, 9
GWTG-HF	Get With The Guidelines-Heart Failure, 11
HF	Heart Failure, 2
KNNs	K-nearest Neighbors, 7
LAD	Left Atrial Dimension, 10
LR	Logistic Regression, 11
LSTM	Long Short-Term Memory, 7
MAGGIC	Meta-Analysis Global Group in Chronic, 11
ML	Machine Learning, 2
ReLU	Rectified Linear Unit, 8
RETAIN	REverse Time AttentIoN Model, 9
RF	Random Forest, 8
RNN	recurrent Neural Networks, 7
ROI	Regions of Interests, 8
RPM	Remote Patient Monitoring, 5
SVM	Support Vector Machine, 7
TAN	Tree-augmented Naive Bayesian, 11

Chapter 9

AF	Atrial Fibrillation, 9
AFL	Atrial Flutter, 10
AUC	Area Under the Roc Curve, 8
BN	Bayes Network, 31
CART	Classification and Regression Trees, 15
CFS	Correlation-based Feature Selection, 31
CMR	Cardiac Magnetic Resonance, 6
CNN	Convolutional Neural Network, 9
CTCA	Computed Tomography Coronary Angiography, 6
DL	Deep Learning, 8
DNN	Deep Neural Network, 9
DUNs	Deep Unified Networks, 20
ECG	Electrocardiogram, 6
EF	Ejection Fraction, 5
EFFECT	Enhanced Feedback for Effective Cardiac Treatment, 10
EHR	Electronic Health Record, 8
ELM	Extreme Learning Machine, 10
ESC	European Society of Cardiology, 6
GDS	Generalized Discriminant Analysis, 16
GLM	Generalized Linear Model, 23
HF	Heart Failure, 1
HFmrEF	HF with Mid-range or Mildly Reduced EF, 5
HFpEF	Heart Failure with Preserved Ejection Fraction, 5
HFrEF	Heart Failure with Reduced Ejection Fraction, 5
HRV	Heart Rate Variability, 9
K-NN	K-nearest Neighbor, 8
LGE	Late Gadolinium Enhancement, 6
LMT	Logistic Model Trees, 31
LR	Logistic Regression, 8
LS-SVM	Least Square SVM, 9
LSTM	Long Short-term Memory, 9
MAGGIC	Meta-analysis Global Group in Chronic, 24
ML	Machine Learning, 7
MLP	Multilayer Perceptron, 8
NB	Naïve Bayes, 34
NLP	Natural Language Processing, 16
NN	Neural Network, 8
NRD	Nationwide Readmissions Database, 21
NYHA	New York Heart Association, 5
RBF	Radial Basis Function, 18
RDW	Red Blood Cell Distribution Width, 26
RF	Random Forest, 9
RNN	Recurrent Neural Network, 8

ROT	Rotation Forest, 16
RS	Rough Set, 8
RSA	Random Search Algorithm, 10
SAE	Sparse Auto-encoder, 9
SGD	Stochastic Gradient Descent, 9
SVM	Support Vector Machines, 8

Chapter 10

AI	Artificial Intelligence, 1 bp Blood Pressure, 11
CAD	Coronary Artery Disease, 15
CT	Computed Tomography, 15
CVDs	Cardiovascular Diseases, 1
DL	Deep Learning, 12
ECG	Electrocardiogram, 1
EIS	Electrochemical Impedance Spectroscopy, 4
IoT	The Internet of Things, 11
MRI	Magnetic Resonance Imaging, 2,13
RI	Refractive Index, 6

Chapter 11

BMI	Body Mass Index, 9
CHF	Chronic Heart Failures, 2
CIHM	Chronicle Implantable Hemodynamic Monitor, 19
CRT	Cardiac Resynchronization Therapy, 19
HCG	Human Chorionic Gonadotropin, 21
IASD	Inter Atrial Shunt Device, 22
LA	Left Atrial, 17
LAP	Left Atrial Pressure, 18
MCT	Mobile Cardiac Telemetry, 6
NYHA	New York Heart Association, 19
PA	Pulmonary Artery, 17
PAM	Patient Advisory Module, 20
RV	Right Ventricle, 17

Chapter 12

AI	Artificial Intelligence, 3
ANN	Artificial Neural Networks, 4
AUC	Area Under Curve, 6
CNN	Convolutional Neural Network, 4
CRT	Cardiac Resynchronization Therapy, 6
DL	Deep Learning, 3
DNN	Deep Neural Network, 5
ECG	Electrocardiographic, 5

HF	Heart Failure, 1
k-NN	k-Nearest Neighbors, 5
LVAD	Left Ventricular Assist Device, 7
ML	Machine Learning, 3
PPGs	Photoplethysmograms, 8
RF	Random Forest, 4
RNN	Recurrent Neural Network, 5
RV	Right Ventricular, 2
RVF	Right-ventricular Failure, 7
RVFRS	Right Ventricular Failure Risk Score, 7
SVM	Support Vector Machine, 4

Chapter 13

ABP	Arterial Blood Pressure, 4
AF	Atrial Fibrillation, 11
CAD	Coronary Artery Diseases, 19
CardioMEMS	Cardio-Microelectromechanical system, 3
CRT	Cardiac Resynchronization Therapy, 18
CRT-D	Cardiac Resynchronization Therapy Defibrillator, 4
CVDs	Cardiovascular Diseases, 3
ECG	Electrocardiogram, 2
FDA	Food and Drug Administration, 13
HF	Heart Failure, 1
hour	Heart Rate, 13
ICDs	Implantable Cardioverter-defibrillators, 5
LAP	Left Atrial Pressure, 5
LVAD	Left Ventricular Assist Device, 18
MI	Myocardial Infarction, 14
NSTEMI	Non-ST-elevation Myocardial Infarction, 18
NYHA	New York Heart Association, 10
OHRM	Optical Heart Rate Monitor, 9
PAP	Pulmonary Artery Pressure, 3
PD	Photodiode, 9
PPG	Photoplethysmogram, 4
RR	Respiration Rate, 13
STEMI	ST-elevation Myocardial Infarction, 18
SVM	Support Vector Machine, 18
VF	Ventricular Fibrillation, 11

Acknowledgment

This publication was supported by Qatar University Internal Grant No. IRCC-2020-013 and Sultan Qaboos University through Grant # CL/SQU-QU/ENG/20/01, respectively. The findings achieved herein are solely the responsibility of the authors.

1

Invasive, Non-Invasive, Machine Learning, and Artificial Intelligence Based Methods for Prediction of Heart Failure

Hidayet Takcı

1.1 Introduction

Heart diseases are the deadliest in the world. Of the many diseases included in the category of heart disease, the most prominent is coronary artery disease (CAD), which causes heart attacks. CAD, high blood pressure, and many other heart diseases cause heart failure (HF). With HF being a consequence of heart disease, the prediction of HF is related to the prediction of diseases categorized as heart disease.

In this chapter, the diagnosis of HF is discussed in terms of invasive/non-invasive and artificial intelligence/machine learning techniques. Invasive and non-invasive techniques are distinct in the way the patient is treated. Invasive methods are usually associated with a physical intervention in the body. This intervention involves operations such as taking blood for blood analysis and not pressing strongly on the abdominal area. Non-invasive methods include physical therapy, taking blood pressure, and temperature measurement. In today's world, where information technologies have evolved in every field, the field of health has also received its share. Computer-aided clinical decision support systems provide the strongest support for diagnostic studies today. The most important components of computer-aided diagnosis are artificial intelligence and machine learning systems that offer a wide range of services from smart assistant applications to imaging techniques. Artificial intelligence and machine learning have a healing role in electrocardiography, echocardiography, and similar invasive and non-invasive techniques.

In the second section of this chapter, HF will be described and its causes, symptoms, and treatment revealed. The third section will explain diagnosis by invasive and non-invasive methods. Computer-aided diagnosis and decision support systems are briefly mentioned in the fourth section. The fifth section looks first at what artificial intelligence is and then presents fields and examples of artificial intelligence supported studies. The sixth section explains machine learning, learning types, machine learning algorithms, and machine learning based diagnostic studies. The chapter's concluding section summarizes studies and comments upon diagnostic studies for HF.

Predicting Heart Failure: Invasive, Non-Invasive, Machine Learning, and Artificial Intelligence Based Methods, First Edition. Edited by Kishor Kumar Sadasivuni, Hassen M. Ouakad, Somaya Al-Maadeed, Huseyin C. Yalcin, and Issam Bait Bahadur.

1.2 Heart Failure

HF belongs to a class of diseases that occur due to several diseases known as heart diseases and can be fatal if left untreated. In this section, HF is defined and the factors causing it, its symptoms, and its treatment are examined.

1.2.1 What is HF?

HF is sometimes known as congestive HF (CHF). HF is not a failure of the heart, but a condition in which the heart muscle cannot pump enough blood. It occurs due to, for example, narrowing of the coronary arteries, cardiovascular diseases, and high blood pressure.

HF can occur at any age, but is more common in older people. Although it is not possible to cure the disease, some of its symptoms can be improved by the correct interventions. Conversely, faulty interventions will make the situation worse than before.

The most common symptoms of HF are shortness of breath after movement or during rest, fatigue and weakness, swelling in the ankles and legs, disturbed heartbeat, persistent cough, and dizziness and the like. Symptoms can develop rapidly (acute HF) or gradually over weeks (chronic HF).

With early intervention for HF, it will be possible for patients to live longer. Some measures such as losing weight, reducing stress, and reducing the amount of salt used will positively affect the quality of life of patients. One way to prevent HF is to prevent and control conditions such as CAD, high blood pressure, diabetes, and obesity.

The activity that will benefit most is diagnosing the disease and conducting studies according to the symptoms. Thus, as in many other diseases, early diagnosis will have a life-saving effect in HF, as will correct diagnosis and determining the type and real cause of the ailment.

1.2.2 Causes of HF

As mentioned, the causes of HF are CAD, high blood pressure, and other heart diseases, and it occurs because of the damage to the heart muscle brought about by these and similar conditions. While oxygen is regularly carried to a normal heart, it is not possible to carry enough oxygen in the case of a damaged heart. Although HF usually occurs on the left side of the heart, it can develop on the right or both sides. Table 1.1 lists multiple HF types and their results.

Some of the prominent causes of HF are:

- **CAD and heart attack**: CAD is the most prominent heart disease and the most common cause of HF. The disease occurs when blood circulation is not normal due to fat deposits, called plaques, in the blood vessels. Heart attacks are divided into mild heart attack and major heart attack. Mild heart attacks occur in a small portion of the heart muscle. However, a mild heart attack should be taken seriously because it can cause a second attack. Major heart attack affects a large part of the heart muscle.

Table 1.1 HF types and their outcomes.

HF Type	Outcome
Left-sided HF	This causes fluid to accumulate in the lungs, which causes shortness of breath in people.
Right-sided HF	Fluid builds up in the abdomen, legs, and feet, which causes swelling in the abdomen and legs.
Systolic HF	This occurs when the heart muscle cannot contract strongly as it should; as a result, blood is not pumped in the normal way.
Diastolic HF	There is insufficient blood filling the area due to the inability of the heart to relax sufficiently.

The blood flow to the heart is completely blocked or there is no blood flow for a long time. Major heart attack can cause cardiac arrest and death.

- **High blood pressure (hypertension)**: High blood pressure is one of the factors that makes it difficult for the heart to pump blood to the body. This strain causes the heart muscle to work more than normal, damaging it.
- **Faulty heart valves**: The function of the heart valves is to keep the blood flowing in the right direction. Failure of heart valves to function is known as heart valve malfunction. Heart valve malfunctions can be caused by genetic factors, old age, and infection. A faulty valve tires the heart, forcing it to work harder and causing it to weaken over time.
- **Damage to the heart muscle (cardiomyopathy)**: Cardiomyopathy can have many causes, such as various diseases, infections, alcohol use, and the toxic effect of drugs like cocaine or chemotherapy drugs. Sometimes it can be due to genetic factors.
- **Heart muscle inflammation**: This is caused by viruses and can lead to left-sided HF.
- **Congenital heart defects**: If the heart and chambers or valves aren't formed correctly, the healthy parts of the heart have to work harder to pump blood, which can lead to HF.
- **Heart arrhythmias:** Abnormal heart rhythms will show heart-damaging output in both fast heartbeat and slow heartbeat. Its rapid beating will tire the heart, and its slow beating will cause problems in circulation.
- **Other diseases**: Diabetes, HIV, hyperthyroid and similar diseases can also cause HF.

Heart diseases and the factors that affect the HF that occur as a result may be genetic, sometimes congenital abnormalities, and sometimes related to our lifestyle. Overweight, having a sedentary life, smoking, and stressful work life are also harmful factors for the heart [1].

1.2.3 What are the Symptoms of HF?

HF may be faced if one or more of the following symptoms are present. For example, if someone is tired earlier than before even though they are doing the same activity, this might be a symptom. This symptom should not be confused with early fatigue due to old age – a 55-year-old person should compare and interpret their symptoms according to their current age, not to what it was at the age of 45 or younger.

Another symptom of HF is loss of appetite, which can be related to other ailments. Therefore, the loss of appetite that occurs without any external cause should be evaluated. Another symptom associated with loss of appetite may be nausea, which can also occur with extreme sensitivity to some foods and certain odors. Due to HF, blood accumulates in the abdomen and presses on the intestinal wall and stomach. This pressure causes loss of appetite and nausea.

HF can also cause shortness of breath, but is not, of course, the only cause of this; severe shortness of breath is possible in the case of advanced bronchitis and asthma, which includes narrowing of the airways and chest, and a wheezing sound from the lungs. Shortness of breath caused by HF occurs due to pulmonary edema. It is accompanied by fatigue and weakness, caused by heart-induced constriction; shortness of breath is caused by bronchitis or asthma and, similarly, often by overweight and obesity. Shortness of breath experienced without an external cause should be taken seriously.

Everyone has a certain gradual transition in weight gain and weight loss. Under normal conditions, this situation does not develop suddenly, so sudden weight gain might be associated with HF. The relationship between HF and weight gain is related to the weakness of some organs in performing their duties due to the inability of the heart. When the calories taken into the body through food are more than the calories consumed by the body, this excess is stored as fat. Insulin resistance develops due to excess fat in the body and one of the diseases caused by insulin resistance is HF. The measurement of excess fat is carried out with the help of the body weight index (BMI). Those with a BMI of 25–29.9 are considered overweight and those with a BMI over 30 are considered obese. In addition, these values change depending on age. While the normal BMI values for 25–35-year-olds are 20–25, this BMI value is 24–29 for those over 65 years old.

One of the most important indicators of possible heart disease is chest pain. Sometimes people may panic due to the sensitivity of the subject. Some problems in the digestive system, such as bloating in the stomach, can cause chest pain and tightness in the chest area. However, it is best not to leave it to chance.

Coughing and related sputum production of pink or white color may also be a harbinger of HF. As will be appreciated, heart disease is not the only cause of a cough, but it is one of its causes.

Interrelated heart palpitations and pulse irregularities are also associated with HF. In addition, swelling of the ankles, legs, and abdomen due to edema can occur as a result of right-sided heart problems. Seeing one or more of these problems can also be viewed as a symptom.

People often find themselves in a state of indolence when they are low in morale. They want to sleep all the time and cannot easily concentrate on any task. The condition that manifests itself as in the body may sometimes indicate a heart problem.

Two other problems with HF are frequent urination at night and the prominence of blood vessels in the neck. The accumulated blood in the abdominal region of HF patients who go into a supine position enters the circulation. As a result, the kidneys detect excess volume and this increases urination. HF can be suspected if blood sugar is normal but there is frequent urination at night.

When at least one of these symptoms is noticed, often by the person themself, the control phase should start and the doctor should be consulted for diagnosis without delay. Even if going to the doctor does not solve the HF, it will contribute to one's survival time and quality of life [2].

1.2.4 HF Treatment

Treatment in HF generally gives effective results, the purpose being a decrease in sudden death and an increase in survival time. Within the scope of treatment are acting to support a healthy life, medication use, medical support, and surgical interventions.

In drug treatment, the patient is generally supported with more than one drug supplement. Medicines are used to strengthen the heart muscle, lower blood pressure, and remove the edema accumulated in the body. Some medicines used in the treatment of HF show blood thinning and cholesterol lowering effects. Many drugs are difficult for the patient, but their use can produce the desired effect.

Surgical methods and medical support devices are other method used in treatment. Surgical methods and medical support aim to eliminate the irregularities that occur in the heart. One of the surgical methods is coronary bypass and another is heart valve replacement surgery. The most known and preferred method in the treatment of HF is undoubtedly heart surgery. Deciding this is itself an important issue. If the heart has become unable to perform its duties, and if medication or a stent are far from being a solution, a heart surgery decision should be made with a physician's recommendation.

The use of pacemakers can also be considered within the scope of surgical methods. The function of pacemakers is to support the heart and, with a solution similar to a pacemaker, the disturbed rhythm of the heart is understood and shock is applied to the heart to eliminate the rhythm disturbance. In addition, placing a heart pump in the chest cavity to support the weakened heart is a method of treatment. One of the most effective and definitive solutions within surgical methods is heart transplantation. The broken heart is removed and a healthy heart is transplanted.

One of the techniques that reduce the risk of heart attack and thus helps treatment is blood thinning. Thinning the blood is a known technique for preventing blood clotting, a significant problem that causes major diseases such as stroke, heart attack, and kidney failure. Pills, subcutaneous injections, or tubes placed in a vein are used to thin the blood. The pill is warfarin; the other methods use heparin.

1.3 Invasive and Non-Invasive Procedures

A detailed clinical examination and patient history are important in diagnosing HF. In a detailed examination, symptoms of high blood pressure, high cholesterol, and high sugar levels should also be examined. In the diagnosis of HF, it should be considered whether the patient has had one of the diseases in the HF class previously. Physical examination is also one of the useful applications in terms of diagnosis, as it can reveal abnormalities in the patient that disrupt the balance of the body.

There are numerous invasive, non-invasive, machine learning, and artificial intelligence based methods for diagnosing HF. While invasive methods roughly refer to the types of studies that can be seen as subcutaneous interventions, non-invasive methods refer to procedures performed outside the body, for example measuring blood pressure.

1.3.1 What are Invasive and Non-Invasive Procedures?

The invasive procedure – also called invasion – involves opening veins that are usually closed, stenting, needle procedures, and the like. Invasive procedures are generally performed by applying a physical effect to the body. For example, operations that cause an incision in the body, such as open surgery, are this type.

Apart from invasive procedures, there are also non-invasive and minimally invasive methods. As a medical term, the invasive procedure is used for situations requiring surgical intervention, while non-invasive procedure is the name given to situations that do not require surgical procedures and do not need any intervention such as cutting or piercing the body. Measurement of a patient's blood pressure and temperature are just two examples of the non-invasive method.

Minimally invasive procedure refers to invasive studies performed in a very narrow area, in a very short time, and with little effect. For example, endoscopic interventions are known as minimally invasive methods and while taking blood from a vein for analysis is invasive, taking blood from a small incision in the tip of the finger is known to be minimally invasive.

1.3.2 Diagnosis by Invasive Procedures

There are many invasive procedures in use, including surgical interventions. Tens of millions of invasive procedures are performed on patients worldwide almost every year [3].

One of the invasive tests for heart conditions is blood tests. Within the scope of blood tests, cardiac enzymes, C-reactive protein (CRP), fibrinogen, homocysteine, lipoproteins, triglycerides, brain natriuretic peptide (BNP), and prothrombin values are checked. Blood tests can confirm whether a heart attack has occurred, the extent of damage can be predicted, future risk can be found, and general information on blood clotting can be obtained [4].

One of the tests that should be considered within the scope of blood tests is the troponin test, which is a method that can determine the risk of heart attack in healthy individuals. What is tested is the amount of troponin protein that is released when the heart muscle is damaged. Based on this measurement, the cases likely to have a heart attack in the coming years can be predicted.

Another invasive technique is known as heart catheterization. The inside of the heart and blood vessels are imaged using special x-rays called angiograms. A thin hollow tube, a catheter, is guided through a blood vessel in the arm, groin, or neck toward the heart. Dye is injected into the blood vessels through the catheter, thus enhancing the image quality of the x-ray. This process takes 2–3 hours on average and, through angiography, can lead to an understanding of what caused the chest pain – angiography can reveal both the obstruction in the vessels and the problem in the heart valves and, in addition, can measure the blood pressure and oxygen content within the heart [4].

Since angiography has some limitations, non-invasive methods such as smart calculation algorithms are also frequently used and better results can sometimes be obtained.

1.3.3 Diagnosis by Non-Invasive Procedures

Pressure examination, hammer examination, ultrasonography are some common examples of non-invasive methods, and there are many non-invasive methods used in HF. Each method will be briefly mentioned in this section.

Electrocardiography is one of the non-invasive methods in HF. It monitors heart rhythm changes by recording the heart's electrical activity and, thus, determines whether a heart attack has occurred from abnormalities in rhythm. Electrocardiography and blood tests are the most common methods used in HF diagnosis and the aim of electrocardiography is to determine the complex factors underlying HF [5].

Sometimes, the heart's activity is recorded throughout the day, not just for a short time. This process is known as Holter monitoring. The method aims to determine how the heart responds during daily activities and the average heart rhythm. Holter monitoring not only detects abnormalities in the heart, but can also help doctors treat them.

Chest x-ray also provides a non-invasive method for diagnosing heart diseases, by taking a picture of the heart, lungs, and rib cage. With the radiological imaging performed, it can be seen if the heart is enlarged after a heart attack or fluid accumulation in the lungs. Systolic and diastolic dysfunction of the heart can be discovered through electrocardiography and chest x-ray [6].

Echocardiography has been used for many years to characterize HF [7]. It uses high frequency sound waves (ultrasound) to produce images of heart size, movement, and structure. The printout of the test gives information about heart health and helps to gather information about heart arrhythmias. Echocardiography outputs have been used with both machine learning algorithms and deep learning algorithms [8].

Computed imaging (tomography) is used to detect other diseases as well as in HF. It creates three-dimensional (3D) images that can show the obstructions in our main vessels with the help of a computer system. Through computed tomography, testing can be performed, especially for aortic disease.

The exercise test works with skin-attached electrodes and a monitor recording a person's heart function while walking on a treadmill. Many aspects of heart function can be checked, including heart rate, breathing, blood pressure, ECG, and how tired someone is while exercising. This test is particularly helpful in diagnosing CAD and is also used to predict heart attack risk. It helps diagnose the possible cause of symptoms such as chest pain (angina).

The last procedure on this subject is known as the thallium stress test. The thallium test is similar to a routine exercise stress test. The difference is that the radioactive thallium material injected into the patient's blood is photographed by special gamma ray cameras when the patient is at the maximum exercise level. Thus, the extent of coronary artery occlusion can be determined and the extent of damage from heart attack can be determined [9].

1.4 Computer-Aided Diagnosis

The number of diseases and patients is increasing daily due to food-related problems, a sedentary lifestyle, and many similar reasons. Factors such as the complexity of the diseases, the increasing number of patients, and the aging of the world population have led to new searches in the field of health. Diseases are not old diseases, and their solution methods cannot be old methods. Being aware of this situation, health professionals and technology workers have joined hands and developed solutions for the health sector. In this context, many studies using technology in the field of health have been carried out [10]. Notably, using internet of things (IoT) sensor technologies, human movements have been monitored and abnormal situations detected [11].

The first solution that comes to mind regarding data collected with the help of IoT sensors is alarm generation resulting from abnormalities in the collected data, and sometimes making diagnoses and patient interventions the patient [12]. Abnormalities in patient movements or blood values are usually associated with a disease. For example, irregular tissue growths are related to cancer, and irregular heartbeats, heart diseases, and balance problems in the body are related to nerve diseases. IoT is a network where physical objects communicate with each other and with central systems. The use of IoT devices in disease diagnosis is carried out with the help of wearable technologies or additional components that make it possible to generate alarms about the patient with the help of systems that collect information, especially heart rate information, from the patient and transmit it to the center. This is carried out according to a method called anomaly detection in the name of alarm generation. An alarm is generated in case of an abnormality by comparing the last state of the patient with their recorded normal state. Thus, an approach similar to anomaly detection in networks provides the background for diagnosis based on IoT systems.

HF is a complex disease that occurs due to many different causes. The complexity of the disease makes its correct diagnosis a challenging problem for doctors. In addition, heart diseases, and especially heart attacks, are diseases that frequently affect people over the age of 65 who choose to live at home rather than a health center, and thus it is not possible to keep the patient's condition under control. Due to the increase in cardiac diseases and the inability of patients to be under continuous control, studies to detect abnormalities in the heart before the onset of a crisis should be carried out earlier [13]. Early diagnosis is important as it affects the early intervention for the patient.

In the diagnosis of HF, the risk of HF is estimated based primarily on the patient's clinical history, current symptoms, physical examination, and ECG. If all the measurements mentioned are normal, there is probably no risk, otherwise more detailed analysis should be done for diagnosis. Performing analyses allows specialists to identify patients who need echocardiography [14]. Diagnosis can be made with clinical methods, and decision support systems based on machine learning algorithms. From a machine learning perspective, HF diagnosis is a binary classification problem, a type of classification in which samples are assigned to one of two groups. For the diagnosis of HF, there would be two classes: "heart failure" and "no heart failure."

Thanks to machine learning, it can be understood whether the person being controlled has HF.

1.4.1 Clinical Decision Support Systems

There is a need to develop a system in order to collect patient data and make diagnoses based on them. These systems are generally called decision support systems. Decision support systems work by analyzing the data collected from the terminal units in accordance with the needs in the center to support decision making and presenting the results. Decision support systems can sometimes be developed for the field of health and sometimes for another field. Regardless of the field, the task of decision support systems is to infer with the help of the collected data and the rules at hand.

Decision support systems developed specifically for the health field are often referred to as clinical decision support systems. Clinical decision support systems sometimes help experts diagnose disease and recommend treatment methods based on health information. The concept of computer-aided clinical decision making came to the fore many years ago [15]. The working principle of clinical decision support systems is simply as follows: information such as blood values and enzyme values of the patient is obtained, this information is evaluated according to the knowledge base of the health institution, and an inference is made about the patient. When a direct relationship can be established between the inputs and the final decision during inference, this is known as an open box decision support system; when the correct relationship cannot be established between the inputs and the final decision, it is called a closed box decision support system [16].

A decision support system is a software that helps decision making and works based on the ruleset. The rule set can be in the form of simple IF-THEN rules or a more complex structure. Rule sets can be created with the help of expert knowledge or with models that learn from data. Comparing the event that occurred with the rules in the rule set determines which rule triggered the situation. Thus, whichever rule is triggered by the situation to produce the result, the output of the decision support system will be consistent.

Decision support systems are systems that help to decide about a situation. A system that will decide on HF takes the patient's measurements as input and provides information about the risk of HF as output. The system's inputs are sometimes the information coming from the IoT devices and sometimes the data that has been entered manually. For example, based on heart rate and blood values, it will be possible to predict whether there will be HF. At this point, we come across systems based on machine learning and knowledge. In machine learning based systems, data classification is carried out with the help of models trained with historical data. As a result of the classification, there might or might not be an indicated risk of HF.

1.5 Diagnosis with Artificial Intelligence Methods

One of the techniques that can be used to diagnose of HF is artificial intelligence and machine learning.

1.5.1 Introduction to Artificial Intelligence

Artificial intelligence is the name of the general discipline that combines software and hardware studies. It includes designing systems that act like a human, learning and making decisions like humans. Scientists have been curious about artificial intelligence since the 1950s and there is increasing interest in it. It has become an even more important discipline with the developments in information technologies. The focus on developing systems that exhibit human-like behavior has already attained this goal in some areas. Examining the recent history of artificial intelligence shows that machine learning algorithms and then deep learning algorithms have led to striking developments. For example, thanks to natural language processing, systems that produce and understand language have been developed; with the help of image processing techniques, systems close to human vision have been developed; systems that imitate human learning, systems that extract information, systems that establish connections have been developed; and studies that reveal abnormal situations have been conducted.

The main reason artificial intelligence-powered solutions have come to the fore is their ability to exploit many advantages of information technologies. Cheaper storage units, the increase in the capacities of the processing units, and advances in artificial intelligence algorithms make the field more popular every day. The cheaper storage units and the increase in their capacity have enabled more patient data to be stored. The increase in capacity and speed in processor units makes it possible to analyze data in a way not possible in the past. In fact, data collection and transfer possibilities from remote units have increased due to the developments in network technologies. All developments favor artificial intelligence and data science, and many jobs have become fulfilled with the help of artificial intelligence and data science.

The developments have also contributed to artificial intelligence programming skills. With artificial intelligence, it has become possible to solve many problems that could not be solved with classical programming skills, and while complex data relationships cannot be solved with classical methods, recently relationships between data have become easily inferred.

One of the areas most supported by artificial intelligence is computer-aided decision making, thanks to its various capabilities, notably diagnosis and prediction. Artificial intelligence-based diagnostic systems can be seen as an example of a non-invasive procedure, because there is no interference with the body in artificial intelligence supported clinical decision support systems, in which expert systems make decisions based on both expert opinions and machine learning systems' modeling from past case examples. These systems, which are sometimes used separately, are used together in some places. With the increase in the studies on artificial intelligence, its subfields have emerged. There are many artificial intelligence subdomains, each with different characteristics. Among these subareas, machine learning, deep learning, expert systems, and image processing in particular provide auxiliary features in computer-aided decision making.

1.5.1.1 Expert Systems

Expert systems are based on imitating human expertise with machines [17]. They are considered among the first successful applications of artificial intelligence. An expert system is often used in decision support systems development. In addition, the expert system has two components: the knowledge base and the inference engine.

1.5.1.2 Machine Learning

Machine learning is the most prominent area among the artificial intelligence subareas. It is a field focused on developing systems that learn with the help of historical data. As a result of learning, they can classify new data, cluster, establish similarities between data, and capture other relationships. Although supervised and unsupervised learning algorithms are often prominent in machine learning algorithms, semi-supervised and reinforced learning methods are also supported. The main purpose of machine learning algorithms is to aid decision making [18].

1.5.1.3 Deep Learning

Deep learning is a sub-branch of machine learning. It is also recognized as the most powerful alternative to machine learning. It can perform more complex operations with fewer data. In addition, while feature selection is performed manually in traditional machine learning algorithms, this process is automatic in deep learning. The working principle of deep learning algorithms is the working principle of the brain. It is based on densely multilayered neural networks, but constrained Boltzman machines and probabilistic graph models are also associated with deep learning. These are the methods that work with large amounts of data and reach the final output by further improving the results in each layer. It is supervised, unsupervised, or semi-supervised in terms of the type of education. Its prominent algorithms are convolutional neural network (CNN) and recurrent neural network (RNN). Deep learning models have found use in many areas from natural language processing to image processing.

1.5.1.4 Image Processing

Image processing is one of the most important application areas of artificial intelligence. With the help of image processing techniques, visual features are converted into numerical features and thus diagnostic studies are carried out. It refers to studies based on finding the patterns in the images. Especially with the help of 3D image processing, the borders of the diseased areas can be determined (Figure 1.1). Yang et al. [19] conducted a study of the 3D reconstruction of coronary vessels from angiography images, thus providing the possibility of better diagnosis of CAD. In the study, an aperture camera model and optimization methods were used.

1.5.2 Artificial Intelligence Supported HF Diagnostic Studies

With the use of artificial intelligence in health and especially in heart diseases, it has been possible to estimate the risk, diagnoses, and work flows and to apply sensitive treatment methods [21]. Thanks to artificial intelligence techniques, it has been possible to interpret large-sized data sets and thus obtain a more precise diagnosis. Within the artificial intelligence discipline, machine learning, image processing, robotics, and even

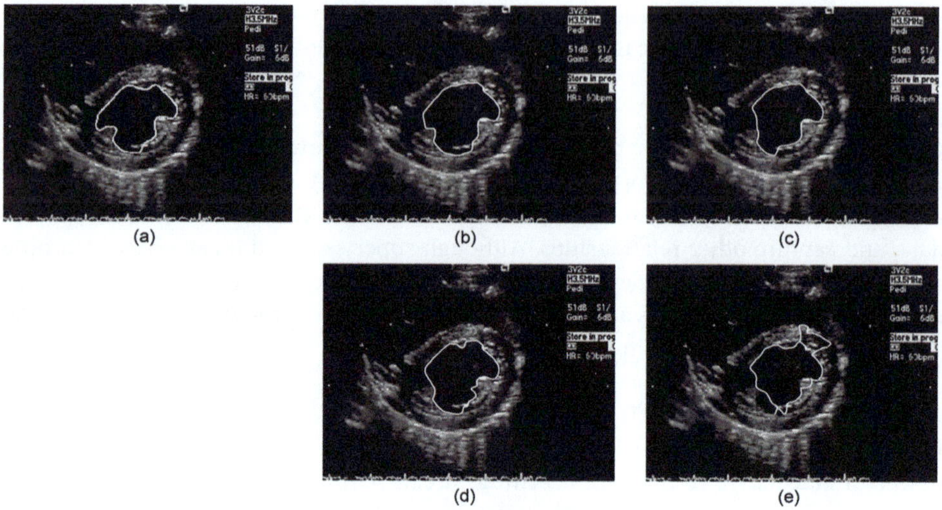

Figure 1.1 Images for boundary detection in different views of heart, with permission from Springer Nature [20].

natural language processing artificial intelligence techniques will be able to participate in the early detection and diagnosis of HF as well as outcome prediction and prognosis evaluation [22].

In a proposed study to help clinicians diagnose HF at an early stage, a scoring model based on a support vector machine (SVM) has been proposed. According to this model, samples were divided into three groups as healthy group, HF prone group, and HF group. The overall accuracy of the model in classification was 74.4% [23].

A study by Guidi et al. [24] was designed to help non-field experts make decisions in the analysis of HF. The system is based on three functional parts: diagnosis (severity assessment), prognosis, and follow-up. Four artificial intelligence techniques are used in the diagnostic function: artificial neural network (ANN), SVM, decision tree, and a fuzzy system with genetic algorithm support. A new technique for identifying HF patients using spectral analysis and neural networks was investigated in a study by Elfadil et al. [25]. A data set was used in the study, with 17 of the 53 samples being normal and the rest being patients. HF patients were divided into four groups with an accuracy of 83.65%.

Gharehchopogh et al. [26] presented a decision support model to help physicians in the study. The model, based on an ANN, was able to detect the presence or absence of HF with 85% accuracy. The study is within the scope of medical data mining.

Candelieri et al. developed a decision tree to determine patient stabilization [27] (with 88% accuracy). Pecchia et al. used decision tree techniques to classify patients into three severity groups using heart rate variability (HRV) measurements (HF: Healthy = 96% accuracy; Severe–Moderate = 79.3% accuracy) [28].

1.6 Machine Learning Supported Diagnosis

Invasive and non-invasive methods offer a wealth of diagnostic information. However, the interpretation of the available information can only be possible with the help of a physician. The increase in heart patients and the increase in patient data in parallel make it difficult to evaluate the data and extract information from them day by day. The intersection of the symptoms of heart disease with the symptoms of other diseases also makes the diagnosis of the disease a difficult problem. For this reason, there is a need to evaluate the data obtained with the help of invasive and non-invasive techniques with intelligent analysis tools in order to increase the diagnostic accuracy. Artificial intelligence and machine learning will assist physicians in intelligent analysis. Machine learning models trained with past patient data can be used to diagnose future cases. With the diagnostic capabilities to be gained by the machines, it will sometimes be possible for them to diagnose more precisely and more sensitively than the physicians. Supporting decision support systems working in expert systems logic with machine learning models will enable them to give better results.

1.6.1 Introduction to Machine Learning

Disease prediction and diagnosis can be made with the help of machine learning models. Disease diagnosis applications have been developed and used extensively, especially with controlled machine learning techniques. This technique has enabled models to be created from historical data and these models have sometimes been used in diagnosis and treatment. Developing a system based on machine learning is not just about developing machine learning algorithms, but rather it is done by working on data step by step from start to finish in a way similar to the data mining process. For example, determining which variables are important and which are not important in the solution of a problem directly affects the quality of the solution. This process, called feature selection, determines which parameters will be used in the system to be installed. The feature selection process is often achieved by establishing the correct relationships between targeted data and predictive data.

The feature selection phase is followed by feature transformation. Data transformation, which is a method that improves data quality, has recently emerged as feature engineering, which includes feature studies performed to increase prediction success. Like feature selection, feature engineering will also affect the success of the result. Both feature selection and feature engineering also solve the problem of high dimensionality in data. Loss of data and methods of combating loss are also important. The fight against lost values is sometimes carried out by estimating the lost value and sometimes by replacing it with other values.

It is also important to choose the learning models to be used when creating machine learning systems. There are four basic learning methods under the title of machine learning: supervised learning, unsupervised learning, semi-supervised learning, and reinforced learning. The latter two methods, semi-supervised learning is a type of learning that occurs with the combination of supervised and unsupervised techniques; reinforced learning is an agent-based learning technique where the decision is made according to the rewarding mechanism, and it is used to reveal the most possible solution to a subject that we did not have any previous knowledge about.

The most prominent techniques – supervised and unsupervised learning – will be explained in the following paragraphs.

1.6.2 Machine Learning Algorithms

There are many machine learning algorithms developed to date. To understand algorithms, the two learning methods of supervised learning and unsupervised learning (see Figure 1.2) need to be understood.

Supervised learning algorithms are often used in machine learning and perform two basic tasks: classification and regression. The output of classification operations is a nominal value, while the output of regression operations is usually a continuous value. Although supervised learning algorithms are often used to diagnose diseases, the field of machine learning is, as we have seen, wider and includes the additional methods we have mentioned, which are used for jobs where supervised learning is insufficient.

1.6.2.1 Supervised Learning

Supervised learning consists of two basic steps: creating a model with labeled data and testing with untagged data, the two prominent techniques in the category of supervised learning algorithms. Classification, one of the two prominent techniques in the category of supervised learning algorithms, is a supervised learning technique in which the target variable is of categorical type, while regression, the other prominent technique, is of the numerical type of the target variable. Operations are performed based on a model in which the target variable calculated from predictive variables is estimated. The purpose of classification is to assign records seen for the first time to one of the predefined categories. Identification and modeling of categories takes place with the help of training data. Training data and machine learning algorithms come together to form machine learning models. Machine learning models also match the records to the classroom that suits

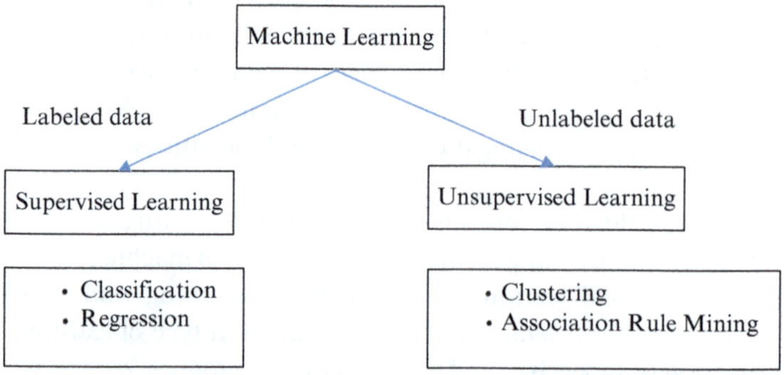

Figure 1.2 Supervised and unsupervised machine learning.

them best.The most important feature that distinguishes supervised learning from unsupervised learning is label information in supervised data. It is the class label in the data that provides the control. Although the output of both methods is different, the goal is to estimate the value of the output variable based on input variables.

1.6.2.1.1 Decision Trees

One of the prominent algorithms related to the classification task is the decision tree. The model presented with the tree data structure is learned directly from the data. Through the tree induction process, the characteristics of the training data are processed on the tree. The decision tree algorithm we often use and are used to seeing is the C4.5 algorithm [29]. Since the C4.5 algorithm is suitable for working with both numerical and categorical input variables, it can be used in many data sets.

1.6.2.1.2 Naive Bayes

The Naive Bayes classifier is a probability-based classifier. It is an algorithm that tries to find the final probabilities P (Cj I A) of the test data with the help of the preliminary probabilities P (A I Cj) learned from the training data. The algorithm is based on the Bayes' theorem [30]. According to Bayes' theorem, events are interrelated and there is a relationship between probabilities P (A I C) and P (C I A), P (A), P (C). Therefore, while calculating the value of P (A I C) with the help of Bayes, we use the equation P (C I A) = (P (A I C) P (C)) / (P (A)). The Naive Bayes approach is used to solve the zero probability problem of Bayesian approach. Thanks to the naive approach, it is assumed that there is no relationship between the events and the process is shortened. Thus, it is possible to get rid of sparsity in the data relatively.

1.6.2.1.3 Support Vector Machines

SVMs were first introduced by Vapnik [31]. The technique uses what we call support vectors to distinguish between data points belonging to different classes. The method aims to find the hyperplane that will best distinguish (margin maximization) different classes from each other. In its simplest form, it distinguishes two-class spaces from each other with the help of two equations $w^Tx + b = + 1$ and $w^Tx + b = -1$. SVMs were first developed in accordance with linear classification and, later, kernel functions for nonlinear spaces were developed. Kernel functions express a transformation between linear and nonlinear spaces. There are types such as linear, polynomial, radial basis function, and sigmoid. Depending on the nature of the data used, kernel functions can be superior to each other.

1.6.2.1.4 K-Nearest Neighbor

The k-nearest neighbor (k-NN) algorithm is a distance-based classifier, which looks at the neighbors of the data point to classify a data object whose class is unknown. A majority vote is made for the classification decision. The two prominent parameters for the algorithm are the k (neighbor) number and the distance (distance) function. There is no exact method for determining the number of neighbors, so the ideal k value is often found after trials. The cosine similarity, Manhattan, Euclidian, or Chebyshev distance is used as the distance function. One of the problems with the k-NN algorithm is the scale problem. When the method based on operating in geometric space gives a scale problem, the problem is solved by feature engineering.

1.6.2.1.5 Neural Nets

An ANN is a machine learning method that emulates human learning. ANNs, which are frequently used in classification problems, are also used in clustering and optimization processes. Although the simplest neural network model is perceptron, multilayer perceptron is often used in classification problems. Deep learning methods, which have been used in many important tasks recently, are based on ANNs. The adaptability and parallel processing capability of ANNs make them a powerful option for many problems.

1.6.2.2 Unsupervised Learning

Unsupervised learning works with untagged data and its purpose is to create clusters based on the characteristics of the data. Unlike supervised learning, untagged data is used instead of labeled data. After the data are divided into groups according to their similarity or distance, labeling is done with the help of an expert. Two applications that stand out in unsupervised learning are clustering and association rule mining. Clustering is the assignment of data points to groups called clusters. It has two types: partitioned and hierarchical methods. In partitioned clustering, a data point can only be in one cluster. In hierarchical clustering, a point can be hierarchically located in more than one cluster. In association rules mining, association rules focused on finding rules based on relationships between events are used in mining relationships between attributes.

1.6.2.2.1 K-Means

The K-means segmentation clustering algorithm was first developed in 1967 by MacQueen [32]. The purpose of the algorithm is to divide the data into K clusters. Each cluster is presented with a center of gravity named centroid. The K value is determined by the user. An iterative method is used to divide the data into clusters. The distance function obtains the point to which each data point will be assigned.

1.6.2.2.2 Apriori Algorithm

The apriori algorithm is the prominent algorithm in association rules mining. It finds common patterns in the transaction database and performs rule generation [33]. With the help of the obtained rules, the occurrence of another event can be predicted after an event occurs. It is a frequently preferred algorithm especially because it helps to establish relationships between events.

1.6.3 Machine Learning Supported HF Studies

Machine learning, the most common application of artificial intelligence, reveals patterns in data by continuously improving the ability to learn from data and the prediction and diagnosis of cardiovascular disease [34]. When the machine learning based diagnosis system of HF is considered as input, process, and output modules, the modules can be presented as follows. The input module contains data to be used by the decision support system, such as physical examination data, laboratory results, clinical data, ECG monitoring data, and electrocardiography data. The transaction module is the module that contains machine learning algorithms, which are mainly supervised and unsupervised learning algorithms. In diagnosing HF the machine learning algorithms currently used include nearest neighbor, self-organizing maps, multilayer perceptron, classification and regression trees, random forests, SVMs, neural networks, logistic regression, decision trees, clustering, and fuzzy-genetic and neuro-fuzzy expert systems. In the output module, information such as the presence of HF, risk of HF events, evaluation of left ventricular deterioration, response to advanced therapies, and risk of death is attempted to be determined.

When the literature on machine learning methods (Table 1.2), which is an important option in diagnosing HF, is examined, it will be seen that the use of HRV stands out in many studies. In one of the case studies, Yang et al. [35] used a scoring method to diagnose HF. In the study, with the help of two SVM models, it was first checked whether the person has HF. If the result was normal, the second SVM model came into play and classified the person being examined as healthy or prone to HF. The scores were matched with the SVM model outputs and diagnostic outputs were obtained according to the score ranges.

The aim of the study by Son et al. [36] was to distinguish between CHF and shortness of breath problems. The study was initially made with 72 features; rough sets and logistic regression techniques were used to reduce the number of variables. The accuracy of the classification obtained according to the features selected with the help of coarse clusters was 97.5%, and the classification accuracy obtained with the features selected based on logistic regression was measured as 88.7%.

Masetic et al. 2016 [37] applied the random forest algorithm to ECG time series to detect CHF. The features on the ECG were extracted using the autoregressive Burg method. In the study, apart from the random forest algorithm, C4.5, SVM, ANN, and k-NN classifiers were used with the random forest algorithm giving the best performance.

Wu et al. [38] studied detecting HF prior to clinical diagnosis. Information such as electronic health records, health behavior, demographic data, clinical diagnosis, and clinical precautions were used to detect the disease in advance. SVM, boosting, and logistic regression were used for early detection of the disease. In addition, the contribution of feature selection to success was observed.

Aljaaf et al. [39] proposed a multilevel risk assessment for developing HF. With the help of the C4.5 classifier, estimates were made according to five different risk levels (1: No risk; 2: Low risk; 3: Moderate risk; 4: High risk; 5: Extremely high risk). The Cleveland heart disease data set was used in the study. A 10-fold cross-validation procedure was followed to evaluate the C4.5 classifier.

Zheng et al. [40] proposed a computer-aided diagnostic system for diagnosing HF. This system uses least-squares SVM (LS-SVM). The LS-SVM classifier gave better results than neural nets and hidden Markov models.

Pattekari et al. [41] designed a Naive Bayes-based smart system and developed a decision support system for HF prediction. With the web-based application, users were asked predefined questions and the estimation process was carried out by comparing their answers with the database.

Table 1.2 Literature summary for artificial intelligence and machine learning techniques in HF.

Author	Method	Study
Guidi et al. [24]	ANN, SVM, decision tree, fuzzy genetic algorithm	Clinical decision support system for HF
Elfadil et al. [25]	Neural nets and spectral analysis	HF patients grouping
Gharehchopoghi et al. [26]	ANNs	Decision support system for HF
Candelieri et al. [27]	Decision tree	To determine patient stabilization
Pecchia et al. [28]	Decision tree	To classify patients
Yang et al. [35]	SVM models	Heart attack prediction
Son et al. [36]	Logistic regression models	Distinguish between CHF and shortness of breath problems
Masetic et al. [37]	Random forest, C4.5, SVM, ANN, k-NN	Detect CHF
Wu et al. [38]	SVM, boosting, logistic regression	Detect HF
Aljaaf et al. [39]	C4.5	Risk assessment for HF
Zheng et al. [40]	LS- SVM	HF diagnosis
Pattekari et al. [41]	Naive Bayes	HF prediction
Takcı [42]	12 classification algorithms	Heart attack detection

Takcı [42] introduced a framework for the diagnosis of heart attack. In his study, in which the most successful classifier combination was sought with 12 different algorithms and four different feature selection methods, the most successful classifier was SVM using the linear kernel and the most successful feature selection method was the ReliefF algorithm. The obtained classification accuracy was reported as 84.81%.

Non-invasive techniques, such as electrocardiography, or invasive techniques, such as blood tests, which are used to diagnose HF, also measure irregularities in values. Imbalances and anomalies are measured with artificial intelligence techniques, such as the process performed with existing diagnostic techniques. Previously used conventional diagnostic techniques work by increasing capacity with the support of artificial intelligence. For example, it will be possible to increase the accuracy of diagnosis thanks to electrocardiography supported by artificial intelligence.

1.7 Conclusion and Future Directions

The heart is a vital organ for human beings. When it cannot healthily fulfill its duty it affects the quality of life and may even cause death. The inability of the heart to fully perform its functions, especially due to a heart attack, is called "heart failure." There are several types and many causes of HF. High blood pressure, abnormal heart valves, and damage to the heart muscle are just a few of these causes.

Because of the importance of HF, its diagnosis is also very important. With timely diagnosis, heart patients are more likely to improve their quality of life and survive longer. Invasive and non-invasive procedures are classically used to diagnose the disease. Artificial intelligence and machine learning techniques have also been used for exploratory purposes due to the excessive causes of disease, the increasing number of patients, and patient data. Expert systems, image processing, machine learning, deep learning, and others, which are important fields of study of artificial intelligence, have been used extensively in this field recently. Artificial intelligence based methods both obtain data that could not be obtained before, and analyze previously obtained data more intelligently. Modeling of experiences with the help of machine learning and the use of models in diagnosing new patients have led to a striking development.

The most valuable contribution of artificial intelligence, especially machine learning techniques, to this field is their role in clinical decision support systems. Decision support systems, which were previously developed based on knowledge, now work based on data, thanks to machine learning. Machine learning models trained with disease data and previously given class information have become able to diagnose automatically. Clinical decision support systems, which have reached a certain stage with machine learning systems, have also reached a higher level with deep learning algorithms. Increasing data, complicated algorithm structures, and data relationships that could not be seen before are developing this field.

With a data-oriented and integrated clinical support system, a holistic medicine approach will now be applicable and the relationship between heart diseases and other diseases and even behavioral styles will be revealed. Diagnoses will become faster and more accurate through a more powerful data highway to be achieved thanks to 5G, the wider data holding capacity of cloud systems, more processing power from distributed processing architecture, and more complex and powerful algorithms with deep learning.

References

1 Mayo Clinic. *Heart Failure*. https://www.mayoclinic.org/diseases-conditions/heart-failure/symptoms-causes/syc-20373142, Access date: May 1, 2021.

2 MedicalPark, Kalp Yetmezliği Nedir? Belirtileri nelerdir? https://www.medicalpark.com.tr/kalp-yetmezligi/hg-2209. Access date: April 23, 2021.

3 Cousins, S., Blencowe, N.S., and Blazeby, J.M. (2019). What is an invasive procedure? A definition to inform study design, evidence synthesis and research tracking. *BMJ Open* 9 (7): e028576. https://doi.org/10.1136/bmjopen-2018-028576.

4 Invasive Tests and Procedures. Heart Attack and Stroke Symptoms. https://www.heart.org/en/health-topics/heart-attack/diagnosing-a-heart-attack/invasive-tests-and-procedures. Access date: April 23, 2020.

5 Hannun, A.Y., Rajpurkar, P., Haghpanahi, M., et al. (2019). Cardiologistlevel arrhythmia detection and classification in ambulatory electrocardiograms using a deep neural network. *Nature Medicine* 25 (1): 65.

6 Shamsham, Fadi, M.D. and Mitchell, Judith, M.D. (2000). Essentials of the diagnosis of HF. *AFP Journal*. Mar. 1, 2000. https://www.aafp.org/afp/2000/0301/p1319.html.

7 Ponikowski, P., Voors, A.A., Anker, S.D., et al. (2016). ESC guidelines for the diagnosis and treatment of acute and chronic HF: The Task Force for the diagnosis and treatment of acute and chronic HF of the European Society of Cardiology (ESC). Developed with the special contribution of the HF Association (HFA) of the ESC. *European Journal of Heart Failure* 18 (8) (2016): 891–975.

8 Attia, Z.I., Kapa, S., Lopez-Jimenez, F., et al. (2019). Screening for cardiac contractile dysfunction using an artificial intelligence–enabled electrocardiogram. *Nature Medicine* 25 (1) (2019): 70.

9 Non-Invasive Tests and Procedures. Heart Attack and Stroke Symptoms. https://www.heart.org/en/health-topics/heart-attack/diagnosing-a-heart-attack/noninvasive-tests-and-procedures. Access date: May 20, 2021.

10 Haider, D., Yang, X., and Abbasi, Q.H. (2019). Post-surgical fall detection by exploiting the 5 G C-Band technology for eHealth paradigm. *Applied Soft Computing* 81: 105537.

11 Sahoo, S.P. and Ari, S. (2019). On an algorithm for human action recognition. *Expert Systems With Applications* 115: 524–534.

12 Li, C., Hu, X., and Zhang, L. (2017). The IoT-based heart disease monitoring system for pervasive healthcare service. *Procedia Computer Science* 112: 2328–2334. (2017).

13 Yahaya, S.W., Lotfi, A., and Mahmud, M.A. (2019). Consensus novelty detection ensemble approach for anomaly detection in activities of daily living. *Applied Soft Computing* 83: 105613.

14 Tripoliti, E.E., et al. (2017). Heart Failure: Diagnosis, severity estimation and prediction of adverse events through machine learning techniques. *Computational and Structural Biotechnology Journal* 15: 26–47.

15 Ledley, R.S. and Lusted, L.B. (1959). Reasoning foundations of medical diagnosis: Symbolic logic, probability, and value theory aid our understanding of how physicians reason. *Science* 130: 9–21.

16 Shortliffe, E.H. and Sepulveda, M.J. (2018). Clinical decision support in the era of artificial intelligence. *JAMA* 320: 2199–2200.

17 Jackson, P. (1998). *Introduction to Expert Systems* (3rd ed.). Addison Wesley.

18 IBM Cloud Education. Machine Learning... https://www.ibm.com/cloud/learn/machine-learning. Access date: 15 July 2020.

19 Yang, J., Wang, Y., Liu, Y., Tang, S., and Chen, W. (2009). Novel approach for 3-D reconstruction of coronary arteries from two uncalibrated angiographic images. *IEEE Transactions on Image Processing* 18 (7): 1563–1572.

20 SainiSai, S, K., Dewal, M., and Rohit, M. (2011). A fast region-based active contour model for boundary detection of echocardiographic images. *Journal of Digital Imaging: The Official Journal of the Society for Computer Applications in Radiology* 25: 271–278. doi:10.1007/s10278-011-9408-8.

21 Krittanawong, C., Zhang, H., Wang, Z., Aydar, M., and Kitai, T. (2017). Artificial intelligence in precision cardiovascular medicine. *Journal of the American College of Cardiology* 69 (2017): 2657–2664.

22 Murdoch, T.B. and Detsky, A.S. (2013). The inevitable application of big data to health care. *Journal of the American Medical Association* 309 (13): 1351–1352. 2013.

23 Yang, G., Ren, Y., Pan, Q., and Ning, G. (2010). A HF diagnosis model based on support vector machine. *IEEE International Conference on Biomedical Engineering and Informatics* Vol. 3: 1105–1108.

24 Guidi, G., Iadanza, E., Pettenati, M.C., Milli, M., Pavone, F., and Biffi Gentili, G. (2012). Heart failure artificial intelligence-based computer aided diagnosis telecare system. In: *Impact Analysis of Solutions for Chronic Disease Prevention and Management*, 7251 (ed. M. Donnelly, C. Paggetti, C. Nugent, and M. Mokhtari), ICOST 2012. Lecture Notes in Computer Science. Berlin, Heidelberg: Springer. https://doi.org/10.1007/978-3-642-30779-9_44.

25 Elfadil, N. and Ibrahim, I. (2011). Self organizing neural network approach for identification of patients with congestive HF. *International Conference on Multimedia Computing and Systems (ICMCS)* 1–6.

26 Gharehchopogh, F.S., Mohammadi, P., and Hakimi, P. (2012). Application of decision tree algorithm for data mining in healthcare operations: A case study. *International Journal of Computer Applications (IJCA)* 52 (6): 21–26. August 2012.

27 Candelieri, A. and Conforti, D. (2010). A hyper-solution framework for SVM classification: Application for predicting destabilizations in chronic HF patients. *The Open Medical Informatics Journal* 4: 136–140.

28 Pecchia, L., Melillo, P., and Bracale, M. (2011). Remote health monitoring of HF with data mining via CART method on HRV features. *IEEE Transactions on Bio-Medical Engineering* 58: 800–804.

29 Quinlan, J.R. (1993). *C4.5: Programs for Machine Learning*. San Mateo, CA: Morgan Kaufmann.

30 Joyce, J. (2003). Bayes' Theorem. In: *The Stanford Encyclopedia of Philosophy (Spring 2019 ed.)* (ed. E.N. Zalta). Metaphysics Research Lab. Stanford University. Retrieved Jan. 17, 2020.

31 Vapnik, V.N. (1995). *The Nature of Statistical Learning Theory*. New York, NY, USA: Springer-Verlag.

32 MacQueen, J.B. (1967). Some methods for classification and analysis of multivariate observations. In: *Proceedings of 5th Berkeley Symposium on Mathematical Statistics and Probability*, 1, 281–297. University of California Press.

33 Agrawal, R. and Srikant, R. (1994). Fast algorithms for mining association rules. In: *Proceedings of the 20th International Conference on Very Large Data Bases*, 487–499. Santiago, Chile: VLDB. September 1994. .

34 Johnson, K.W., Soto, J.T., Glicksberg, B.S., Shameer, K., Miotto, R., Ali, M., Ashley, E., and Dudley, T.D. (2018). Artificial intelligence in cardiology. *Journal of the American College of Cardiology* 71: 2668–2679.

35 Yang, G., Ren, Y., Pan, Q., Ning, G., Gong, S., Cai, G., et al. (2010). A heart failure diagnosisodel based on support vector machine. *2010 3rd International Conference on Biomedical Engineering and Informatics (BMEI)* 3 (2010): 1105–1108. http://dx.doi.org/10.1109/BMEI16828.2010.

36 Son, C.-S., Kim, Y.-N., Kim, H.-S., Park, H.-S., and Kim, M.-S. (2012). Decision-making model for early diagnosis of congestive HF using rough set and decision tree approaches. *Journal of Biomedical Informatics* 45 (2012): 999–1008. http://dx.doi.org/10.1016/j.jbi.2012.04.013.

37 Masetic, Z. and Subasi, A. (2016). Congestive heart failure detection using random forest classifier. *Computer Methods and Programs in Biomedicine* 130 (2016): 54–64. https://doi.org/10.1016/j.cmpb.2016.03.020.

38 Wu, J., Roy, J., and Stewart, W.F. (2010). Prediction modeling using EHR data: Challenges, strategies, and a comparison of machine learning approaches. *Medical Care* 48 (2010): S106–113. http://dx.doi.org/10.1097/MLR.0b013e3181de9e17.

39 Aljaaf, A.J., Al-Jumeily, D., Hussain, A.J., Dawson, T., Fergus, P., and Al-Jumaily, M. (2015). Predicting the likelihood of HF with a multi-level risk assessment using decision tree. In: *Third International Conference on Technological Advances in Electrical*. Beirut, Lebanon. 2015.

40 Zheng, Y., Guo, X., Qin, J., and Xiao, S. (2015). Computer-assisted diagnosis for chronic HF by the analysis of their cardiac reserve and heart sound characteristics. *Computer Methods and Programs in Biomedicine* I22 (2015): 372–383. http://dx.doi.org/10.1016/j.cmpb.2015.09.001.

41 Pattekari, S.A. and Asma, P. (2012). Prediction system for heart disease using Naïve Bayes. *International Journal of Advanced Computer and Mathematical Sciences* 3 (3): 290–294.

42 Takci, H. (2018). Improvement of heart attack prediction by the feature selection methods. *Turkish Journal of Electrical Engineering & Computer Sciences* 26: 1–10. https://doi.org/10.3906/elk-1611-235.

2

Conventional Clinical Methods for Predicting Heart Disease

Aisha A-Mohannadi, Jayakanth Kunhoth, Al Anood Najeeb, Somaya Al-Maadeed, and Kishor Kumar Sadasivuni

2.1 Introduction

The heart is the most essential organ of the human body located at the center of the chest in between the lungs and is mainly responsible for pumping blood across the blood vessels of the cardiovascular system. The blood is pumped through a network of arteries, delivering oxygenated blood and other nutrients to different cells of the body. The two large veins (superior vena cava and inferior vena cava) carry carbon dioxide as well as other metabolic waste products to the lungs for purification via pulmonary arteries. Unhealthy life habits may lead to high blood pressure and cholesterol which may affect the proper functioning of the heart thus causing serious heart diseases. The unhealthy life habits which can affect the heart's health are a sedentary lifestyle, smoking, overweight or obesity, poor eating habits, and excessive alcohol consumption. Smoking can raise the heart rate, tighten arteries, and cause irregular heart rhythm. Moreover, smoking can lead to atherosclerosis, where fat and cholesterol are deposited in the arteries. The deposit of fat and cholesterol is called plaque. This plaque narrows the arteries and blocks the blood flow. A sedentary lifestyle and poor eating habits can lead to overweight or obesity and high levels of bad cholesterol and triglycerides, leading to hypertension as well as the formation of plaque in arteries. Excessive drinking of alcohol can elevate blood pressure and weaken the heart's muscles. Elevated blood pressure and weakened muscles can cause stroke or heart failure. Apart from unhealthy habits, congenital disorders can also affect the proper working of the heart and even cause mortality. Heart diseases such as coronary artery disease, arrhythmia, angina pectoris, and cardiomyopathy can often result in cardiac arrest leading finally to death. Having a well-balanced diet, proper medication, and early diagnosis of symptoms at an early stage can greatly reduce the chances of getting heart disease.

The common symptoms of heart diseases include chest pain, tightness in the chest, dyspnea, palpitations, fainting, as well as collapse. Dyspnea is a condition where the patient suffers from shortness of breath and feels suffocation as well tightness in the chest; palpitation is the condition that refers to irregular and rapid heartbeats, which can also lead to shortness of breath. Individuals who are frequently experiencing these symptoms are advised to contact the physician as early as possible. Other physical symptoms

Predicting Heart Failure: Invasive, Non-Invasive, Machine Learning, and Artificial Intelligence Based Methods, First Edition. Edited by Kishor Kumar Sadasivuni, Hassen M. Ouakad, Somaya Al-Maadeed, Huseyin C. Yalcin, and Issam Bait Bahadur.

that can be seen in patients suffering from heart disease are unexpected color changes in the face and nails, and unexpected movements of the eyeballs. Moreover, patients suffering from coronary heart diseases experience chest pain called angina when involved in heavy exercise or heavy labor. Heart valve disease, cardiomyopathy, and heart failure conditions can cause swellings in the legs, ankles, or feet. In acute cases, these conditions can also lead to swellings in organs. Tiredness is also a common symptom for patients suffering from heart valve disease and heart failure conditions. Patients with heart infections experience severe fever and tiredness. Even though these symptoms are warning signs of heart disease, other mild health conditions apart from heart disease can also cause similar symptoms in the human body. Because of that, a clinical examination is extremely necessary in order to differentiate heart diseases from false alarms. A prudent and comprehensive examination is essential to analyze health conditions and assess the reason for as well as the intensity of symptoms. A detailed examination conducted in the clinic by a licensed physician or cardiologist can detect whether heart disease is the cause of underlying symptoms. If it is, they can refer the patient for further advanced examination to assess the individual risk of heart disease and provide immediate medication.

The physician or cardiologist initially explores the patient's family history, past medical history, and lifestyle along with examining the symptoms being experienced by the patient. Further examination includes inspection of cyanosis (bluish discoloration commonly found in nails), and scrutiny of faces to look for unexpected color changes and movement of the eyeballs. The examination is then extended to check blood pressure and perform blood tests, along with advanced procedures including electrocardiography, echocardiography, chest roentgenography, etc.

This chapter briefly describes the various clinical examination methods traditionally used by cardiologists in detecting heart diseases. It also explains various symptoms and physiological factors related to heart diseases and their clinical significance. In addition, the chapter also discusses the works in the literature that have integrated artificial intelligence and machine learning methods along with the clinically observed physiological values for improved detection of heart disease conditions.

2.2 Physical Assessments

As in past years, experts and doctors rely on many physical techniques as a path to early diagnosis of heart diseases. Physical assessments for diagnosing heart diseases include the technique, palpation, auscultation, electrocardiography, treadmill test, and cardiac biomarker examination. Each type of examination is chosen based on the result observed in the previous type. Usually, the inspection technique is conducted first and, based on its results, the licensed physician or cardiologist further proceeds with other types of examination.

2.2.1 Inspection Examination

This technique focuses on the visual appearance of the human patients, where the skin color, general health, face expressions, and nutritional status of the patient are taken into consideration. For instance, sweatiness, paleness, or cyanosis can be the initial signs of a possible heart attack in an acutely ill patient. Cyanosis is a medical condition where a bluish discoloration is seen in the lips, ears, nose, fingernails, as well as toenails. This condition is usually known as "blue hands or feet" due to hypoxemia. Hypoxemia is a condition where oxygen levels are lower than normal in the blood. The bluish color is caused by the excess amount of deoxyhemoglobin in the blood when various heart-related conditions prevent blood flow from tissues to the heart and backward. Excess amounts of deoxyhemoglobin in the blood can be due to various heart-related diseases including heart failure, myocardial infections, congenital heart diseases, valvular heart conditions, etc. Moreover, malar flush, corneal arcus, xanthomata, and proptosis are manifestations in the face of the patient suffering from heart disease. Malar flush is a facial manifestation where the cheeks turn a plum-red color. The malar flush symptom is closely related to valvular heart disease called mitral stenosis. Mitral stenosis is a condition where the mitral valve's area is less than 2 cm^2 (the normal area is about 5 cm^2) during diastole. Reduction in the area causes carbon dioxide retention and leads to vasodilation (widening of blood vessels) of the arterioles present in the cheek. In the xanthomata condition, the eyes, palms, or tendons will experience a yellowish deposit of lipids. The excess yellowish deposit is due to high-level blood lipids and fats. The tendon xanthomata is a sign of high-level LDL (low-density lipoprotein) cholesterol in the blood as well as atherosclerosis. Proptosis refers to a change in the eyeball movement, especially to a protruded eyeball. In non-acute patients, one important sign is cachexia, as it is a clear sign for the prognosis of heart failure [1]. Cachexia is a wasting disorder where the patient experiences severe weight loss as well muscle loss.

2.2.2 Palpation Examination

Palpation examination involves pulse tracing of patients' jugular veins, arterial pulses, precordial impulses, etc. This includes examination using the fingers or hands to test patients. Jugular veins can be tested by evaluating the internal jugular veins located in the patient's neck. Whereas arterial pulse examination involves assessing the arteries located either in the hands or legs, assessment of the hand arteries can be measured by examining how fast or slow the heart rate is. This is done by placing fingers on the arteries located in the patient's wrist and comparing the timing along with the consistency of the impulses. The physician can use their other hand to palpate the subjec patient's other wrist to confirm the measurements. The heart rate is determined by counting the radial pulse for 30 seconds and then multiplying it by 2. This can give an accurate result except in the case of irregular rhythm.

2.2.3 Auscultation Examination

Auscultation means listening carefully to the heart sounds or murmurs through a stethoscope. The stethoscope tool consists of two parts: the bell and the diaphragm. Each part has its particular features, with the bell focusing on low-pitched sounds and detecting murmurs of aortic valve stenosis or carotid bruits, and the diaphragm focusing on high-pitched sounds that can detect valve closures or systolic clicks. During auscultation examination, the physician makes the patient lie in four different positions (shown in Figure 2.1): supine, upright, left lateral decubitus, and upright leaning forward [2]. The physician should be looking for irregular murmurs or heart sounds and identifying their location, duration, intensity, and pitch. This will all help in diagnosing heart conditions. Although irregular murmurs or heart sounds are not always linked with underlying heart conditions, they can, however, in certain conditions be an early warning of heart diseases.

2.2.4 Electrocardiogram (ECG)

This ECG is generated by a method called electrocardiography, where several electrodes are placed on the patient's heart, legs, and arms and monitor the pulses for around 10 minutes. The technique measures the electrical activity of each heartbeat resulting in an electrocardiogram that shows the heart's functionality. The electrocardiogram generated during the electrocardiography technique is a graph that depicts the characteristic of voltage versus time of the heart's electrical activity. During each cardiac cycle, these electrodes detect the minor electrical changes that occur as a result of cardiac muscle depolarization and repolarization. Several cardiac anomalies, such as cardiac rhythm disruptions (e.g. atrial fibrillation and ventricular tachycardia), insufficient coronary artery blood flow (e.g. myocardial ischemia and myocardial infarction), and electrolyte disturbances (e.g. hypokalemia and hyperkalemia) cause changes in the usual ECG pattern. An illustration of the ECG test is shown in Figure 2.2. An ECG test is required only if the patient has any risk factors, such as hypertension, or physical discomforts, such as angina or palpitations including irregular heartbeats or rapid heartbeats. Patients with an existing history of heart disease are required to do the ECG test. Moreover, healthy individuals with a family history of heart disease are advised to do the ECG test if they are going to begin any heavy exercise routine or heavy labor routine.

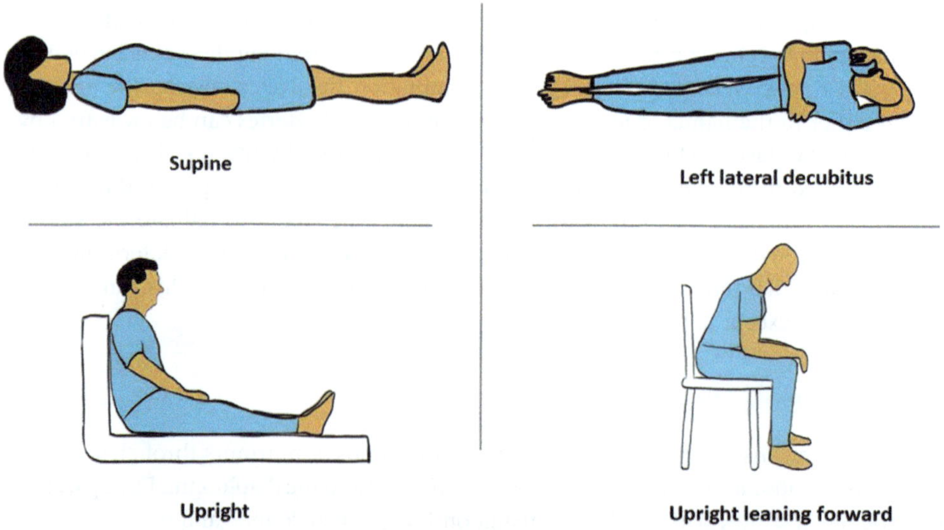

Figure 2.1 Supine, left lateral decubitus, upright, and upright leaning forward positions.

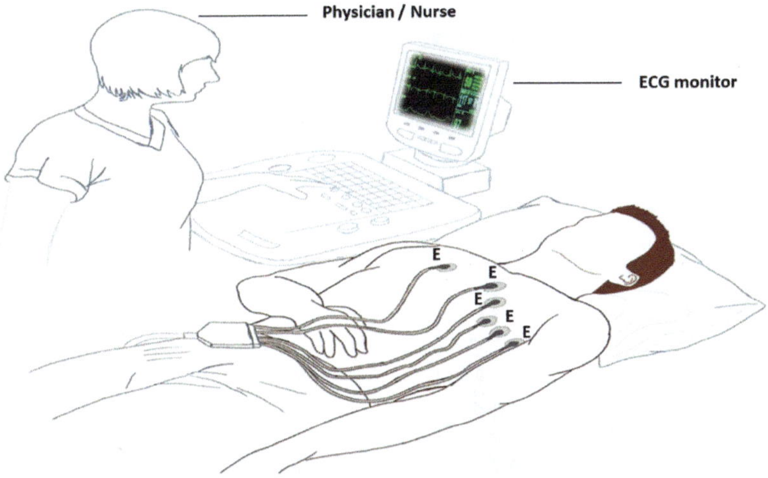

Figure 2.2 ECG. E denotes electrodes placed for detecting the small electrical changes induced by cardiac muscle depolarization. The graph of voltage versus time of the heart's electrical activity is showing in the ECG monitor. A physician/nurse is assigned to supervise the ECG test.

The major waves of a single ECG pattern and the normal values of ECG signals for normal heart rate are given in Figure 2.3. Arrhythmia is detected by verifying against the intervals shown in the table.

2.2.5 Treadmill Test

The treadmill test is done by making patients walk briskly on a treadmill, which makes their hearts pump fast. The treadmill test is conducted to identify how well the heart of a patient handles their work and exercise capacity. During the test session, the heart rhythm, breathing, and blood pressure of the patient are monitored to detect abnormalities. The test is normally done after detecting signs or symptoms of coronary heart disease. It can assist the physician in understanding the severity of heart disease. Generally, the treadmill test is safe and devoid of any risks. However, patients suffering from low

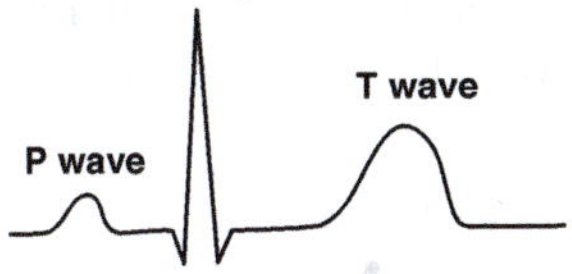

Major waves of single ECG signal

Amplitude	P-Wave	0.25 milli volt
	R-wave	1.60 milli volt
	Q-wave	25% of R wave
	T-Wave	0.1 to 0.5 milli volt
Duration	P-R interval	120-200 milli seconds
	Q-R interval	350-440 milli seconds
	P-Wave interval	110 milli seconds
	QRS interval	90 milli seconds

Normal values of ECG signal

Figure 2.3 Major waves of a single ECG signal and the normal values of ECG signals.

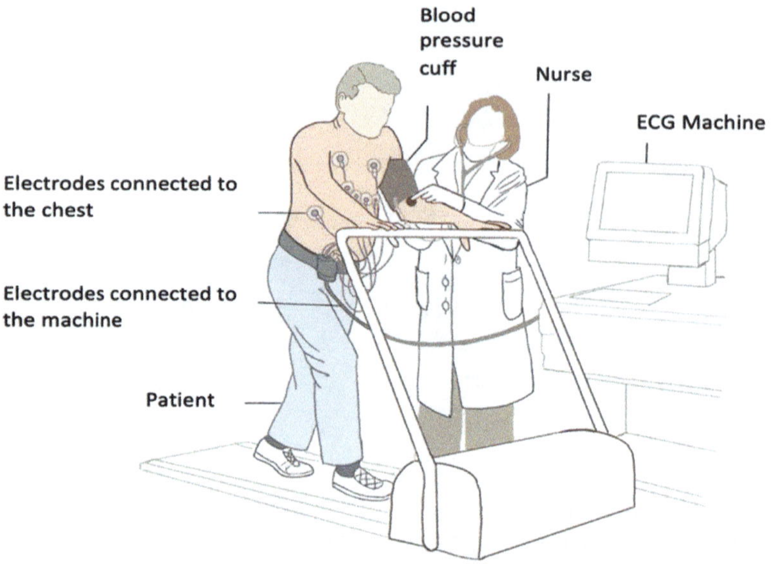

Figure 2.4 Treadmill assessment.

blood pressure can feel dizzy or faint due to the impact of the exercise. Figure 2.4 shows a patient running on a treadmill under the supervision of a nurse; their blood pressure is being monitored as is their heart rate via ECG electrodes placed on their chest.

A treadmill test is required for individuals who have been experiencing angina or other heart disease symptoms. Specifically, the treadmill test is preferred for patients with symptoms of myocardial ischemia, acute chest pain, valvular heart disease, etc. Moreover, the treadmill test is preferred for patients with cardiac arrhythmias to evaluate the chronotropic competence.

Chronotropic competence is the capability of the heart to raise its rate when the body demands or during increased activity. The purpose of the test is to determine whether the patient's heart is receiving enough oxygen as well as proper blood flow under stressed conditions, such as exercise or vigorous activities.

The target heart rate is calculated by the equation: target heart rate $= 0.85 \times (220\text{-Age})$. If the patients feel chest pain or severe arrhythmia the test result is considered positive. Furthermore, ECG recorded during the treadmill test is analyzed to evaluate the condition of the patient. If the ST-segment changes are greater or equal to 1 mm then the test is considered positive. In addition, changes in T-wave and a prolonged QT interval indicate abnormalities with the heart. These abnormalities are not usually found in resting ECG.

2.2.6 Cardiac Biomarker Examination

Cardiac biomarkers are the enzymes released into the blood when the heart experiences any discomfort or defects, such as stress or impairments. The quantity of cardio enzymes in the blood can be utilized to detect heart diseases, especially acute coronary syndrome (ACS) and cardiac ischemia. The test is done by taking a sample of the patient's blood and analyzing it to measure the level of cardiac biomarkers in their blood. It can detect low oxygen intake conditions or injuries in the heart. Myoglobin, troponin, and creatine kinase are the three cardiac biomarkers or enzymes. Among these, the most commonly used cardiac biomarker is troponin due to its highest sensitivity [3]. Usually, the quantity of cardiac markers in the blood is measured in nanogram/milliliter (ng/ml) units. The normal measure of troponin in the blood ranges from 0 to 0.4 ng/ml. The high-sensitivity troponin test can detect a very small level of troponin. The normal range value is 14 ng/l for troponin during cardiac biomarker examination (high-sensitivy troponin test). Anything above 14 ng/l is considered abnormal.

2.2.7 Chest Roentgenography

Despite the increasing number of modern diagnostic imaging techniques accessible to clinicians, chest roentgenography remains a straightforward, low-cost, and highly insightful examination. A roentgenogram, also known as an x-ray image is a photograph of internal structures made by moving x-rays through the body and forming a shadow image on specially sensitized film. Roentgenography was named after Wilhelm Conrad Röntgen, a German physicist who invented it in 1895. The chest x-ray is a reliable method for predicting pulmonary hemodynamic events in patients without chronic obstructive pulmonary disease and offers a fair estimation of pulmonary venous and arterial pressures. Unfortunately, the pulmonary vascular distribution of patients with chronic obstructive pulmonary disease may be substantially altered. This complicates roentgenographic assessment.

2.3 Physiological Values and Characteristics Considered for Clinical Examination

Apart from analyzing the symptoms and manifestations in the face, the physician or cardiologist examines several physiological values as well as characteristics to detect the presence of heart disease. This section briefly describes the physiological attributes/characteristics and values that aid the physician or cardiologist in diagnosing heart disease.

2.3.1 Exercise Capacity

Exercise capacity, also known as cardiorespiratory endurance, is the total amount of physical effort that a person can bear without discomfort. A precise evaluation of workout capacity requires the patient to exert maximal physical effort for an adequate enough time to reflect the stable effect on the circulation. The exercise capacity evaluation is one of the key characteristics for assessing the condition of the patient. Lower exercise capacity is linked with various risks including hypertension, cardiovascular disease, heart failure, etc. Many studies have shown the correlation between lower exercise capacity and acute health conditions [4]. Furthermore, the response of the cardiovascular system during exercise can identify heart diseases as well as mortality [5, 6].

The exercise capacity of an individual can be assessed either by a face-to-face interview or by using laboratory methods based on the available facilities in the clinic. In the face-to-face interview with the patient, the cardiologist will ask about any unprecedented events experienced during various daily activities, such as walking, running, or exercise. On the other hand, the laboratory methods include multiple tests, such as an exercise stress test, a cardiopulmonary exercise test, a 6-minute walk test, a submaximal treadmill test, etc.

2.3.2 Chest Pain or Discomfort

Chest pain or discomfort is the most common symptom found in adults for several reasons either serious or trivial. It occurs due to many causes, such as muscle strain, peptic ulcers, gastroesophageal reflux disease (GERD), asthma, etc. The pain or discomfort generated in the chest can be an important indication of possibly genuine cardiac or cardiovascular disorders. Proper care and treatment should be done early to identify the underlying cause of the chest pain and prevent it worsening. Regular exercise and healthy eating habits can greatly avoid getting chest pain.

Self-diagnosing chest pain based merely on symptoms is quite difficult. However, the frequency of pain and accompanying symptoms may help to shed light on the possible cause to some extent. The pain that arises from mild health issues including muscle strain, GERD, and asthma can last only for a few seconds and affect a specific point on the chest. Moreover, the pain is often relieved when the chest area is massaged, or after taking medication or a deep breath. Specifically, chest pain related to muscle strain gets better with massage and gets worse with sharp and sudden inhalation. Gastroesophageal reflux can cause chest pain which may be experienced shortly after a meal or consumption of alcohol. Sudden and intense pain that lasts longer than a few minutes can be an indicator of heart disease.

2.3.3 Palpitations

Palpitation generally refers to irregular and rapid heartbeats and can arise for a multitude of reasons. It can be caused by certain harmless conditions, such as strenuous exercise, lack of sleep, stress, anxiety, fear, etc., or it can be an alarming indication of certain illnesses relating to the heart, such as cardiac arrhythmia, which involve changes in heart rate and the contraction pattern. It can give the sensation that the heart has skipped, stopped, or added an extra beat, making us more aware of our heartbeat. Heart palpitations can become a significantly diagnosable characteristic in persons already diagnosed with heart failure or defective heart valves.

2.3.4 Dyspnea, Orthopnea, and Paroxysmal Nocturnal Dyspnea

Dyspnea is a condition where the patient suffers from shortness of breath or sometimes difficulty in breathing. Labored breathing, tightness in the chest, heart palpitations, and wheezing are often the indications of a person experiencing dyspnea. It can occur after intense exercise or from traveling to a high altitude. However, it can be directly related to severe health conditions such as pneumonia, heart failure, or low blood pressure. Dyspnea on exertion can be a normal occurrence unless it accompanies an activity that can be considered to be within the tolerance limits of the individual.

Since dyspnea is often characterized by the subjective experience or sensation reported by the patient, it is quite distinguishable from tachypnea, hyperventilation, and hyperpnea, which refer to respiratory variations. The latter conditions exist irrespective of the patients' subjective sensations. Tachypnea is an increase in the respiratory rate, which is indicated by rapid shallow or deep breathing, often unnoticed by the patient. Hyperventilation is the increased and rapid breathing that occurs due to an unbalance between inhalation and exhalation. The increased exhalation results in reduced carbon dioxide levels in the blood, which in turn leads to the symptoms such as dizziness, shortness of breath, etc. Hyperpnea is also a condition of deep breathing but not necessarily faster. The forced respiration causes the inhalation of an increased air volume and the respiratory rate can even stay within normal limits. This is an indication of the body's demand for more oxygen. These medical conditions might not always be associated with dyspnea.

The sensation of breathlessness that occurs only in the specific posture of lying down is referred to as orthopnea. It can result in tightness in the chest that makes breathing uncomfortable. However, it subsides when the patient stands upright or sits down. Still, it might be a symptom of heart or lung disease. The presence of increased heart rate, wheezing, or nausea along with orthopnea is an indicator for heart failure. A condition that is closely related to orthopnea is paroxysmal nocturnal dyspnea. It is a sensation of shortness of breath that makes the patient wake up after 1 or 2 hours of sleep. Similar to orthopnea, this condition is usually relieved after getting back to the upright position.

Apart from the aforementioned conditions of breathing difficulties, there are two uncommon types of breathlessness: trepopnea and platypnea. Trepopnea is typically dyspnea or breathlessness in either lateral decubitus position. The shortness of breath when lying on the left side can be attributed to chronic heart diseases. On the other hand, breathlessness experienced while lying on the right side may be due to a lung disease or a major bronchus. Platypnea is the reverse condition of orthopnea. This refers to breathlessness that occurs in the upright position (sitting or standing) and gets improved when lying down.

2.3.5 Claudication

Claudication is a pain, cramp, or sense of fatigue that results from the lower blood flow to the muscles during exercise. This affects the muscle group of the lower extremities and causes pain in the legs depending on the pace and duration of the walk. It is relieved promptly within a few minutes of rest in positions such as standing evenly on both feet. This condition can occur anywhere in the body, but is predominantly in the legs. Even though the pain is not constant and subsides with rest, it can be a symptom of peripheral artery disease.

2.3.6 Recording History of Heart Disease

In many heart patients, mostly adults, the heart disease or discomfort related to the heart won't begin suddenly in a day. A detailed study about the history of any chest discomfort or heart disease experienced by the patient in the past can provide additional information about the underlying disease for the cardiologist. The history recording procedure investigates whether the patient has suffered any heart attack or coronary artery diseases, whether they have undergone any heart surgery in the past, their medication history, etc. The cardiologist will also ask when an incident happened, how it was diagnosed, about the patient's lifestyle after that incident, etc. Furthermore, the history recording procedure will inquire into whether the patient was healthy during their childhood, whether they were very active and took part in soft or vigorous sports activities, etc.

2.3.7 Family History

The cardiologist enquires about the family history of the patient including whether any cases of heart attacks, strokes, coronary artery diseases, acute heart diseases, and early death linked to heart disease have occurred in the patient's family. The family history of heart disease recording is based on the fact that, if family members have suffered from any heart or cardiovascular disease, then the patient is more likely to have the heart disease. The brothers or sisters of a patient with heart disease are 40% more likely to suffer heart disease in the future, while the offspring of patients with early heart disease are 60 –75% more prone to heart diseases [7].

2.3.8 Blood Pressure and Pulse

The amount of force used by the heart to pump blood across the body is referred to as blood pressure; in other words, the pressure generated when the heart pumps blood into the circulatory system. Blood pressure is measured using a sphygmomanometer or blood pressure monitor in millimeters of mercury unit (mmHg). There will be two components for each reading of blood pressure, the systolic and diastolic pressures. The force exerted on the walls of arteries by the heart during systole is called systolic pressure. The systole is a short span where the ventricles of the heart are contracted, and it happens in between the first and second heart sound. Diastolic pressure is the force exerted on the walls of arteries between the beats. Generally, blood pressure levels between 120 and 80 mmHg are considered normal. Blood pressure level measurement has significant importance in the heart disease examination procedure. Several studies have found that high blood pressure levels have a clear link with the risk of strokes as well heart diseases in individuals irrespective of their ages [8]. However, a study [9] conducted in different age groups of the Framingham heart study participants observed that in individuals aged less than 50 the diastolic blood pressure levels are a clear indicator for predicting heart disease. On the other hand, systolic pressure levels along with pulse pressure levels are the clear predictor of heart diseases in individuals over 50 years old.

The heart rate, or the cumulative number of times the heart beats in a minute, is referred to as pulse. If the person is resting, 60–100 beats per minute are considered natural. The heart rate can elevate up to 150 if the person is involved in any highly vigorous activity. If the resting heart rate of an individual is less than 60, then it is called bradycardia and, if it is greater than 100/120, then it is called tachycardia. Bradycardia is often linked with underlying heart diseases such as heart failure. Similarly, tachycardia can be an early symptom of heart failure or stroke.

2.3.9 Total Cholesterol, Triglycerides, and Associated Lipid Profiles

The lipid fraction of the human body is made up of cholesterol, triglycerides, and high-density lipoproteins (HDLs). Elevated cholesterol levels in the human body can increase the chances of developing heart diseases and stroke. The cholesterol level of a human body is measured by drawing blood samples. The cholesterol level examination generates the measurement of four types of fats (lipids) in the blood: total cholesterol; HDL cholesterol; low-density lipoprotein (LDL) cholesterol; and triglycerides. The overall amount of cholesterol in the blood is known as total cholesterol. HDL cholesterol is known as the "good" cholesterol as it aids in the removal of LDL cholesterol, allowing arteries to remain open and blood to circulate freely. A higher amount of HDL in the blood lowers the rate of heart disease risk [10]. LDL cholesterol is known as "bad" cholesterol since a higher amount of LDL in blood induces atherosclerosis, which is the accumulation of fatty deposits (plaques) in arteries. These plaques may hinder blood flow and cause a heart attack or stroke. Therefore, a higher LDL level represents a higher risk of heart disease [11]. Triglycerides are a type of fat that occurs naturally in the body. Extra calories consumed over the total energy expenditure of a body get converted into triglycerides. These triglycerides are contained in fat cells and are later released into the blood when the body requires energy to do any activity. The elevated level of triglycerides in the blood is due to many reasons, such as obesity, thyroid or liver disease, and genetic conditions. High triglyceride levels are linked to the increased risk of heart disease [12]. A bad diet that includes a significant amount of butter, oil, and excess sugar can cause an increase in the level of triglycerides in the body. Eating a lot of foods rich in carbohydrates or sugar and drinking excessive amounts of alcohol lead to high triglycerides levels in the human body. Apart from food, the main cause of increased triglyceride levels is a sedentary lifestyle. Certain types of food should be avoided or limited if the patient has high triglyceride levels: the intake of starchy vegetables like corn and peas should be limited, while canned fish or beef packed in oil should be avoided. Baked foods that contain a high level of saturated fat should also be avoided and the consumption of butter or margarine should be limited or replaced with olive oil. Lean meats should be preferred over high fat meats such as beef or pork. Moreover, all processed meats are bad for patients with higher levels of triglycerides and should be avoided.

2.3.10 Bruits and Hums of the Head and Neck

A bruit refers to the vascular sound associated with turbulent blood flow. This will be audible and detected with a stethoscope. These auscultatory sounds originating in the heart and radiating to the neck are considered to be cardiac valvular murmurs. A carotid bruit is the sound heard over the cervical arteries and can indicate the underlying arterial occlusive pathology which can lead to a stroke. The carotid artery bruit can also be caused by atherosclerotic stenosis in adults. The cervical venous hum is often felt over the internal jugular cervical veins and is due to the combined effects of gravity on the blood flow and the partial compression of the vein by the transverse process of the atlas. These sounds, especially venous hum, are more common in children than adults and are quite normal. Cranial and orbital bruits, vibrations resulting from turbulence in intracranial or extracranial vessels, are less serious and normally occurring in the younger population. However, cranial-orbital bruits present in the adult category, are usually pathologic and indicate an underlying abnormality such as arteriovenous fistulas, arteriovenous malformations, and intracranial hemangiomas. In addition, an orbital bruit can occur rarely as a result of the atherosclerosis of the arteries in the neck.

2.3.11 Jugular Venous Pressure

The jugular venous pressure or jugular venous pulse estimation is a method for assessing central venous pressure. The central venous pressure alters with a change in the amount of blood flowing back to the heart as well as an increase or decrease in the capability of the heart to drive blood back to the circulatory system. The jugular venous pressure assessment procedure includes making the patient lie in a semi-recumbent position, turning the head of the patient to the left side (normally jugular venous pressure is assessed from the right side of the neck), and jugular venous pressure is measured by estimating the distance between the top point of the internal jugular vein and sternal angle. An elevated jugular venous pressure is linked with abnormal functioning of the right heart, heart failure conditions [13], and hypotension.

2.3.12 Carotid Pulse and Precordial Impulse

The carotid pulse is commonly a pressure signal sensed over the carotid artery when it passes near the neck. This pulse signifies the variations in the arterial blood pressure and volume with each heartbeat. It appears as a smooth rapid upstroke and a gradual downstroke with a brief interruption at the pulse peak. The abnormalities of the carotid pulse can be identified as an alteration in either pulse peak amplitude or a distortion of the upstroke or downstroke or both. These variations in carotid pulse contour reflect underlying cardiac abnormalities, such as aortic stenosis. However, it is generally confirmed only after detecting abnormal cardiac impulse or murmur.

Precordial impulses generally originate from the heart or great vessels visible or palpable on the anterior chest wall. All the precordial impulses including apex impulse, parasternal impulse, and pulmonary artery pulsation are observed and consideration is taken into account of the relevant location, size, and character, which including the duration, force, and contour.

2.3.13 Heart Sounds and Murmurs

Discrete bursts of auditory vibrations that differ in intensity (volume), frequency, quality, and duration are known as heart sounds, the sounds for a normal heartbeat being first heart sound (called lub) and second heart sound (called dub). The first heart sound consists of multiple high-frequency elements where only the first two among them can be heard normally. These two normally audible sound waves occur simultaneously when the mitral and tricuspid valves close. The first heart sound indicates the beginning of ventricular systole and the end of mechanical diastole. The second heart sound is described as a discrete burst of vibration that occurred due to the immediate closure of the aortic valve and pulmonic valve. The second heart sound consists of two components – the aortic component and the pulmonic component – with the aortic valve and pulmonic valve being the sources of the second heart sound. The second heart sound is produced at the end of ventricular contraction and it indicates the beginning of ventricular diastole and the end of mechanical systole.

Apart from the normal first and second heart sounds, unusual third and fourth heart sounds are found in healthy as well as unhealthy individuals. The third heart sound, or ventricular gallop, is an additional unusual sound produced after the first and second heart sound. It is generated when a large amount of blood strikes the left ventricle and happens when the mitral valves open after the second heart sound, allowing passive blood flow to the left ventricle. The fourth heart sound, or atrial gallop, is a low-pitched sound that occurs before the first heart sound as the ventricle fills late in its diastole due to atrial contraction. The fourth heart sound results from vibrations produced within the ventricle, and it is also known as the atrial sound because its development requires an effective atrial contraction.

Generally, the cardiologist examines the heart sound by cardiac auscultation technique using a stethoscope. The unusual pattern of heart sound can indicate a serious underlying heart condition. The first and second heart sound are common, while the third and fourth are unusual in healthy individuals. However, while the third heart sounds *can* be audible in healthy individuals below 40 years of age [14] and pregnant women [15], in people younger than 40 they are considered abnormal and a possible early indication of heart diseases including heart failure. The fourth heart sound is very rare in healthy individuals, but common in patients with heart diseases.

Heart murmurs are the type of abnormal sound generated in the heart as a result of the turbulent flow of blood. These murmurs are generated either by blood flow through an abnormal valve or by abnormalities in the internal chamber of the heart. In most cases, the murmurs are not serious and do not require quick medication or a hospital visit. However, in a few cases, the abnormal murmurs are due to heart valve problems present at birth, or caused by cardiac shunts or septal defects.

2.4 Evolution of the Devices for Conventional Clinical Cardiac Examination

Multiple devices have been used by physicians and paramedical experts to diagnose the existence of any heart defects or disease. Further, they continuously witness the evolution of these devices each year, in terms of size, accuracy, and specificity. This section discusses the very common devices used by the physicians and paramedical experts, and their brief history.

2.4.1 Stethoscope

The stethoscope is one of the common devices used by the physician for auscultation examination. Stethoscopes were first invented by a French physician, René Laënnec, in 1816. The prototype consisted of a rolled paper cone and a wooden tube, the purpose being to hear the heart's sounds. In 1819, it was improved by replacing the wooden tube with a rubber tube. In the following years, many improvements were made to the design, with the introduction of the diaphragm, bell, and binaural version. In 1956, several further improvements were implemented, resulting in the current stethoscope now used by doctors [16]. The evolution of the rubber-based stethoscope is given in Figure 2.5.

The evolution of the stethoscope is not limited simply to design and appearance, but involves functionality, accuracy, and outcome. The first stethoscope only allowed doctors to hear the pumping of the heart through one ear, whereas the binaural stethoscope design, allowed its users to hear and compare sounds of each bell. Then came the stethoscope with its classic design of two sides and one bell, which helped physicians use it for the respiratory and cardiovascular systems. After that, the diaphragm was introduced, helping to distinguish low-pitched and high-pitched sounds for accurate diagnosis.

After several years, the development of digital stethoscopes began. A digital stethoscope (seee Figure 2.6) has the ability to convert acoustic sounds into electronic signals, which can be transmitted to a computer for further processing. The digital stethoscope has three different modules, namely data acquisition, preprocessing, and signal processing. The main benefit of these modules is to enhance the quality of the sound acquired [17]. Other recent improvements include embedded noise reduction and cancelation features that give better accuracy.

2.4.2 Electrocardiogram

The electrical activity of skeletal muscles was first noticed by Dr. Luigi Galvan, a physician in Italy, who pointed out that this activity could be recorded using electrical currents. In 1842, another physicist, Dr. Carlo Matteucci, found the electrical activity or

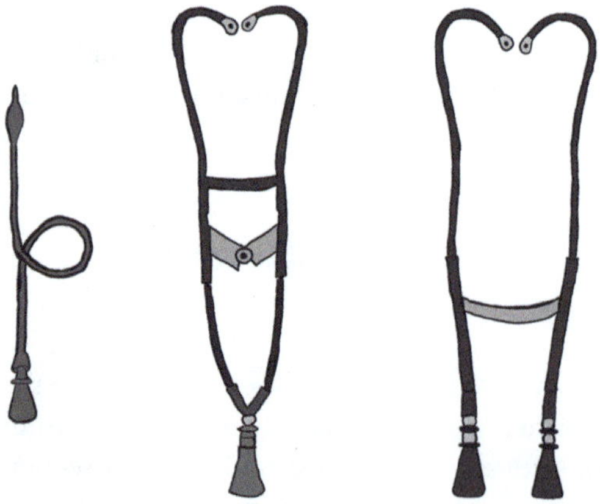

Figure 2.5 Evolution of rubber-based stethoscopes.

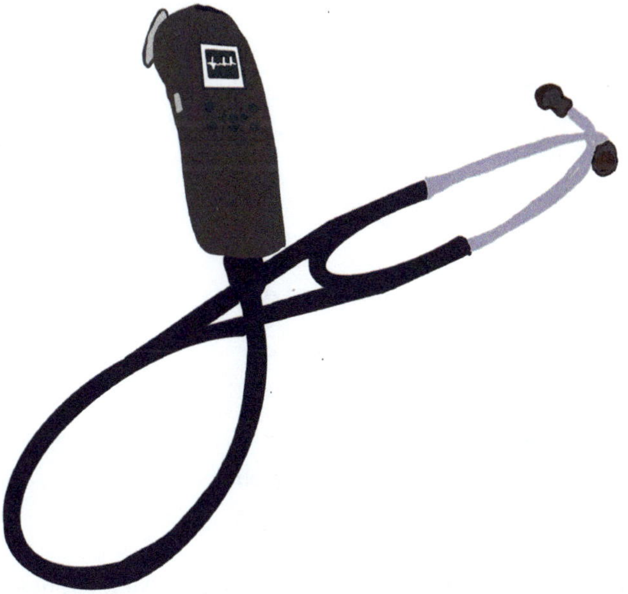

Figure 2.6 A digital stethoscope.

responses for heartbeats in a frog. Several years later, a physiologist from London, Augustus Desiré Waller, showed the first human electrocardiogram, which used a capillary electrometer and electrodes placed on the chest and back. From this experiment, many demonstrations grew, including triphasic electric cardiac activity using improved capillary electrometers, followed by an improvement in refining electrometers by using five measured deflections in the electrocardiograph [18].

The electrocardiogram machine initially had three electrodes forming a triangle. Two were later removed due to the poor yielding. The machine contained cylinders of an electrolyte solution and patients placed their arms and one leg inside these cylinders [18]. Examiners continued to use this machine until a new design was introduced in 1928 which was much lighter than the previous design and had five electrodes. Further improvements consisting of 12 electrodes were then made, giving more accurate measurements.

Today, ECG systems are available in much smaller and portable forms, such as smartwatches, ECG patches, etc., which allow users to place their fingers on them to generate the ECG results within seconds.

2.4.3 Echocardiogram (Ultrasound Devices)

Echocardiogram devices were first introduced in 1950, when the first M-mode echocardiography was developed by two physicists in order to study mitral stenosis and its diagnosis. Their work inspired many cardiologists, as they carried out their work to develop Doppler, two-dimensional (2D), contrast, and transesophageal echocardiograms. The echocardiogram was inspired by stethoscopes, and actually enables users to observe

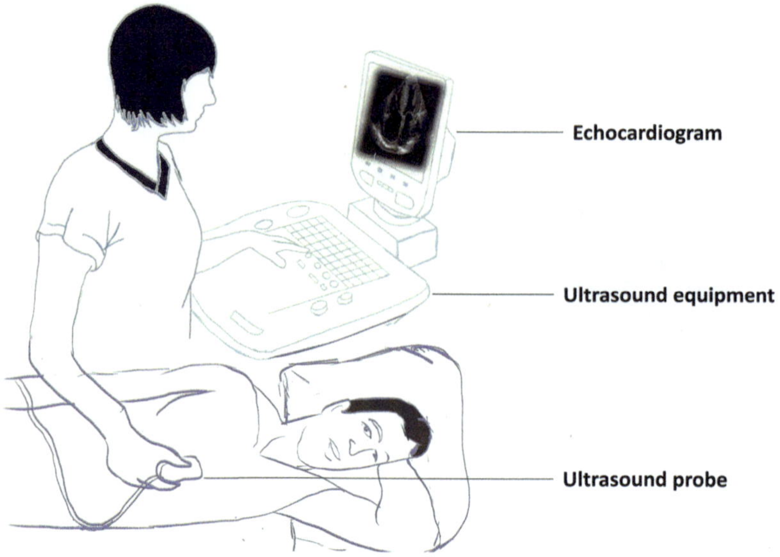

Figure 2.7 The echocardiography method. The patient lies in the left lateral decubitus position, and the ultrasound probe generates sound waves, receives an echo from body tissues, and sends the results to the ultrasound processing unit/computer to create a sonogram image.

what occurs underneath the human skin [19]. The general setup of the echocardiography method is given in Figure 2.7.

The echocardiogram is an ultrasound of the heart that provides moving pictures capable of identifying the structure and function of the heart. It is more effective and efficient than ECG for detecting heart disease. ECG mainly provides information on the rhythm of the heart and involves a lengthy procedure compared to the an echocardiogram which involves a quick test that can be done in 5 minutes. An echocardiogram helps to visualize the heart beating and pumping blood, and aids the identification of heart disease. Providing information about heart functioning by measuring heart rate and rhythm, ECG is the preliminary test for detecting heart problems; any abnormality found here demands further diagnostic tests like an echocardiogram. Moreover, defects in heart valves are often undetected by ECG and the echocardiogram is the more preferred method for detecting valvular heart diseases. The echocardiogram is more efficient, but expensive compared to ECG.

2.5 Artificial Intelligence for Assisting Clinical Cardiac Examination

Artificial intelligence (AI) is the ability of the computer to make human-like decisions based on previous learning to solve problems, recognize an object, or respond to languages. Currently, AI is widely used in various sectors, such as business, agriculture, and health. In recent years, the various AI methods such as machine learning and deep learning have been predominantly used in the health sector in applications such as development assistive systems [20] and automated disease diagnosing systems for various chronic health disorders, such as cancer [21] and coronary heart disease [22].

In the case of cardiac examination, AI is mostly integrated for processing the physiological readings obtained from echocardiography, electrocardiography, and cardiac computed tomography (CT). Various image processing, signal processing, and computer vision algorithms are utilized in the literature to predict the cardiac condition using physiological values obtained in these three procedures.

2.5.1 AI in Echocardiography

The role of ultrasound devices is vital in the early diagnosis of cardiovascular diseases (CVDs). In addition, some of the risk factors of CVDs can be due to high blood pressure or high cholesterol, and one of the main causes of such diseases can be the buildup of inflammatory cells known as plaques, which occur in the arterial wall and result in both blood restriction to the heart and lower oxygen intake. This medical condition is known as atherosclerosis. Early prediction of a CVD disease might help in preventing the progression of atherosclerosis as well as possible heart failures. In Figure 2.8, it is shown that plaque formation occurs mostly in the common carotid artery and internal carotid artery.

One of the ways to identify the plaques in the arterial wall is by analyzing the carotid artery, which consists of a pair of blood vessels and has several parts, namely internal, external, and common parts. Plaques occur in the internal section as well as in the common blood vessels of the carotid artery. Hence, plaques create a thicker wall in these vessels, and can be measured as intima-media thickness (IMT). Thus, carotid IMT is used as a risk marker for early heart disease prediction. It can be done by

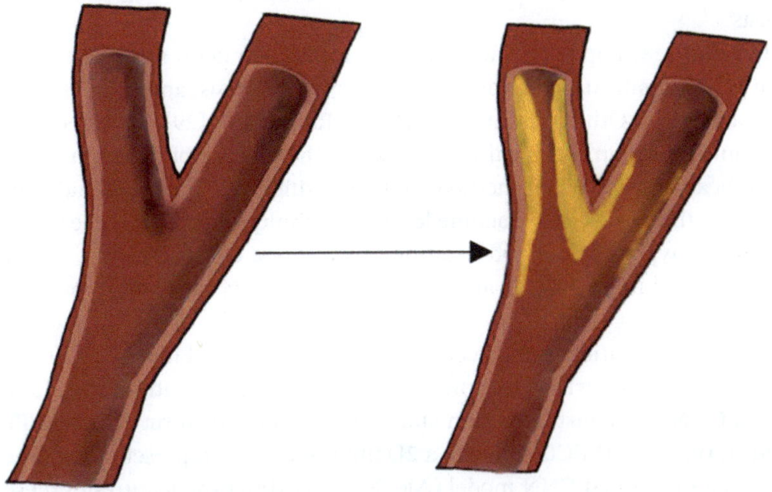

Figure 2.8 Formation of plaques in the common carotid artery and internal carotid artery.

measuring the difference between the lumen-intima (LI) and media adventitia (MA) walls [23].

Recently, many applications regarding ultrasound image segmentation using machine learning and deep learning techniques have been implemented to detect atherosclerosis. The work proposed in Nagaraj [24] used support vector machines (SVM) to train and segment IMT using a dataset of 49 images and resulted in 93% accuracy. Other researchers (see Biswas, Saba, et al. [25]) have worked on a screening tool that integrates a two-stage AI model for IMT and carotid plaque measurements, and consists of a convolutional neural network (CNN) and a fully convolutional network (FCN). The system goes through two deep learning models. The first divides the common carotid artery from the ultrasound images into two categories: the rectangular wall and non-wall patches. Then, the region of interest is analyzed and fed to the second stage, which identifies features in order to calculate the carotid IMT and the plaque total.

The work in Biswas, Kuppili, et al. [26] combined both the CNN algorithm and the machine learning based regression technique for IMT segmentation. Further, Menchón-Lara and colleagues [27] implemented an autoencoder model for segmenting IMT. Their method included regions of interest (ROI) prediction and then LI interface (LII) and MA interface (MAI) walls predictions in the predicted ROI. The authors reported that they used extreme learning machines along with autoencoders to distinguish between the block included in the ROI and the excluded from the ROI. The LII and MAI recognition was done using pixel classification.

2.5.2 AI in Electrocardiography

Electrocardiography has a high impact in detecting abnormalities in heart rhythm. Most of the existing machine learning applications based on ECG focus on classification of electrical signals to spot abnormal activity in the heart. With today's availability of ECG in small portable devices such as smartwatches, AI integration helps patients to monitor their heartbeat levels and detect any abnormalities that might require seeing a doctor or having further tests.

The work of Li et al. [28] applied a multichannel, multiscale deep neural network model to perform ECG classification of normal and abnormal signals, and their method achieved 96.02% accuracy. Other research work by Rajput el. [29] developed an automated ECG signal detection specifically for detecting the severity of hypertension, a high-risk factor for heart disease. Their method included using a two-band optimal biorthogonal wavelet bank filter as well as machine learning techniques to classify the wavelets into low, high-risk hypertension, and healthy. The average classification accuracy for this method was found to be 99.95%, and highlights the ability of this system to be deployed in clinics.

A method for ECG identification and detection of congestive heart failure (CHF) and arrhythmia (ARR) using deep learning techniques is that proposed by Eltrass et al. [30]. It mainly uses both CNN and constant-Q non-stationary Gabor transform (CQ-NSGT), which mainly transforms the 1D ECG signal to a 2D time-frequency representation. The output is then fed to a pretrained CNN model (AlexNet) to extract the features of these signals and then the features are used to diagnose the case by either classifying it as CHF, ARR, or normal sinus rhythm (NSR). The work achieved 98.82% accuracy, 98.87% sensitivity, 99.21% specificity, and 99.20% precision.

In the work by Moridani et al. [31], the authors experimented with multiple machine learning algorithms for ECG signal classification. They concentrated on performing preprocessing techniques for the initial signal and then applying feature extraction for both linear and nonlinear features for the heart rate variability as well as the application of statistical characteristics for the signal. Afterward, they used multilayer perceptron (MLP) and SVM, along with all features as well as optimal features to classify normal and abnormal signals in separate experiments. Their outcomes highlighted the performance of the SVM model that was able to get the highest accuracy while using all features and optimal features. For the optimal features, it achieved 98.3% accuracy, 99.10% sensitivity, and 97.5% specificity.

2.5.3 AI in CT

CT scans are mainly used to view parts of the body in detail. In the case of a cardiac CT scan, it displays the heart and the blood vessels clearly which helps experts to diagnose or detect any abnormality. CT scans can detect the early signs of heart disease by scanning the heart's arteries for any calcified plaque formation to create a coronary artery calcium (CAC) score, which has been proven to be a strong predictor for CVDs (Figure 2.9).

The data captured by a CT scan generates a 3D model of a patient's heart. Cardiac segmentation in chest CT images facilitates partitioning the entire chest CT image into

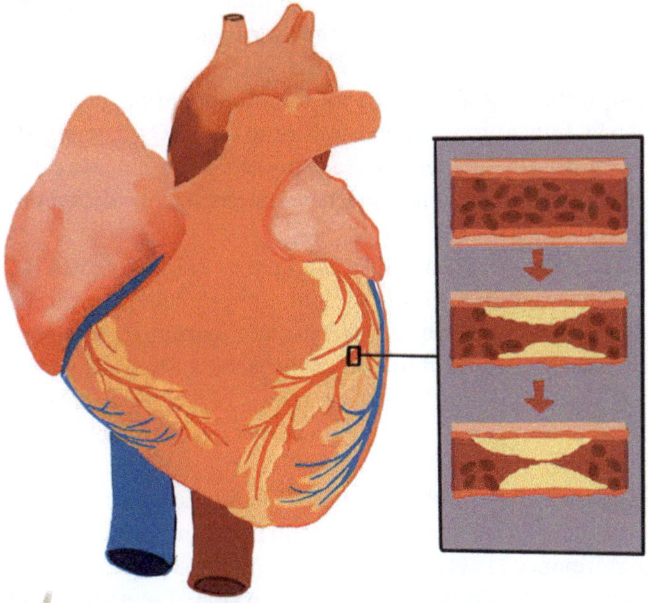

Figure 2.9 Plaque formation in the heart arteries.

numbers of anatomically significant regions that focus on the four chambers of the heart. The manual process of segmentation is becoming replaced by computer-aided techniques such as graph-based segmenting, mean-thresholding, fuzzy clustering methods, and the latest deep learning approach, which has shown promising results. The deep learning system can be trained to identify and quantify coronary artery calcium. This makes an effective early detection device for coronary calcification from atherosclerosis as it detects calcification before symptoms develop. This forms a powerful predictor of future heart problems.

One of the works proposed in the literature regarding CAC was about developing an algorithm that excludes CT scans with negative CAC scores and segments CAC in cases where positive scores are found. The segmented region can further proceed to radiologists for accurate detection. The proposed method highly reduces the workload of radiologists [32]. The proposed method utilized an integrated architecture model which consists of two CNNs where one is for classification and the other for segmentation. The model was able to exclude 86% of the negative cases and segmentation achieved a Dice coefficient of 0.63 and 0.84, for internal and external validation, respectively.

Another research group developed a deep learning model for CAC classification and segmentation [33]. The group focused on calcium quantification of chest CT scans and compared it to manual evaluation. The model was a combination of CNNs along with a ResNet architecture for image feature extraction, as well as an FCN for spatial coordinate features. Their method displayed a high correlation with the manual evaluation for detecting the presence of calcification, with results of 91% sensitivity and 92% specificity. In the case of calcium volume determination, the AI model was able to produce an excellent correlation with the manual determination with no significant difference found. The method proved to be fully automated, reducing the time for evaluation while optimizing clinical calcium scoring.

The work by Zhang et al. [34] utilized deep learning for calcium quantification from CT scan images. They developed a fully automated framework to detect CAC, using 3D CT scans as input for the model and extracting features to apply segmentation and calcification. The obtained results of the proposed method have no significant difference compared to the manual method.

Dekker et al. [35], implemented the deep learning technique to calculate the CAC score during myocardial perfusion imaging (MPI) assessment. They defined a threshold for CAC scores where it was low (<400) and high (≥ 400). The deep learning model used in the proposed method was previously validated in other approaches. The outcomes of the research work highlighted that high CAC scores presented higher accumulative event rates. They also proved that their method could progress risk stratification leading to customized treatments for patients.

In conclusion, AI methods showed better automation and higher accuracy in diagnosis in some applications. Some of the outcomes are even open to further enhancement which could lead to higher performance. This could help to reduce the effort of physicians and radiologists in diagnosing heart disease in the future. AI based methods can't replace clinical methods such as ECG, EEG, or CT scans; however, they can automate the decision-making task.

2.6 Conclusion

Heart diseases are very common nowadays and are one of the major contributors of world mortality rate. The prompt diagnosis of heart disease can reduce the casualty as well as mortality associated with the risk of heart disease to a great extent. Today, due to the technological advancement in signal processing, medical imaging, sensors, etc., diagnosis of heart disease and finding the underlying specific reasons is not hard. Future versions of the medical devices, including the stethoscope and ECG machines, will utilize AI technologies for efficient detection of heart abnormalities in hospitals and clinics. However, conventional methods will also be used alongside advanced methods, with most of the former, including inspection and palpation, being cost-effective and not requiring any advanced devices or sensors. Recent advancements that enabled the development of neural network-based stethoscopes will reduce the effort of physicians to perform conventional auscultation examinations.

This chapter has briefly discussed the various conventional clinical methods for heart disease prediction and has presented several physiological attributes considered by the physician for diagnosing heart disease. The clinical significance of psychological attributes has also been discussed and we provided a brief history of the devices utilized by cardiologists, physicians, and radiologists for heart examination. The chapter ended by providing a brief discussion on how AI can assist physicians as well as a radiologists in cardiovascular examination.

References

1 NCBI Bookshelf. (2004). Cardiology explained: Cardiovascular Examination. A service of the National Library of Medicine, National Institutes of Health.

2 Malik, M.B. and Gopal, S. (2020). Cardiac exam. StatPearls.

3 Jacob, R. and Khan, M. (2018). Cardiac biomarkers: What is and what can be. *Indian Journal of Cardiovascular Disease in Women WINCARS* 03 (04). https://doi.org/10.1055/s-0039-1679104.

4 Peterson, P.N., Magid, D.J., Ross, C., Ho, P.M., Rumsfeld, J.S., Lauer, M.S., Lyons, E.E., Smith, S.S., and Masoudi, F.A. (2008). Association of exercise capacity on treadmill with future cardiac events in patients referred for exercise testing. *Archives of Internal Medicine* 168 (2). https://doi.org/10.1001/archinternmed.2007.68.

5 Cole, C.R., Foody, J.A.M., Blackstone, E.H., and Lauer, M.S. (2000). Heart rate recovery after submaximal exercise testing as a predictor of mortality in a cardiovascularly healthycohort.*AnnalsofInternalMedicine*132(7).https://doi.org/10.7326/0003-4819-132-7-200004040-00007.

6 Jouven, X., Empana, J.-P., Schwartz, P.J., Desnos, M., Courbon, D., and Ducimetière, P. (2005). Heart-rate profile during exercise as a predictor of sudden death. *New England Journal of Medicine* 352 (19). https://doi.org/10.1056/nejmoa043012.

7 Kolber, M.R. and Scrimshaw, C. (2014). Family history of cardiovascular disease. *Canadian Family Physician* 60 (11).

8 Benjamin, E.J., Blaha, M.J., Chiuve, S.E., Cushman, M., Das, S.R., Deo, R., De Ferranti, S.D., Floyd, J., Fornage, M., Gillespie, C., Isasi, C.R., Jim'nez, M.C., Jordan, L.C., Judd, S.E., Lackland, D., Lichtman, J.H., Lisabeth, L., Liu, S., Longenecker, C.T., and Muntner, P. (2017). Heart disease and stroke statistics – 2017 Update: A report from the American Heart Association. *Circulation* 135 (10). https://doi.org/10.1161/CIR.0000000000000485.

9 Franklin, S.S., Larson, M.G., Khan, S.A., Wong, N.D., Leip, E.P., Kannel, W.B., and Levy, D. (2001). Does the relation of blood pressure to coronary heart disease risk change with aging?: The Framingham heart study. *Circulation* 103 (9). https://doi.org/10.1161/01.CIR.103.9.1245.

10 Rader, D.J. and Hovingh, G.K. (2014). HDL and cardiovascular disease. *The Lancet* 384 (9943). https://doi.org/10.1016/S0140-6736(14)61217-4.

11 Fernandez, M.L. and Webb, D. (2008). The LDL to HDL cholesterol ratio as a valuable tool to evaluate coronary heart disease risk. *Journal of the American College of Nutrition* 27 (1). https://doi.org/10.1080/07315724.2008.10719668.

12 Navar, A.M., Pagidipati, N., Mulder, H., Aberra, T., Philip, S., Granowitz, C., and Peterson, E. (2019). Triglycerides as a risk factor for coronary heart disease: What measure and what cutoff? *Journal of the American College of Cardiology* 73 (9). https://doi.org/10.1016/s0735-1097(19)32471-4.

13 Chua Chiaco, J.M.S., Parikh, N.I., and Fergusson, D.J. (2013). The jugular venous pressure revisited. *Cleveland Clinic Journal of Medicine* 80 (10). https://doi.org/10.3949/ccjm.80a.13039.

14 Kupari, M., Koskinen, P., Virolainen, J., Hekali, P., and Keto, P. (1994). Prevalence and predictors of audible physiological third heart sound in a population sample aged 36 to 37 years. *Circulation* 89 (3). https://doi.org/10.1161/01.CIR.89.3.1189.

15 Breuer, H. (1981). Auscultation of the heart in pregnancy (author's transl). *MMW, Munchener Medizinische Wochenschrift* 123 (45): 1705–1707.

16 Roguin, A. (2006). René Theophile Hyacinthe Laënnec (1781-1826): The man behind the stethoscope. *Clinical Medicine and Research* 4 (3). https://doi.org/10.3121/cmr.4.3.230.

17 Swarup, S. and Makaryus, A.N. (2018). Digital stethoscope: Technology update. *Medical Devices: Evidence and Research* 11. https://doi.org/10.2147/MDER.S135882.

18 AlGhatrif, M. and Lindsay, J. (2012). A brief review: History to understand fundamentals of electrocardiography. *Journal of Community Hospital Internal Medicine Perspectives* 2 (1). https://doi.org/10.3402/jchimp.v2i1.14383.

19 Singh, S. and Goyal, A. (2007). The origin of echocardiography: A tribute to Inge Edler. *Texas Heart Institute Journal/from the Texas Heart Institute of St. Luke's Episcopal Hospital, Texas Children's Hospital* 34 (4).

20 Kunhoth, J., Karkar, A., Al-Maadeed, S., and Al-Attiyah, A. (2019). Comparative analysis of computer-vision and BLE technology based indoor navigation systems for people with visual impairments. *International Journal of Health Geographics* 18 (1). https://doi.org/10.1186/s12942-019-0193-9.

21 Al Maadeed, S., Kunhoth, S., Bouridane, A., and Peyret, R. (2017). Multispectral imaging and machine learning for automated cancer diagnosis. *2017 13th International Wireless Communications and Mobile Computing Conference, IWCMC 2017*. https://doi.org/10.1109/IWCMC.2017.7986547.

22 Masetic, Z. and Subasi, A. (2016). Congestive heart failure detection using random forest classifier. *Computer Methods and Programs in Biomedicine* 130. https://doi.org/10.1016/j.cmpb.2016.03.020.

23 Molinari, F., Meiburger, K.M., Saba, L., Rajendra Acharya, U., Ledda, M., Nicolaides, A., and Suri, J.S. (2012). Constrained snake vs. conventional snake for carotid ultrasound automated IMT measurements on multi-center data sets. *Ultrasonics* 52 (7). https://doi.org/10.1016/j.ultras.2012.03.005.

24 Nagaraj, Y., Teja, A.H.S., and Narasimhadhan, A.V. (2019). Automatic segmentation of intima media complex in carotid ultrasound images using support vector machine. *Arabian Journal for Science and Engineering* 44 (4). https://doi.org/10.1007/s13369-018-3549-8.

25 Biswas, M., Saba, L., Chakrabartty, S., Khanna, N.N., Song, H., Suri, H.S., Sfikakis, P.P., Mavrogeni, S., Viskovic, K., Laird, J.R., Cuadrado-Godia, E., Nicolaides, A., Sharma, A., Viswanathan, V., Protogerou, A., Kitas, G., Pareek, G., Miner, M., and Suri, J.S. (2020). Two-stage artificial intelligence model for jointly measurement of atherosclerotic wall thickness and plaque burden in carotid ultrasound: A screening tool for cardiovascular/stroke risk assessment. *Computers in Biology and Medicine* 123. https://doi.org/10.1016/j.compbiomed.2020.103847.

26 Biswas, M., Kuppili, V., Araki, T., Edla, D.R., Godia, E.C., Saba, L., Suri, H.S., Omerzu, T., Laird, J.R., Khanna, N.N., Nicolaides, A., and Suri, J.S. (2018). Deep learning strategy for accurate carotid intima-media thickness measurement: An ultrasound study on Japanese diabetic cohort. *Computers in Biology and Medicine* 98. https://doi.org/10.1016/j.compbiomed.2018.05.014.

27 Menchón-Lara, R.M., Sancho-Gómez, J.L., and Bueno-Crespo, A. (2016). Early-stage atherosclerosis detection using deep learning over carotid ultrasound images. *Applied Soft Computing Journal* 49. https://doi.org/10.1016/j.asoc.2016.08.055.

28 Li, D., Zhang, J., Zhang, Q., and Wei, X. (2017). Classification of ECG signals based on 1D convolution neural network. *2017 IEEE 19th International Conference on E-Health Networking, Applications and Services, Healthcom 2017, 2017-December*. https://doi.org/10.1109/HealthCom.2017.8210784.

29 Rajput, J.S., Sharma, M., Tan, R.S., and Acharya, U.R. (2020). Automated detection of severity of hypertension ECG signals using an optimal bi-orthogonal wavelet filter bank. *Computers in Biology and Medicine* 123. https://doi.org/10.1016/j.compbiomed.2020.103924.

30 Eltrass, A.S., Tayel, M.B., and Ammar, A.I. (2021). A new automated CNN deep learning approach for identification of ECG congestive heart failure and arrhythmia using constant-Q non-stationary Gabor transform. *Biomedical Signal Processing and Control* 65. https://doi.org/10.1016/j.bspc.2020.102326.

31 Moridani, M.K., Abdi Zadeh, M., and Shahiazar Mazraeh, Z. (2019). An efficient automated algorithm for distinguishing normal and abnormal ECG signal. *IRBM* 40 (6). https://doi.org/10.1016/j.irbm.2019.09.002.

32 Van Den Oever, L.B., Cornelissen, L., Vonder, M., Xia, C., Van Bolhuis, J.N., Vliegenthart, R., Veldhuis, R.N.J., De Bock, G.H., Oudkerk, M., and Van Ooijen, P.M.A. (2020). Deep learning for automated exclusion of cardiac CT examinations negative for coronary artery calcium. *European Journal of Radiology* 129. https://doi.org/10.1016/j.ejrad.2020.109114.

33 Van Assen, M., Martin, S.S., Varga-Szemes, A., Rapaka, S., Cimen, S., Sharma, P., Sahbaee, P., De Cecco, C.N., Vliegenthart, R., Leonard, T.J., Burt, J.R., and Schoepf, U.J. (2021). Automatic coronary calcium scoring in chest CT using a deep neural network in direct comparison with non-contrast cardiac CT: A validation study. *European Journal of Radiology* 134. https://doi.org/10.1016/j.ejrad.2020.109428.

34 Zhang, N., Yang, G., Zhang, W., Wang, W., Zhou, Z., Zhang, H., Xu, L., and Chen, Y. (2021). Fully automatic framework for comprehensive coronary artery calcium scores analysis on non-contrast cardiac-gated CT scan: Total and vessel-specific quantifications. *European Journal of Radiology* 134. https://doi.org/10.1016/j.ejrad.2020.109420.

35 Dekker, M., Waissi, F., Bank, I.E.M., Isgum, I., Scholtens, A.M., Velthuis, B.K., Pasterkamp, G., De Winter, R.J., Mosterd, A., Timmers, L., and De Kleijn, D.P.V. (2021). The prognostic value of automated coronary calcium derived by a deep learning approach on non-ECG gated CT images from 82Rb-PET/CT myocardial perfusion imaging. *International Journal of Cardiology* 329. https://doi.org/10.1016/j.ijcard.2020.12.079.

3

Types of Biosensors and their Importance in Cardiovascular Applications

S. Irem Kaya, Leyla Karadurmuş, Ahmet Cetinkaya, Goksu Ozcelikay, and Sibel A. Ozkan

3.1 Introduction

Cardiovascular disease (CVD) is a general nomenclature given to the group that includes diseases of the heart or blood vessels and describes any disease that affects the circulatory system. CVDs include heart attacks, congenital heart disease, rheumatic heart disease, hypertension, cerebrovascular disease, peripheral artery disease, and heart failure. Although there are several causes of CVD, the most common causes are atherosclerosis and/or hypertension which are the leading cause of death worldwide. Hypertension can be very dangerous because in most cases there can be no apparent symptoms at the early stages that will prompt patients to seek medical care. Although it is a disease with a fairly silent course, a few symptoms including headache, ringing in the ears, nosebleeds, and visual impairment can be warning signs [1]. In the last two decades, mortality rates from CVDs have decreased in high-income countries. Still, morbidity and mortality rates have increased surprisingly rapidly in low- and middle-income countries. More than 17 million people die from CVDs each year, which is around 31% of all deaths worldwide. 75% of CVD deaths occur in low- and middle-income countries and occur almost equally in men and women. If the current situation is allowed to persist, it is estimated that, by 2030, an estimated 23.6 million people will die from CVD [2–5].

Although these diseases are generally seen in older adults, primary prevention efforts should begin early in life, especially since atherosclerosis dates back to childhood. Therefore, there is increasing emphasis on eliminating risk factors through, for example, healthy eating, exercise, and smoking avoidance in atherosclerosis prevention. There are many causes of CVDs, and the main reasons are tobacco use, physical inactivity, unhealthy diet, and the harmful use of alcohol. Many studies have proven that dietary habits are directly related to CVDs. Inadequate intake of whole grains, high consumption of salt, saturated fatty acid, and fried food in the diet of individuals are important parameters that increase the risk of CVDs. Changes that can be made in lifestyle habits, such as increasing fruit and vegetable consumption, adopting a diet that includes regular consumption of olive oil, fish, whole grains, and milk and dairy products, and walking for about 40 minutes daily to support this, as well as exercises to be determined according

Predicting Heart Failure: Invasive, Non-Invasive, Machine Learning, and Artificial Intelligence Based Methods, First Edition. Edited by Kishor Kumar Sadasivuni, Hassen M. Ouakad, Somaya Al-Maadeed, Huseyin C. Yalcin, and Issam Bait Bahadur.

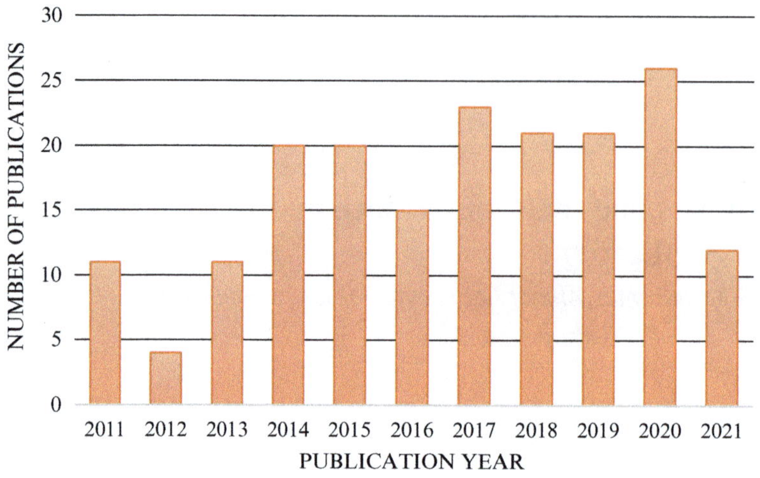

Figure 3.1 Statistics of the number of publications per year related to cardiovascular biomarkers.

to age and risk status all improve the quality of individuals' lives and reduce the risk of CVDs [6–9]. CVDs place a heavy burden on the economies of individuals and countries. People with CVD or at high cardiovascular risk need appropriate early detection and management [10, 11].

There is an increasing demand for the design of fast, portable, and low-cost biosensing devices for the treatment and early diagnosis of CVD. Biosensors can play a significant role in the early diagnosis of CVD as an alternative to time-consuming and expensive laboratory analysis. In recent years, many biosensors have been improved to determine cardiac markers. One of the biggest challenges in CVD is estimating an individual's risk of suffering from CVD. There is great attention in research to find early diagnostic biomarkers that can be detected in the blood and predict CVD risk. The best known of these biomarkers is C-reactive protein (CRP), followed by cardiac troponin (cTn) I or T, interleukin-6, interleukin 1, myoglobin, lipoprotein-associated phospholipase A (2), tumor necrosis factor-alpha, myeloperoxidase, and low-density lipoprotein. In this chapter, the available biosensor platforms for detecting various CVD markers are explained in detail, and the publications on this subject are given in tables [12–16]. Biosensors constitute a large proportion of cardiovascular biomarkers detection research over the last 10 years, as presented in Figure 3.1. Troponin I and CRP diagnosis are gaining attraction. Also notable is the stability in the last 5 years in the usage of electrochemical-based biosensors. This chapter will focus on these recent developments in biosensors used to detect cardiovascular biomarkers.

3.2 Specific Biomarkers for Cardiovascular Research

Nowadays, different reasons, such as particular lifestyles and dietary habits, cause an increase in the risk factors and incidence of CVDs. In addition, individual risk factors, such as age and other diseases, play an essential role for patients [17].

Biomarkers are biological materials found in bodily fluids, and they indicate the normal or pathological processes or responses of the body [18]. Biomarkers are critical tools for diagnosing and monitoring many diseases. CVDs involve various disorders, both acute and chronic. The effective, accurate, and rapid diagnosis of acute conditions with biomarkers in the short term can be life-saving [19]. Besides this, for evaluating long-term risks related to CVDs, which can occur in the later stages of patients' lives, biomarkers are widely used to improve patient's life quality. Cardiovascular research with biomarkers includes, in addition to diagnostic studies, post-disease risk and damage monitoring, such as evaluation of damages after stroke, the severity of cardiac damage, and cardiac arrest-related brain injury in Figure 3.2 [20].

There are various biomarkers available for cardiovascular research that have been used for years and are emerging and new. In Table 3.1, the most significant and specific biomarkers for cardiovascular research are classified.

It is possible to categorize biomarkers based on the physiologic processes. For example, inflammation-related biomarkers are CRP, sST2, GDF-15, TNF-α, etc. LDL and MPO are related to oxidative stress [24]. Considered from another angle, lipid-based biomarkers (HDL, LDL, etc.), CRP, and cTnI are considered widely used traditional biomarkers, while sSTN2, TNF-α, Gal-3, and GDF-15 are emerging biomarkers. Copeptin is another promising biomarker for cardiovascular research, and there are ongoing studies on copeptin that demonstrate its use as a diagnostic biomarker for MI, in addition to the well-known and clinically established biomarkers such as myoglobin and cTnI [22, 34]. Stability and ease of measure of copeptin are considered an alternative biomarker. However, the changes on the levels of copeptin during the perioperative course should be monitored for establishing copeptin as a guiding biomarker [34, 35]. On the other hand, myoglobin, H-FABP, and MPO are add-on biomarkers that are more valuable with a multibiomarker approach [30].

Essentially, an ideal cardiovascular biomarker should be highly specific with definite reference limits in order to provide valuable information for clinical assessment [24].

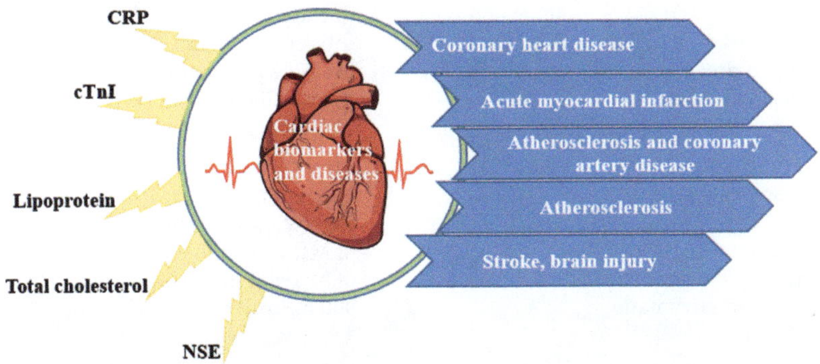

Figure 3.2 A schematic representation of some cardiac biomarkers and diseases.

Table 3.1 Specific biomarkers for the evaluation of CVDs.

Biomarker	Description	Related CVD	Clinical Assessment	Reference
C-reactive protein (CRP)	CRP is a hepatic, acute-phase protein that is related to systemic inflammation; it is used for the early-stage detection of CVDs	Coronary heart disease, thrombotic complications, atherosclerosis, and acute coronary syndrome	Elevated CRP levels indicate a higher risk for adverse cardiovascular events (CRP < 1 mg/L low risk, $1 <$ CRP < 3 mg/L moderate risk, CRP > 3 mg/L high risks)	[12, 17, 21, 22]
Cardiac troponin I (cTnI)	cTnI inhibits actomyosin ATPase, and is released by necrosis of cardiac muscle cells	Acute myocardial infarction and ischemic stroke	Increased cTnI levels are related to the acute phase of acute myocardial infarction and ischemic stroke	[20, 23, 24]
Procalcitonin (PCT)	PCT is an acute phase reactant and a circulating neurohumoral biomarker	Acute heart failure and acute decompensated heart failure	Higher PCT levels are associated with the characterization and early diagnosis of heart failure	[18, 24, 25]
Brain natriuretic peptide (BNP)	BNP is a peptide structured neurohormone, and it has vasodilator, lusitropic and antiproliferative effects	Acute and chronic heart failure, ventricular hypertrophy, cerebral infarction, and cardioembolic stroke	BNP blood level higher than 20 pg/mL is associated with a serious risk of future CVDs. BNP levels are monitored to evaluate cardiac response to treatment	[26–29]
Neuron-specific enolase (NSE)	NSE is a glycolytic enzyme that is specific to the brain. Normally, it is present at negligible levels	Stroke, brain injury after cardiac arrest	Evaluation of infarct volume and integrity of the blood-brain barrier	[20]
Copeptin	Copeptin is an emerging and novel biomarker, which is also a precursor peptide of arginine vasopressin	Heart failure and acute coronary syndrome	Copeptin level is used to exclude myocardial infarction (MI) and evaluate perioperative myocardial injury risk	[17, 18, 22, 30]
Myoglobin	Myoglobin is responsible for binding, transporting, and storing oxygen, and is a non-enzymatic protein	Acute MI	Most reliable and efficient biomarker for early-stage diagnosis of MI; very high levels of myoglobin (up to 900 ng/mL) during MI	[21, 31]

(Continued)

Table 3.1 (Continued)

Biomarker	Description	Related CVD	Clinical Assessment	Reference
Myeloperoxidase (MPO)	MPO is an enzyme that is involved with lipid peroxidation and the production of reactive oxidant species	Atherosclerosis, acute coronary syndrome, and coronary artery disease	MPO provides early phase diagnosis of coronary artery disease, and causes damage in atherosclerotic tissues	[18, 26, 29]
Micro RNAs (miRNAs)	miRNAs, as non-coding RNA sequences, participate in gene expression regulation by inhibiting protein translation	Coronary artery disease, acute MI, heart failure, and stroke	miRNAs can be released from protein complexes such as HDL, apoptotic bodies, exosomes, and microvesicles to peripheral blood; elevated blood levels of circulating miRNAs are associated with CVDs	[26, 31, 32]
Growth differentiation factor (GDF-15)	GDF-15 is secreted as a protection against stress factors such as oxidative stress, cellular ischemia, and myocardial overload	Atrial fibrillation, acute coronary syndrome, heart failure	Elevated GDF-15 levels indicate the renal injury associated with cardiovascular stress	[17, 18, 22, 29]
Galectin-3 (Gal-3)	Gal-3 is involved in inflammatory and fibrotic processes of the body	Hypertrophied hearts, heart failure, and outflow tract tachycardias	Higher Gal-3 levels indicate a higher risk of mortality in end-stage heart failure patients	[17, 24, 30]
Heart fatty acid-binding protein (H-FABP)	H-FABP is one of the fatty acid-binding proteins that is released from myocardial tissue during myocardial ischemia	Atherosclerosis, acute coronary syndrome, and MI	H-FABP is a significant early clinical biomarker to exclude MI probability	[17, 18, 30]
Tumor necrosis factor-alpha (TNF-α)	TNF-α is a proinflammatory cytokine and is involved in inflammatory pathways in cells	Atherosclerosis, arteriosclerosis, platelet activation, and vascular dysfunction	TNF-α is used for the prediction of postoperative complications	[17, 22, 26]
Interleukin-6 (IL-6)	IL-6 belongs to the immune cytokine family, and it is associated with CRP activation and acute phase inflammation	Atherothrombosis and obesity	IL-6 levels are used for the evaluation of cardiovascular risks of patients	[17, 18, 28]

(Continued)

Table 3.1 (Continued)

Biomarker	Description	Related CVD	Clinical Assessment	Reference
Fibrinogen	Fibrinogen is associated with clotting, platelet aggregation, and plasma viscosity processes	Thrombotic diseases and acute coronary syndrome	Fibrinogen is used for the risk assessment of acute coronary syndrome	[17, 18]
Soluble suppressor of tumorgenicity 2 (sST2)	sST2 is involved with cellular inflammatory pathways, and is released after the stretching of cardiac myocytes or fibroblasts	Acute and chronic heart failure	sST2 is clinically used for the risk assessment and future prediction of acute and chronic heart failure	[18, 22, 29, 30]
Total cholesterol	Total cholesterol is one of the traditional lipid-based biomarkers, and it is described as the total amount of LDL and HDL	Atherosclerosis	Evaluation of cardiovascular risks, mortality, and morbidity	[17, 18, 22]
Low-density lipoprotein (LDL)	LDL is responsible for cholesterol transport in the body Peroxidation of LDL results with the foam cell formation	Atherosclerosis and coronary artery disease	Elevated levels of LDL are associated with a higher risk of CVDs	[22, 26, 33]
High-density lipoprotein (HDL)	HDL provides the disruption of very-low-density lipoprotein and chylomicrons	Atherosclerosis and coronary artery disease	Lower HDL levels are associated with a higher risk for CVDs	[17, 33]
Triglycerides (TG)	TG is responsible for the transfer of glucose and adipose fat from the liver	Atherosclerosis, MI, and coronary heart disease	Elevated levels are associated with a higher risk of CVDs	[17, 18, 33]
D-dimer	D-dimer is formed by the fibrin degradation of blood clots	Thrombosis, ischemic heart disease, chronic heart failure, and acute aortic dissection	Elevated levels are associated with cardiovascular mortality	[17, 18, 26]

3.3 Types of Biosensors for Cardiovascular Biomarkers Detection

3.3.1 Electrochemical Biosensors

The basic principle of electrochemical biosensors is based on the generated electrical signal resulting from the electrochemical redox reaction between the biorecognition element and analyte [36]. The analyte concentration is directly proportional to the measured electrochemical response, which allows the quantitative analysis [37]. Three electrode electrochemical cell systems can use various transducers based on voltammetric, potentiometric, conductometric, and impedimetric techniques [38].

Electrochemical biosensors are label-free, affordable, easily applicable, and highly sensitive with a low limit of detection (LOD) value, and offer accurate, rapid, and robust analysis [39, 40]. They are also easy to miniaturize and apply to devices that use small sample volumes to detect more than one analyte simultaneously [37, 40]. Electrochemical biosensors include the following:

Amperometry-based electrochemical biosensors measure the current flow changes at a constant potential, and they are the most widely used biosensors [36, 38]. They are suitable for mass production, and provide more sensitive analysis than potentiometry-based biosensors [38].

Voltammetry-based electrochemical biosensors determine the current change as a function of the applied potential. They are highly specific, sensitive sensors with noise-free and reproducible measurements [37, 41].

Potentiometry-based electrochemical biosensors' measurement principle is based on the potential difference at a zero current flow [38]. They are used for the determination of both ions and biological molecules [42].

Impedance-based electrochemical biosensors focus on the changes of resistance and capacitance generated by various biomolecular interactions between proteins or antigen and antibody etc. [36, 42].

Conductometry-based electrochemical biosensors focus on electrical conductivity changes, but are not widely preferred for enzymatic analysis [36, 38].

3.3.2 Piezoelectric Biosensors

Piezoelectricity is the ability of some materials to produce an electric potential, charge, or field after mechanical stress [38, 43]. Crystals and certain ceramics, such as bone, quartz, lithium niobate, polylactic acids, zinc oxide, aluminum nitride and phosphate, and polyvinylidene fluoride, are examples of the most common piezoelectric materials [41, 43, 44]. In a piezoelectric biosensor, biorecognition material is immobilized on the piezoelectric surface that consists of a gold electrode coated quartz crystal. When an electric potential is applied due to the interaction between analyte and biorecognition material, an elastic deformation and mass change occur, resulting in a mechanical vibration effect [38, 42, 43]. The frequency of oscillation and crystal mass are related, and increased mass due to analyte absorption can cause a change in the oscillation frequency [38]. Quantitative determination with piezoelectric biosensors is based on the ratio between analyte amount and oscillation frequency [44].

Piezoelectric biosensors are advantageous because they offer easy, rapid, label-free, and low-cost analysis [41]. Nonetheless, issues about the regeneration of crystal surface, incubation time, and multiple immobilization steps may cause setbacks [41].

Piezoelectric biosensors are used to determine a wide variety of materials, such as drugs, pesticides, nucleic acids, bacteria, proteins, pesticides, etc. [45].

3.3.3 Thermal/Thermometric Biosensors

Thermal biosensors are not very commonly used biosensors. In thermal biosensors, a reaction that results in heat production or absorption occurs between the biorecognition element and the analyte [42]. A thermistor is used for the measurement of temperature changes. It is highly sensitive and can detect changes between 0.0001 and 0.05 ^{0}C [38]. Thermal biosensors are able to measure concentrations as low as 10^{-5} M without frequent recalibration [36, 38]. However, they do not show sensitivity for electrochemical and optical characteristics of the analyte [38].

3.3.4 Optical Biosensors

Optical biosensors are biosensors whose transduction principle is based on optical processes. The interaction between analyte and biorecognition elements is changed into an output signal by optical transducers [46]. The measurement of the change in optical characteristics of materials such as polarization, amplitude, frequency, and radiation phase is used for quantitative determination [47]. Changes in the optical characteristics resulting from the molecular interactions between biological elements affect the measured output signal. For example, luminescent biosensors focus on the changes of luminescence related to the produced radiation due to the biomolecular interaction [47]. Optical biosensors can be either label-free or fluorescent-based. In fluorescent-based biosensors, the labeling of biomarkers with fluorescent tags provides a highly sensitive analysis. On the other hand, fluorescent signal bias is considered an issue [44]. Label-free biosensors are capable of rapid and real-time analysis with an ultra-small sample volume [42, 44].

Optical biosensors can employ different techniques such as surface plasmon resonance (SPR), surface plasmon resonance imaging (SPRi), localized surface plasmon resonance (LSPR), surface-enhanced Raman scattering (SERS), laser light scattering, reflection spectroscopy, and chemiluminescence, etc. [38, 47]. All of them have their advantages and disadvantages. Which is preferred is based on the analyte and characteristics. Nevertheless, SPR is considered the most effective and most preferred technique which is affordable and highly selective with the ability to detect various interactions [37, 48].

Optical biosensors offer significant advantages over other biosensors: in addition to being highly selective, they are sensitive and biocompatible, provide a minimally invasive method for in vivo applications, and overcome the electromagnetic interference issue [42].

3.3.5 Wearable/Implantable Biosensors

Biosensor technology is one of the most popular areas continuously being developed and studied intensively. In addition to biosensors' existing advantages, research and studies to improve traditional diagnosis and health monitoring methods have recently developed wearable/implantable biosensors. [49]. Both wearable and implantable sensors provide continuous and remote monitoring for patients without clinical procedures [50]. Implantable biosensors are implanted in the body, while wearable biosensors are worn on the body, such as in clothes, contact lenses, watches, rings, etc. [51].

In classical biosensors, pretreatment steps are often required after sampling, and carrying the samples near the devices/sensors is also required. Although the wearable/implantable biosensors utilize the same transducers as classical biosensors such as optical, electrochemical, and thermal, miniaturization and wearability are the features that make them differ from other biosensors. These new technology biosensors offer unique advantages over other classical biosensors: real-time and continuous data acquirement, saving money and time, reducing the waste of disposable medical materials, and more efficient and quality measurements [52]. Increases and changes in patients' and professionals' healthcare demands have also been significant in developing this type of biosensors. Wearable/implantable biosensors, which can also be integrated with devices such as smartphones, can evaluate the data they measure and provide information to emergency services or patient relatives in critical situations (Figure 3.3) [53]. They are used in CVDs to detect heart rate, electrocardiography, and blood pressure [53].

However, some potential technical issues include biocompatibility, biofouling, errors in measurements with small volume samples, and challenges with analysis of saliva, tears, and sweat [49]. Analysis of biological fluids has always been challenging because of the complexity of the medium. Clinical tests based on blood samples are reliable but involve invasive strategies that can be uncomfortable for patients. Saliva, tears, and sweat are examined as non- or minimally invasive biosensor options for diagnostics. Problems such as contamination of saliva samples with foods and the presence of several metabolites with concentration correlation issues – although they can be detected in sweat samples – demonstrate the improvement requirements for wearable sensors [49].

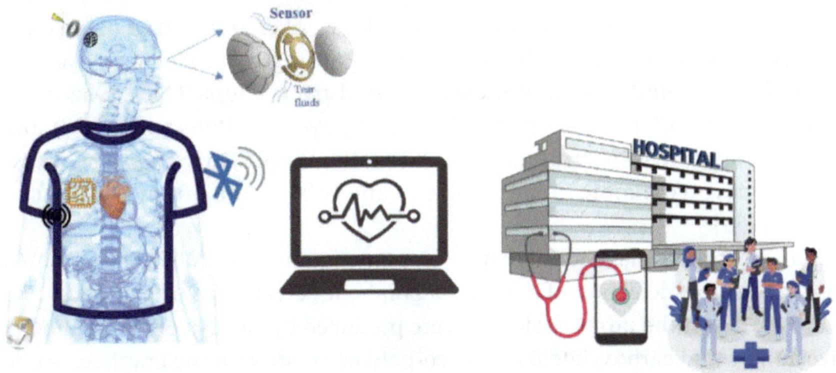

Figure 3.3 Application of wearable/implantable biosensors for healthcare monitoring.

3.4 Applications of Biosensors for Cardiovascular Research

In the last decade, various electrochemical studies investigated the biodetection of biomarkers related to CVDs. Some of these studies examined the biosensor, nanomaterial, molecularly imprinted polymers, and aptamer-based approaches, while others focused on methods of detecting cardiac biomarkers. Reviewing recently published studies on different aspects of electrochemical methods, there is considerable research on the application of electrochemical techniques to detect cardiovascular biomarkers. Table 3.2 provides extensive information on electrochemical biosensing of cardiac biomarkers and diverse electrode modification techniques.

Chi and co-workers have developed a label-free photoelectrochemical (PEC) immunosensor using a CdS:Mn sensitized graphene (G)/Cu_2MoS_4 composite detection probe for the quantification of cTnI. The superior sensitivity of the immunosensor and the large electrochemical behavior of G/Cu_2MoS_4 allowed cTnI to be determined effectively. Consequently, cTnI was found at a concentration of 0.18 pg.mL^{-1} in phosphate buffer conditions [60]. Nandini et al. also reported an electrochemical biosensor based on nanohybrid containing functionalized graphene oxide modified graphite electrode for cholesterol biosensing. The proposed Gr/GO-SH/AuNs/ChOx shows a detection limit of 0.2 nM with a linear range from 0.05 mm to 11.45 mm. Conclusively, the proposed sensor has been effectively applied for the determination of cholesterol in real samples [93]. In another study, Tertis et al. presented a sensitive and selective multipulse amperometric sensor for the determination of interleukin 6 in human serum based on AuNPs and PPy-NPs. The linear concentration range for interleukin 6 was from 1.0 pg.mL^{-1} to 15 μg.mL^{-1} with the detection limit (S/N = 3) of 0.33 pg.mL^{-1} at the optimized conditions (0.1 M Tris–HCl, pH 7.2) [122]. In the electrochemical aptasensor suggested by Taghdisi et. al, the detection was based on the Y-shape structure of DApt-CS conjugate using screen-printed gold electrodes (SPGEs). Differential pulse voltammetry displayed that the aptasensor is able to find out 27 p.m. of myoglobin in a linear range of 100 pM-40 nM. The results demonstrated that the DApt-CS-modified electrodes show excellent selectivity, accuracy and are very selective in myoglobin determination [141]. These comb structured gold microelectrode arrays (CSGMs) were characterized using electrochemical techniques by Kongsuphol et al. The resulting biosensor was used for the detection of TNF-α under optimum experimental parameters. TNF-α was measured and allowed the LOD of 1.0 pg.mL^{-1} by using cyclic voltammetry (CV) and electrochemical impedance spectroscopy (EIS). Finally, this CSGM/Magnetic beads/Ab sensor can achieve a dynamic range between 1 and 1000 pg.mL^{-1} from non-diluted serum samples [155].

Karimi and co-workers have designed a biomimetic nanomolecularly imprinted polymer for the sensitive detection of cTnT via a graphene screen-printed electrode. The cavities created to detect the target molecule were produced by electropolymerization of a conductive aniline and carboxylated aniline co-polymer matrix on the graphene oxide (GO) electrode by cyclic voltammetry. The best MIP surface was achieved at an aniline/

Table 3.2 Latest biosensor applications for cardiovascular research.

Compound	Sensor	Technique	Linear Range	LOD	RSD (%)	Buffer or Media	Real Sample	References
cTnI	N-prGO/COOH/PEG-aptamer/GCE	DPV	0.001–100 pgL^{-1}	0.88 fgL^{-1}	4.3	PBS (0.1 M, pH 7.4)	Human blood and serum	[54]
cTnI	BSA/APTES/nZrO_2/ITO	CV	0.1-100 pgL^{-1}	0.1 pgL^{-1}	NR	PBS (pH 7.0)	-	[55]
cTnI	PrGO/GCE	CV-EIS	0.1-10 pgL^{-1}	70 fgL^{-1}	NR	PBS (0.1 M, pH 7.4)	Human-cTnI protein	[56]
cTnI	Au/Fc-SiNPs/Aptamer	SWV	0.024–24 pgL^{-1}	24 fgL^{-1}	NR	PBS (pH 7.4)	Human serum	[57]
cTnI	Au/2-ABA/f-GN	LSV	0.01–1.0 pgL^{-1}	10 fgL^{-1}	7.27	PBS (1.0 M, pH 7.4)	Human blood	[58]
cTnI	G-MWCNT/GCE	EIS	0.001–10 pgL^{-1}	0.94 fgL^{-1}	9.0 >	PBS- KCl (0.1 M, pH 7.4)	Human serum	[59]
cTnI	ITO/G/Cu_2MoS_4@ CdS:Mn	EIS	0.005–1000 pgL^{-1}	0.18 fgL^{-1}	1.5-2.0	PBS	Human serum	[60]
cTnI	CMWCNT-WNFs/GCE	CV	0.5-100 pgL^{-1}	0.04 fgL^{-1}	3.54	PBS (0.01 M, pH 7.4)	Human serum	[61]
cTnI	Fc-COOH-CIL-HCNTs/GCE	DPV	0.01–600 pgL^{-1}	0.006 pgL^{-1}	6.0 >	PBS (0.1 M, pH 7.4)	Human serum	[62]
cTnI	Au SPE/Au nanodumbbells/Apt Au disc/Triangular	DPV	0.05–500 pgL^{-1}	8.0 fgL^{-1}	12.0	Tris-HCl (0.02 M, pH 7.4)	Human blood	[63]
cTnI	Au disc/Triangular icicle-like Au	DPV	0.01–5 pgL^{-1}	0.9 fgL^{-1}	4.4	Tris-HCl (0.5 M, pH 7.4)	Human serum	[64]
cTnI	Ti disc/AuNPs/Apt	DPV	1-1100 pM	0.18 pM	3.28	PBS (pH 7.0)	Human serum	[65]
cTnI	DNA 3WJ/MB/Apt	CV	NR	1.0 pM	NR	HEPES buffer Tris-HCl (0.04 M, pH 7.4)	Human serum	[66]
cTnI	GCE/N-prGO/Apt	DPV	0.001–100 pgL^{-1}	1.0 fgL^{-1}	4.3	PBS (0.1 M, pH 7.4)	Human serum	[54]

(*Continued*)

Table 3.2 (Continued)

Compound	Sensor	Technique	Linear Range	LOD	RSD (%)	Buffer or Media	Real Sample	References
cTnI	Au SPE/rGO/PEI/Apt	DPV	0.001–10 pgL^{-1}	1.0 fgL^{-1}	5.9	PBS (0.1 M)	Human serum	[67]
cTnI	ITO/rGO-WO3/Ab	DPV	0.01–250 pgL^{-1}	0.01 pgL^{-1}	4.36	PBS (0.05 M, pH 7.4)	Human serum	[68]
cTnI	Au disc/Nafion/DIL-HCNT/Ab	DPV	0.05–30 pgL^{-1}	0.03 pgL^{-1}	7.3	PBS (0.1 M, pH 7.0)	NR	[69]
cTnI	PtCoCuPd HBTPs/GCE	DPV	0.001–100 pgL^{-1}	0.2 fgL^{-1}	4.7	PBS (0.1 M, pH 7.4)	Human serum	[70]
cTnI	Au disc/Chitosan-Ni3V2O8/Ab	CV	0.005–100 pgL^{-1}	5.0 fgL^{-1}	7.43	PBS (pH 7.4)	Human serum	[71]
cTnI	MIPs/MWCNTs/GS/GCE	DPV	0.005–60 $ngcm^{-3}$	0.0008 $ngcm^{-3}$	4.5	Tris-HCl (0.02 M pH 7.5)	Human serum	[72]
cTnI	MIP/BNQDs/GCE	DPV	0.01–5 pgL^{-1}	0.0005 pgL^{-1}	0.47	PBS (0.1 M, pH 7.0)	Plasma samples	[73]
cTnI	Fe_3O_4@UiO-66/Cu@Au nanocomposites	DPV	0.05–100 pgL^{-1}	16.0 fgL^{-1}	4.3	PBS (0.01 M, pH 7.4)	Human serum	[74]
cTnI	Au SPE/DNA NTH/Tro4Apt	DPV	0.01–100 pgL^{-1}	7.5 fgL^{-1}	5.3	Tris-HCl (0.01 M pH 8.0)	Human serum	[75]
cTnI	GCE/Chitosan/Glutaraldehyde/Ab	ASSWV	35.0 $fg.mL^{-1}$-350 pgL^{-1}	0.011 fgL^{-1}	4.9	ABS (0.1 M, pH 5.4)	Plasma samples	[76]
cTnI	GCE/TiO2 NP/PPy/AuNP/Ab	SWV	0.0005–10 pgL^{-1}	0.17 fgL^{-1}	2.22	PBS	Human serum	[77]
cTnI	GCE/AuNPs/Ab	DPV	0.005–20 pgL^{-1}	2.0 fgL^{-1}	3.17	PBS	Human serum	[78]
cTnI	GCE/Au NR@PDA/ Ab	DPV	0.00075–100 pgL^{-1}	0.00025 pgL^{-1}	5.0 >	PBS (0.1 M, pH 7.0)	Human serum	[79]
cTnI Myo CRP	Microelectrodes/VACNFs	DPV	NR	0.020 pgL^{-1} 11 pgL^{-1} 0.020 pgL^{-1}	NR	PBS (0.1 M, pH 7.4)	NR	[80]

cTnI CRP	PDMS-GNP composite film/Carbone fiber WE	DPV	0.01–50 pgL^{-1} 0.5-200 pgL^{-1}	NR	6.3 7.8	ABS (0.1 M, pH 4.5)	Human serum	[81]
cTnI FABP	GCE/GONR/Ab	SWV	0.00005–50 pgL^{-1} 0.00005–50 pgL^{-1}	0.000001 pgL^{-1} 0.000003 pgL^{-1}	4.0 4.4	PBS	Human serum	[82]
cTnT	Au disc/Macroporous Au nanostructure/Apt	DPV	0.05–5 pgL^{-1}	23.0 fgL^{-1}	5.1	Tris-HCl (0.02 M)-KCl (0.5 M)	Human serum	[83]
cTnT	GCE/Nafion/xGnP/AuNP-Hep/Ab	DPV	0.05–0.35 pgL^{-1}	0.016 pgL^{-1}	6.5	PBS (0.01 M, pH 7.4)	Human blood plasma	[84]
cTnT	N-MIP/RGO-SPE	DPV	0.02–0.09 pgL^{-1}	0.008 pgL^{-1}	12.0	PBS (0.01 M, pH 7.4)	Human serum	[85]
cTnT	Carbon SPE/MWCNT/Ab	ch-AMP	0.02–0.32 $ng.mL^{-1}$	0.016 $ng.mL^{-1}$	2.5	ABS (0.1 M, pH 4.8)	Human serum	[86]
Cholesterol	ChOx/NiO/ITO/glass bioelectrodes ChEt-ChOx/NiO/ITO/ glass bioelectrodes	CV-EIS	1.0-12.0 mm 0.12–10.23 mm	0.5 mm 0.1 mm	1.06 1.18	PBS (0.05 M, pH 7.0)	Human serum	[87]
Cholesterol	Au-SPE/Pt/PDA-ChOx	CV	35.3–500 μM	10.5 μM	3.2	PBS (0.1 M, pH 7.4)	Whole blood	[88]
Cholesterol	ChOx-CSPPy-g-$C_3N_4H^+$/GCE	AMP	0.02–5.0 mm	8.0 μM	≤ 3.7	PBS (0.1 M, pH 7.4)	Human serum	[89]
Cholesterol	PTBA/FAD/apo-ChOx/PGE PABA/FAD/apo-ChOx/PGE	AMP	0.8–4.8 μM 0.8–5.6 μM	0.22 μM 0.32 μM	≤ 1.6	PBS (0.1 M, pH 7.0)	Human urine	[90]
Cholesterol	G/Ti(G)-3DNS/CS/ChOx	AMP	0.05–8.0 mm	6.0 μM	≤ 3.4	PBS (0.1 M, pH 7.0)	Human serum	[91]
Cholesterol	ChE/ChO/HRP-AuNPs/c-MWCNTs	CV	0.01 mm-5.83 mm	0.01 mm	NR	PBS (0.01 M, pH 7.2)	Human serum	[92]
Cholesterol	Gr/GO-SH/AuNs/ChOx	CV-EIS	0.05–11.45 mm	0.2 nM	8.6	PBS (0.1 M)	Human serum	[93]
Cholesterol	ChOx/AuNPs/IL/HTNSs/ITO	CV-EIS	8.33–417 nM	6.30 nM	≤ 3.39	PBS (0.2 M)	Human serum	[94]

(*Continued*)

Table 3.2 (Continued)

Compound	Sensor	Technique	Linear Range	LOD	RSD (%)	Buffer or Media	Real Sample	References
Cholesterol	CPE/SnO2 -ChOx/ Nafion	CV-EIS	0.20–4.95 μM	0.04 μM	4.4	PBS (0.05 M, pH 7.4)	Human serum	[95]
Cholesterol	GCE/MWCNT-PANI-Pt nanocomposite/ChOx	AMP	0.002–0.5 mm	8.0 μM	3.9	PBS containing 0.9% NaCl	Human serum	[96]
Cholesterol	GCE/G-Chitosan/ChOx	DPV	0.005–1.0 mm	0.715 μM	≤ 3.7	PBS (0.1 M, pH 7.0)	Human serum	[97]
Cholesterol	SPE/PB/ChOx SPE/ChOx/PTZ	AMP	0.05–0.30 mm 0.015–0.15 mm	3.7 μM 2.3 μM	5.4	PBS (0.05 M, pH 6.8) containing KCl (0.1 M)	Human plasma	[98]
Cholesterol	GCE/PTH/ChOx/HRP	DPV	25–125 μM	6.3 μM	≤ 1.9	PBS (0.05 M, pH 7.0)	Human serum	[99]
Cholesterol	GCE/RGO-nPd-Nafion/ ChOx-ChEt	AMP	0.005–0.14 mm	0.05 μM	≤ 3.45	PBS (0.1 M, pH 7.2)	Human serum,	[100]
Cholesterol	SPE/PANI-PVP-G/ChOx	AMP	50 μM–10 mm	1.0 μM	≤ 5.0	PBS (0.05 M, pH 7.0)	Human serum	[101]
Cholesterol	GCE/MWCNTs-GO-Thionine-Au/ChOx	ECL	0.15–828 μM	50 nM	≤ 7.2	PBS (0.05 M, pH 7.4)	Human serum	[102]
Cholesterol	FC-GO/SPE	AMP	0.5–46.5 μM	0.1 μM	3.0	PBS (0.1 M, pH 7.2)	Human serum	[103]
Cholesterol	Nafion/ChOx/GNPs-MWCNTs/GCE	CV	0.01–5.0 mm	4.3 μM	4.8	PBS (0.1 M, pH 7.0)	Human serum	[104]
CRP	PDA-CRP/$Cu_3(PO4)_2$ nanospheres-GCE	SWV	0.5 fgL^{-1}-1.0 pgL^{-1}	0.13 fgL^{-1}	≤ 3.2	NR	Human serum	[105]
CRP	CRP- Zn^{2+}/Ab/AuNPs @ Si MSs bioconjugates	SWV	0.005–125 pgL^{-1}	0.0017 pgL^{-1}	≤ 5.23	Tris-HCl (0.01 M, pH 7.4) containing NaCl (100 mm) and $CaCl_2$ (10 mm)	Human serum	[106]
CRP	poly(3-ATP)/anti-CRP/4-AAP/GCE	DPV	75 pgL^{-1}-150 ngL^{-1}	7.24 ngL^{-1}	NR	PBS (0.1 M, pH 7.4)	Human serum	[107]
CRP	MoS_2-PANI-GNPs/GCE	DPV	0.2-80 pgL^{-1}	40 fgL^{-1}	4.9	PBS (pH 7.4)	Human serum	[108]

CRP	anti-CRP antibodies/ MPA/rGO- NP/ITO	CV-EIS	1-1000 pgL^{-1}	0.06 pgL^{-1} 0.08 pgL^{-1}	< 7.1	CBS (0.01 M, pH 9.0)	Human serum	[109]
CRP	QDs composition-Bi citrate/CRP/SPE	SV	0.2-100 pgL^{-1}	0.05 pgL^{-1}	< 15.3	PBS (0.02 M, pH 8.6)	Human serum	[110]
CRP	anti-hsCRP-rGO-TEPA-Pb^{2+}/GCE	CV	0.05–100 pgL^{-1}	16.7 fgL^{-1}	< 5.04	PBS (0.1 M, pH 7.4)	Human serum	[111]
CRP	SW/CNF/Ab	CV-EIS	420 pM-42 nM	90 pM	NR	PBS (0.1 M, pH 7.4)	NR	[112]
CRP	SPE(Au)/ HOOC-Magnetic	AMP	0.07–1000 pgL^{-1}	0.021 pgL^{-1}	NR	Tris–HCl (0.1 M, pH 7.0) PBS (0.1 M, pH 7.0)	Human serum	[113]
CRP	Standard polycrystalline GE/Ab	EIS	0.5-50 nM	176 pM	NR	PBS (0.01 M, pH 7.4)	Human serum	[114]
CRP	Glass(Au)/ZnO nanotubes/Ab	PT	10 ngL^{-1}-1.0 mgL^{-1}	1.0 $ng.L^{-1}$	< 5.0	PBS (0.01 M)	NR	[115]
Insulin	Au INCs-Ab_1-Zn_2SiO_4-Pd-Ab_2/GCE	SWV ch-AMP	0.1 fgL^{-1}-50 pgL^{-1}	0.25 $fgmL^{-1}$ 80 $fgmL^{-1}$	< 5.0	PBS	Human serum	[116]
Insulin	SPE/OMC-TPS/Aptamer	DPV	1.0 fM-10.0 pM	0.18 fM	4.9	PBS (0.1 M, pH 7.4)	Human serum	[117]
Insulin	PGE/ Poly-orthophenylene	EIS	1.0-1000 nM	0.27 nM	5.1	PBS (0.1 M, pH 7.4)	Human plasma and urine	[118]
Insulin	Au@Pb-β-CD/ Ab_2CRuSi NPs/GCE	ECL	0.1 fgL^{-1}-10 fgL^{-1}	0.042 fgL^{-1}	2.31	PBS (0.01 M, pH 7.4)	NR	[119]
Insulin	GCE/O-GNs/ AuNPs/ Aptamer	DPV	10 fM-0.5 nM	6.0 fM	3.4	PBS (0.1 M, pH 7.4)	Human serum	[120]
Insulin	MWCNT/Py/PGE	SWV	NR	15 pM	NR	PBS (pH 7.4)	Human serum	[121]
Interleukins	IL-6/MCHApt/ AuNPs/ PPyNPs/SPGE	EIS	1.0 fgL^{-1}-15 ngL^{-1}	0.33 ngL^{-1}	< 4.99	Tris-HCl (0.1 M, pH 7.2)	Human serum	[122]
Interleukins	poly-HRP-anti-TNF-TNFa-anti-TNF-HOOC-Phe-	AMP	0.5-100 fgL^{-1}	0.38 fgL^{-1}	2.7	PBS (0.1 M, pH 7.4)	Human serum	[123]

(Continued)

Table 3.2 (Continued)

Compound	Sensor	Technique	Linear Range	LOD	RSD (%)	Buffer or Media	Real Sample	References
Interleukins	HOOC-MBs/ IL-8 SPdCEs	AMP	241.3-5000 fgL^{-1}	72.4 fgL^{-1}	≤ 8.4	Tris-HCl (0.01 M, pH 8.0) containing EDTA (1.0 mm)	Human serum	[124]
Interleukins	Monothiol-alkane-PEG acid SAM/IL-8/GE	EIS	900 $fgmL^{-1}$-900 $ngmL^{-1}$	90 $fgmL^{-1}$	NR	PBS (0.1 M, pH 7.4)	Human serum	[125]
Interleukins	HRP-Ab2-AuNP-PDA@CNT/IL-6/ITO	AMP	1–40 fgL^{-1}	0.3 fgL^{-1}	7.2	PBS (0.05 M) containing hydroquinone (1 mm)	Human serum	[126]
Interleukins	BSA/anti-IL-6 /ERGO/ AuPdNPs/HCPE	LSV	0.1–100 fgL^{-1}	0.059 fgL^{-1}	< 6.3	PBS (0.01 M, pH 7.4)	Human serum	[127]
Interleukins	GO/PANi/CdSe nanocomposites/GCE	EIS-ECL	0.0005–10 fgL^{-1}	0.17 fgL^{-1}	6.3	PBS (0.1 M, pH 7.4)	Human serum	[128]
Interleukins	CD-R/ Streptavidin poly-HRPc-Ab/IL-6/GE	AMP	10–1300 $fgmL^{-1}$	10 $fgmL^{-1}$	< 2.0	PBS (0.01 M, pH 7.4)	Human serum	[129]
LDL	AAB/NiO/ITO/glass bioelectrode	CV	0.018–0.5 μM	0.015 μM	≤ 2.2	PBS (0.05 M, pH 7.0)	Human serum	[87]
LDL	P/GO/C nanocomposite film electrode	CV	10–120 $mgdL^{-1}$	10 $mgdL^{-1}$	NR	PBS and ABS	NR	[130]
LDL	RGO-NiO NPs/Ab/ITO	CV-EIS	Up to 130 $mgdL^{-1}$	5 $mgdL^{-1}$	≤ 5.6	PBS (0.05 M, pH 7.4)	Human serum	[131]
LDL	BSA-AAB/CdS-NiO/ITO	CV-EIS	5–120 $mgdL^{-1}$	0.05 $mgdL^{-1}$	≤ 6.0	PBS (0.05 M, pH 7.4) containing NaCl (0.15 M)	Human serum	[132]
LDL	ITO/NiO NPs/Ab	CV-EIS	0.018–0.5 μM	0.015 μM	1.06	PBS	NR	[133]
LDL	BSA-AAB/CNT-NiO/ ITO bioelectrode	EIS	5–120 $mgdL^{-1}$	0.63 $mgdL^{-1}$	< 4.3	PBS (0.05 M, pH 7.4)	NR	[134]

LDL	ITO/Chitosan-CNT/Ab	CV-EIS	Up to 120 $mgdL^{-1}$	12.5 $mgdL^{-1}$	NR	PBS (0.05 M, pH 7.4)	NR	[135]
LDL	ITO/NH2 -RGO/Ab/BSA	EIS	50–1200 mgL^{-1}	0.5 mgL^{-1}	4.4	PBS (0.05 M, pH 7.4)	NR	[136]
Myo	RGO/Ru(bpy)$_3$ $^{2+}$ / Sm_2O_3/SPCEs	ECL	0.05–25 nM	12 pM	≤ 4.1	PBS (pH 7.4)	Human serum Human urine	[137]
Myo	ITO/APTES-AuNPs/Ab	CV-EIS	0.02–1 ngL^{-1}	5.5 pgL^{-1}	5.1	PBS (pH 7.4)	Human serum	[138]
Myo	ITO/AuNPs-APTES/Ab	CV-EIS	10 pgL^{-1}-1.0 ngL^{-1}	2.7 fgL^{-1}	≤ 3.6	PBS	Synthetic serum samples	[139]
Myo	GCE/TCPP-G/AuNPs/ Aptamer	DPV	20 pM–0.77 μM	6.7 pM	1.9	PBS (0.1 M, pH 7.4)	Human serum	[140]
Myo	DApt-CS modified electrodes/SPE	DPV	100 pM–40 nM	27 pM	≤ 7.4	PBS (0.01 M, pH 7.4)	Human serum	[141]
Myo	AuNPs@rGO/MbAb/SPE	DPV	1–1400 pgL^{-1}	0.67 pgL^{-1}	NR	SABS (pH 7.0)	Human serum	[142]
Myo	SPE(MWCNT)/Ab	CV-EIS	0.1–90 fgL^{-1}	0.08 fgL^{-1}	≤ 1.5	PBS (0.05 M, pH 7.4)	Human serum	[143]
Myo	Mb/MBA/Au/APTES/ GCE	CV	0.0001–0.15 gL^{-1}	30.9 $ngmL^{-1}$	4.6	PBS	Muscle	[144]
Myo	Pt(MPA)/APTES/ITO	EIS	0.01–1 μgmL^{-1}	1.7 $ngmL^{-1}$	NR	PBS (pH 7.4)	NR	[145]
TN-α	DWCNTs/SPCE	AMP	1–200 fgL^{-1}	0.85 fgL^{-1}	≤ 0.7	PBS	Human serum	[123]
TN-α	ITO/RGO-AuNPs/3-MPA/Ab	EIS	1–1000 fgL^{-1}	0.67 fgL^{-1}	< 4.8	PBS (0.01 M, pH 7.4)	Human serum	[146]
TN-α	ITO/Polymer P3/Ab	CV-EIS	0.01–2 fgL^{-1}	3.7 $fgmL^{-1}$	4.03	PBS (pH 7.0)	Human serum	[147]
TN-α	Fe3O4@AuNP-DNA/ MGCE	SWV	10 fgL^{-1}-100 fgL^{-1}	10 fgL^{-1}	< 6.0	PBS (0.01 M, pH 7.4) containing 0.25 M NaCl	Human serum	[148]
TN-α	SB–EA–anti-TNF-a/ DTSP/AuE	DPV	500 fgL^{-1}-100 pgL^{-1}	60 fgL^{-1}	NR	PBS (0.01 M, pH 7.4)	Human serum	[149]
TN-α	HRP-Ab_2/TNF-α/Ab_1/ PPC-PBA/ITO	ch-AMP	0.01–500 pgL^{-1}	10 fgL^{-1}	≤ 11.7	PBS (pH 7.4)	Whole blood	[150]

(*Continued*)

Table 3.2 (Continued)

Compound	Sensor	Technique	Linear Range	LOD	RSD (%)	Buffer or Media	Real Sample	References
TN-α	ITO/RGO/AuNPs/Ab	CV-EIS	1–1000 fgL^{-1}	0.43 fgL^{-1}	NR	PBS (0.01 M, pH 7.4)	NR	[151]
TN-α	Ag@Pt-CNTs/CS/SPE	DPV	6–60 fgL^{-1}	1.6 fgL^{-1}	≤ 3.4	PBS (pH 7.4)	Human serum	[152]
TN-α	CNTs-C60 -IL/Ab/SPE	DPV	5–75 fgL^{-1}	2.0 fgL^{-1}	≤ 3.6	PBS (pH 7.4)	Human serum	[153]
TN-α	GCE/AuNP/MWCNT/AuNP/IL-CS/Ab_1/Ag	DPV	6–100 fgL^{-1}	2.0 fgL^{-1}	≤ 3.7	PBS (pH 7.4)	Human serum	[154]
TN-α	Magnetic beads/Ab/CSGM electrodes	EIS	1–1000 fgL^{-1}	1.0 fgL^{-1}	NR	PBS	Human serum	[155]
TN-α	Ag/mAb_1/poly(anthranilic acid)/SPE HRP-pAb_2/Ag/mAb_1/ poly(anthranilic acid)/SPE	EIS	Up to 100 fgL^{-1} Up to 100 fgL^{-1}	5.0 fgL^{-1} 3.2 fgL^{-1}	≤ 4.6	PBS (0.1 M, pH 7.4)	Human serum	[156]
TN-α	Fc-Phe/AuNPs//TNF-α/PS-ALP-Ab_2/GCE	SWV	1.0 fgL^{-1}-10 pgL^{-1}	0.5 fgL^{-1}	≤ 5.4	PBS (0.1 M)	Human serum	[157]
TG	Lip-GLDH/AgCNFs/ITO Lip-GLDH/CNFs/ITO	CV	50–400 $mgdL^{-1}$ 100–400 $mgdL^{-1}$	10.6 $mgdL^{-1}$	≤ 1.67	PBS (0.05 M, pH 7.0)	NR	[158]
TG	PGE/GPONPs/GKNPs/LIPNPs	CV	0.1 mm–45 mm	0.1 nM	NR	PBS (0.1 M, pH 7.0)	Human serum	[159]
TG	PDA/AuNPs-enzyme/SCE	CV	1.0–25 mm	0.075 mm	≤ 7.35	PBS (0.1 M, pH 7.0)	NR	[160]
TG	GE/GPONPs/GKNPs/LIPNPs	CV	1.0–100 $mgdL^{-1}$ 100–500 $mgdL^{-1}$	1.0 μgmL^{-1}	NR	PBS (0.1 M, pH 7.0)	Human serum	[161]
TG	ITO/RGO/LIP	CV-EIS	50–300 $mgdL^{-1}$	25 $mgdL^{-1}$	NR	PBS (0.05 M, pH 7.0)	NR	[162]
TG	ITO/Chitosan-Nano	CV	0.25–4 $mgmL^{-1}$	155 μgmL^{-1}	NR	PBS (0.1 M, pH 7.4)	Human serum	[163]

TG	ITO/RGO-PdNPs/ LIP-GLDH	CV-EIS	25–400 $mgdL^{-1}$	25 $mgdL^{-1}$	NR	PBS (pH 7.4)	NR	[164]
TG	Lipase-GK-GPO/GM/ GCE	AMP	12–100 $mgdL^{-1}$	12 $mgdL^{-1}$	NR	PBS (0.1 M, pH 7.0)	Artificial serum samples	[165]
TG	Glass/ITO/AuNPs@ PDA/LIP	CV	50–300 $mgdL^{-1}$	0.84 $mgdL^{-1}$	NR	PBS (0.05 M, pH 7.4)	Human serum	[166]

NR: Not reported, **Myo:** Myoglobin, **TN-α:** Tumor necrosis factor-α, **Mb:** Cardiac myoglobin, **TG:** Triglyceride, **Ab:** Antibody, **LDL:** Low-density lipoprotein, **Apt:** Aptamer, **MIP:** Molecularly imprinted polymer, **cTnI:** Cardiac troponin I, **PEG:** Polyethylene glycol, **cTnT:** Cardiac troponin T, **APTES:** 3-aminopropyl triethoxy silane, **$nZrO_2$:** Nanostructured zirconia, **CRP:** C- reactive protein, **BSA:** Bovine serum albümin, **PrGO:** Porous graphene oxide, **PCB:** Printed circuit board, **Fc:** Ferrocene, **2-ABA:** 2-aminobenzyl amine, **SiNPs:** Silica nanoparticles, **G:** Graphene, **MWCNT:** Multi-walled carbon nanotube, **CdS:Mn:** Manganese doped CdS, **LIG:** Laser-induced graphene, **N-GNRs:** N-doped graphene nanoribbons, **FABP:** Human heart-type fatty-acid-binding protein, **Fe-MOFs:** Fe-based-Metal-organic frameworks, Fc-COOH: Ferrocenecarboxylic acid, **CIL:** Carboxyl-terminated ionic liquid, **WNFs:** Whiskered nanofibers, **PDMS:** Poly(Dimethylsiloxane), **CMWCNT:** Carboxylated multi-walled carbon nanotube, **MB:** Methylene blue, **PGE:** Pencil graphite electrodes, **N-prGO:** Nitrogen-doped reduced graphene oxide, **SPE:** Screen printed electrode, **WE:** Working electrode, **GE:** Gold Electrode, **ITO:** Indium tin oxide, **rGO:** Reduced graphene oxide, **WO3:** Tungsten oxide, **PEI:** Polyethyleneimine, **xGnP:** Exfoliated graphite nanoplatelets, **Hep:** Heparin, **CuNPs:** Copper nanoparticles anchored, **GN:** Graphene nanoplatelets, **f-GN:** Amine functionalized graphene, **DIL:** Dialdehyde-functionalized ionic liquid, **MWCNT:** Multi-walled carbon nanotube, **QDs:** Quantum dots, **VACNFs:** Vertically aligned carbon nanofibers, **DPV:** Differential pulse voltammetry, **CV:** Cyclic voltammetry, **SWV:** Square wave voltammetry, **ch-Amp:** Chronoamperometry, **ASSWV:** Anodic stripping square wave voltammetry, **EIS:** electrochemical impedance spectroscopy, **LSV:** Linear sweep voltammetry, **SV:** Stripping voltammetry, **PT:** Potentiometric technique, **ECL:** Electrochemiluminescence, **3WJ:** 3 way-junction, **HCNT:** Helical carbon nanotube, **HRP:** Horseradish peroxidase, **ChOx:** Cholesterol oxidase, **apo-ChOx:** apo-cholesterol oxidase, **ChEt:** Cholesterol esterase, **HCNTs:** Helical carbon nanotubes, **GCE:** Glassy carbon electrode, **PTH:** Polythionine, **AuNPs:** Gold nanoparticles, **PDA:** Polydopamine, **PPy:** Polypyrrole, **RGO:** Reduced graphene oxide, **AuNR:** Au nanorod, **CNF:** Carbon nanofiber, **CSPPy:** Cylindrical spongy shaped polypyrrole, **PANI:** Polyaniline, **PB:** Prussian Blue, **MB:** Methylene blue, **TEPA:** Tetraethylene pentamine, **MPA:** 3-mercaptopropionic acid, **NTH:** Nanotetrahedron, **AuINCs:** Gold icosahedra nanocrystals, **AuNS:** Gold nanospike, **OMC:** Ordered mesoporous carbon; **TPS:** 1,3,6,8-pyrenetetrasulfonate, **Pb-ß-CD:** Pb(II)-ß-cyclodextrin, **CRu:** $Ru(bpy)_3{}^{2+}$, **ITO:** Indium tin oxide, **Py:** Pyrenebutyric acid frameworks, **DWCNTs:** Double-walled carbon nanotubes, **PS:** Polystyrene, **TCPP:** Meso-tetra (4-carboxyphenyl) porphyrin, **PPC:** Phenyl phophorylcholine, **PBA:** Phenyl butyric acid, **ALP:** Alkaline phosphatase, **CSGM:** Comb structured gold microelectrode arrays, **CNT:** Carbon nanotube, **LIP:** lipase, **GLDH:** Glycerol dehydrogenase, **N-MIP:** Nano-molecularly imprinted polymer, **GK:** Glycerol kinase, **ALP:** Alkaline phosphatase, **PS:** Polystyrene sphere, **C:** Chitosan, **GM:** Gelatin membrain, **GO:** Graphene oxide, **GPO:** Glycerol-3-phosphate oxidase, **PBS:** Phosphate buffer solution, **ABS:** Acetate buffer solution, **CBS:** Carbonate buffer solution, **SABS:** Sodium acetate buffer solution carboxylated aniline ratio of 1:4. Techniques such as cyclic voltammetry (CV), differential pulse voltammetry (DPV) and scanning electron microscopy (SEM) were used for surface characterization of the sensor. The linear range of sensor was in the range of 0.02 to 0.09 ng/mL, with the detection limit of 0.008 ng/mL [85].

A new immunosensor based on bismuth citrate-modified graphite screen-printed electrodes (SPEs) has been fabricated for the voltammetric detection of CRP using quantum dots (QDs) tags in human serum by Kokkinos et al. The modified SPE was used both as a biological recognition element and as a QDs reader. Quantification of the target protein was achieved by the acidic dissolution of PbS QDs and anodic stripping voltammetric detection of released Pb(II). Determination was performed at bismuth nanodomains formed on the sensor surface during the electrolytic preconcentration step, as bismuth citrate was reduced to metallic bismuth simultaneously with the deposition of Pb on the surface of the immunosensor. The result was linear over the range 0.2–100 ng mL − 1 CRP and the limit of detection was 0.05 ng mL − 1 CRP in the optimum conditions [110].

Nanoparticles (NPs) of commercial lipase from Candida rugosa, glycerol kinase (GK) from Cellulomonas species, and glycerol-3-phosphate oxidase (GPO) from Aerococcus viridans were prepared with a pencil graphite electrode (PGE) by Narwal and Pundir. The characterization of PGE before and after co-immobilization of enzyme nanoparticles (ENPs) was achieved by SEM, CV, and EIS. A linear relationship was obtained between a wide range (0.1 –45 mm) in the optimum conditions within 2.5s at a pH 7.0 and a temperature of 35 °C [159].

In addition to these, there are other biosensors technologies such as fluorimetric, SPR, and chemiluminescence for the determination of CVD biomarkers. For example, in CRP analysis, fluorimetric biosensors can offer affordable and accurate analysis but their lower sensitivity is a drawback [167]. CRP is a significant biomarker in CVDs and is much studied. In a study, a chemiluminescence based biosensor was developed for CRP detection using and improving conventional enzyme-linked immunosorbent assay (ELISA) [168]. SPR biosensors are popular optical techniques and details of their applications on cardiovascular biomarkers such as cTnI and myoglobin are available in the literature [169, 170].

3.5 Future Outlook

Further research is needed to work on novel biomarkers and to offer multimarker strategies for better early treatment protocols. The application of novel detection biosensors, such as electrochemical biosensors, piezoelectric biosensors, thermometric biosensors, and optical biosensors, is still in the developmental stages, and there is the potential for rapid growth. Turning these discoveries into clinical practice will be critical for reducing the incidence of CVDs. Point-of-care devices provide ease of application for patients and medical staff through user-friendly diagnostic and monitoring kits. User-friendly devices will likely become commonplace in the future. Smartphone health applications are attracting attention from scientists, focusing on their integration with apps and biosensor systems. Wearable sensors will also make life easier in the future and, thus, many patients' lives will be saved thanks to the early detection of CVDs.

3.6 Conclusion

Coronary and peripheral artery disease, congenital heart disease, heart failure, hypertension, and stroke are responsible for an extremely high mortality rate. CVDs are known as the most common disease in the world. The use of cardiac biomarkers is one of the best tools for early diagnosis of the disease, monitoring the disease stage, determining the treatment protocol, and so on. Early-stage biomarkers of CVDs can potentially save many lives and help to fight against CVDs in clinical trials. Troponin I, CRP, and lipoproteins (LDH, HDL) are evaluated traditional biomarkers, and these types of biomarker biosensors have developed extensively in the last 10 years.

Biosensors are obtained from a combination of biological affinity material and transducer. The analyte is recognized from the bioreceptor, analyzed with a transducer, and then evaluated after signal processing. In this chapter, cardiovascular biosensors have been evaluated under five different subtitles. Electrochemical biosensors are widely used for the determination of cardiac biomarkers. The advantages and challenges of biosensors are evaluated within the framework of short- and mid-term related healthcare applications.

The many current biomarkers are used clinically for the detection of last-stage disease. The discovery of new potential biomarkers for CVDs along with current ones has increased the importance of fully validated cardiac biomarker biosensors and has led to new approaches for CVDs-based research.

References

1 Olin, B.R. and Pharm, D. (2018) Hypertension : The Silent Killer : Updated JNC-8 Guideline Recommendations.

2 WHO (2017) Cardiovascular Diseases: The Solution. https://www.who.int/nmh/publications/fact_sheet_cardiovascular_en.pdf.

3 Schettler, G. and Brisse, B. (1980). Cardiovascular diseases. *Munchener Medizinische Wochenschrift* 122 (Suppl. 1): 6–9.

4 Liu, M.B. (2014). Cardiovascular diseases. *Chinese Medical Journal* 127: 6–7.

5 Leonard, E.A. and Marshall, R.J. (2018). Cardiovascular Disease in Women. *Primary Care: Clinics in Office Practice* 45: 131–141 .

6 Boraita, A., Adamuz, C., Alcocer Ayuga, M., Carro, A., Díaz González, L., Heredia, J.R., Madaria, Z., Masiá, M.D., Rossi, M., Sánchez Testal, M., Trias de Bes, J., Azcárate, P., Barriales, R., Benito, B., Calvo-Iglesias, F., Fuertes Moure, Á., de la Guía, F., Martínez, A., Martínez Alday, J., Moñivas, V., Peiró Molina, E., Vera, T.R., de la Rosa, A., Avanzas, P., Congost, G.B., Boraita, A., Bueno, H., Calvo, D., Campuzano, R., Delgado, V., Dos, L., Ferreira-González, I., Gómez Doblas, J.J., Pascual Figal, D., Sambola Ayala, A., Viana Tejedor, A., Ferreiro, J.L., and Alfonso, F. (2021). Comments on the 2020 ESC guidelines on sports cardiology and exercise in patients with cardiovascular disease. *Rev. Española Cardiol. (English Ed.* 74 (6): 488–493.

7 Riccardi, G., Vitale, M., and Vaccaro, O. (2020). Are Europeans moving towards dietary habits more suitable for reducing cardiovascular disease risk? *Nutrition, Metabolism & Cardiovascular Diseases* 30 (11): 1857–1860.

8 Zampelas, A. and Magriplis, E. (2020). Dietary patterns and risk of cardiovascular diseases: A review of the evidence. *The Proceedings of the Nutrition Society* 79 (1): 68–75.

9 Keung, V., Lo, K., Cheung, C., Tam, W., and Lee, A. (2019). Changes in dietary habits and prevalence of cardiovascular risk factors among school students in Macao, China. *Obesity Research & Clinical Practice* 13 (6): 541–547.

10 Balakumar, P., Maung-U, K., and Jagadeesh, G. (2016). Prevalence and prevention of cardiovascular disease and diabetes mellitus. *Pharmacological Research : The Official Journal of the Italian Pharmacological Society* 113: 600–609.

11 Reamy, B.V., Williams, P.M., and Kuckel, D.P. (2018). Prevention of Cardiovascular Disease. *Primary Care* 45 (1): 25–44.

12 Qureshi, A., Gurbuz, Y., and Niazi, J.H. (2012). Biosensors for cardiac biomarkers detection: A review. *Sensors and Actuators, B Chemicals* 171–172: 62–76.

13 Yang, Z. and Min Zhou, D. (2006). Cardiac markers and their point-of-care testing for diagnosis of acute myocardial infarction. *Clinical Biochemistry* 39 (8): 771–780.

14 Satoh, K. and Shimokawa, H. (2018). Recent Advances in the Development of Cardiovascular Biomarkers. *Arteriosclerosis, Thrombosis, and Vascular Biology* 38 (5): e61–e70.

15 Gualandro, D.M., Twerenbold, R., Boeddinghaus, J., Nestelberger, T., Puelacher, C., and Müller, C. (2019). Biomarkers in cardiovascular medicine: Towards precision medicine. *Swiss Medical Weekly* 149: w20125.

16 Simpson, W.G. (2019). Biomarker variability and cardiovascular disease residual risk. *Current Opinion in Cardiology* 34 (4): 413–417.

17 Upadhyay, R.K. (2015). Emerging risk biomarkers in cardiovascular diseases and disorders. *Journal of Lipids* 2015: 1–50.

18 Derosa, G. and Maffioli, P.(2015). Testing Pharmacological Profiles with Biomarkers Relevant to Cardiovascular Profiles. In eds: Patel V., Preedy V., *Biomarkers in Cardiovascular Disease*. Dordrecht: Springer, 1–24.

19 Savonnet, M., Rolland, T., Cubizolles, M., Roupioz, Y., and Buhot, A. (2020). Recent advances in cardiac biomarkers detection: From commercial devices to emerging technologies. *Journal of Pharmaceutical and Biomedical Analysis* 194: 113777.

20 Dolati, S., Soleymani, J., Kazem Shakouri, S., and Mobed, A. (2020). The trends in nanomaterial-based biosensors for detecting critical biomarkers in stroke. *Clinica Chimica Acta* 514 (December 2020): 107–121.

21 Bakirhan, N.K., Ozcelikay, G., and Ozkan, S.A. (2018). Recent progress on the sensitive detection of cardiovascular disease markers by electrochemical-based biosensors. *Journal of Pharmaceutical and Biomedical Analysis* 159: 406–424.

22 Dhir, S. and Dhir, A. (2020). Cardiovascular risk assessment for noncardiac surgery: Are we ready for biomarkers? *Journal of Cardiothoracic and Vascular Anesthesia* 34 (7): 1914–1924.

23 Negahdary, M. (2020). Aptamers in nanostructure-based electrochemical biosensors for cardiac biomarkers and cancer biomarkers: A review. *Biosensors & Bioelectronics* 152 (January): 112018.

24 Dhingra, R. and Vasan, R.S. (2017). Biomarkers in cardiovascular disease: Statistical assessment and section on key novel heart failure biomarkers. *Trends in Cardiovascular Medicine* 27 (2): 123–133.

25 Boonkaew, S., Jang, I., Noviana, E., Siangproh, W., Chailapakul, O., and Henry, C.S. (2021). Electrochemical paper-based analytical device for multiplexed, point-of-care detection of cardiovascular disease biomarkers. *Sensors and Actuators, B Chemicals* 330 (September 2020): 129336.

26 Ghantous, C.M., Kamareddine, L., Farhat, R., Zouein, F.A., Mondello, S., Kobeissy, F., and Zeidan, A. (2020). Advances in cardiovascular biomarker discovery. *Biomedicines* 8 (12): 1–19.

27 Forman, D.E., de Lemos, J.A., Shaw, L.J., Reuben, D.B., Lyubarova, R., Peterson, E.D., Spertus, J.A., Zieman, S., Salive, M.E., and Rich, M.W. (2020). Cardiovascular biomarkers and imaging in older adults: JACC Council perspectives. *Journal of the American College of Cardiology* 76 (13): 1577–1594.

28 Wang, T.J. (2011). Assessing the role of circulating, genetic, and imaging biomarkers in cardiovascular risk prediction. *Circulation* 123 (5): 551–565.

29 Hoeger, C.W. and Hayek, S.S. (2019). Role of cardiovascular biomarkers in the risk stratification, monitoring, and management of patients with cancer. *Cardiology Clinics* 37 (4): 505–523.

30 Ouyang, M., Tu, D., Tong, L., Sarwar, M., Bhimaraj, A., Li, C., Coté, G.L., and Di Carlo, D. (2021). A review of biosensor technologies for blood biomarkers toward monitoring cardiovascular diseases at the point-of-care. *Biosensors & Bioelectronics* 171 (September 2020).

31 Negahdary, M. (2020). Aptamers in nanostructure-based electrochemical biosensors for cardiac biomarkers and cancer biomarkers: A review. *Biosensors & Bioelectronics* 152 (November 2019): 112018.

32 Di Stefano, V., Zaccagnini, G., Capogrossi, M.C., and Martelli, F. (2011). MicroRNAs as peripheral blood biomarkers of cardiovascular disease. *Vascular Pharmacology* 55 (4): 111–118.

33 Ekroos, K., Lavrynenko, O., Titz, B., Pater, C., Hoeng, J., and Ivanov, N.V. (2020). Lipid-based biomarkers for CVD, COPD, and aging – A translational perspective. *Progress in Lipid Research* 78 (February): 101030.

34 Lattuca, B., Sy, V., Nguyen, L.S., Bernard, M., Zeitouni, M., Overtchouk, P., Yan, Y., Hammoudi, N., Ceccaldi, A., Collet, J.P., Kerneis, M., Diallo, A., Montalescot, G., and Silvain, J. (2019). Copeptin as a prognostic biomarker in acute myocardial infarction. *International Journal of Cardiology* 274: 337–341.

35 Holm, J., Szabó, Z., Alehagen, U., Lindahl, T.L., and Cederholm, I. (2018). Copeptin release in cardiac surgery – A new biomarker to identify risk patients? *Journal of Cardiothoracic and Vascular Anesthesia* 32 (1): 245–250.

36 Qazi, S. and Raza, K. (2020). *Smart Biosensors for an Efficient Point of Care (Poc) Health Management*. Elsevier Inc.

37 Sohrabi, H., Kholafazad Kordasht, H., Pashazadeh-Panahi, P., Nezhad-Mokhtari, P., Hashemzaei, M., Majidi, M.R., Mosafer, J., Oroojalian, F., Mokhtarzadeh, A., and De La Guardia, M. (2020). Recent advances of electrochemical and optical biosensors for detection of C-reactive protein as a major inflammatory biomarker. *Microchemical Journal* 158 (April): 105287.

38 Lakshmipriya, T. and Gopinath, S.C.B. (2019). *An Introduction to Biosensors and Biomolecules*. Elsevier Inc.

39 Malhotra, B.D. and Chaubey, A. (2003). Biosensors for clinical diagnostics industry. *Sensors and Actuators, B Chemicals* 91 (1–3): 117–127.

40 Veloso, A.J., Cheng, X.R., and Kerman, K. (2012). *Electrochemical Biosensors for Medical Applications*. Elsevier Masson SAS.

41 Srivastava, K.R., Awasthi, S., Mishra, P.K., and Srivastava, P.K. (2020). *Biosensors/Molecular Tools for Detection of Waterborne Pathogens*. Elsevier.

42 Malhotra, B.D. and Ali, M.A. (2018). Nanomaterials in biosensors. *Nanomaterials for Biosensors* 1–74.

43 Tan, S.N., Wang, W., and Ge, L. (2011). Biosensors based on sol-gel-derived materials. *Comprehensive Biomaterials* 3: 471–489.

44 Rebelo, R., Barbosa, A.I., Kundu, S.C., Reis, R.L., and Correlo, V.M. (2020). Biodetection and Sensing for Cancer Diagnostics. In eds: Subhas C. Kundu, Rui L. Reis, *Materials Today: Biomaterials for 3D Tumor Modeling*. Elsevier, 643–660.

45 Skládal, P. (2016). Piezoelectric biosensors. *TrAC - Trends in Analytical Chemistry* 79: 127–133.

46 Lechuga, L.M. (2005). Optical biosensors. *Comprehensive Analytical Chemistry* 44: 209–250.

47 Kobun, R. (ed.). (2021). Nanotechnology-based optical biosensors for food applications. *Advanced Food Analysis Tools*. Elsevier, 147–165.

48 Rezabakhsh, A., Rahbarghazi, R., and Fathi, F. (2020). Surface plasmon resonance biosensors for detection of Alzheimer's biomarkers; an effective step in early and accurate diagnosis. *Biosensors & Bioelectronics* 167 (August): 112511.

49 Parlak, O., Curto, V.F., Ojeda, E., Basabe-Desmonts, L., Benito-Lopez, F., and Salleo, A. (2019). Wearable biosensors and sample handling strategies. In eds: Parlak O., Salleo A., Turner A., *Materials Today: Wearable Bioelectronics*. Elsevier, 65–88.

50 Córcoles, E.P. and Boutelle, M.G. (2013). Implantable biosensors, In: *Biosensors and Invasive Monitoring in Clinical Applications: SpringerBriefs in Applied Sciences and Technology*. Heidelberg: Springer, 21–41.

51 Reid, R.C. and Mahbub, I. (2020). Wearable self-powered biosensors. *Current Opinion in Electrochemistry* 19: 55–62.

52 Zhang, J.X.J. and Hoshino, K. (2014). Implantable Sensors. *Molecular Sensors and Nanodevices*. Elsevier, 415–465.

53 Zhu, X., Liu, W., Shuang, S., Nair, M., and Li, C.Z. (2017). Intelligent tattoos, patches, and other wearable biosensors. In ed: Narayan R.J., *Medical Biosensors for Point of Care (POC) Applications*. Woodhead Publishing, 133–150.

54 Chekin, F., Vasilescu, A., Jijie, R., Singh, S.K., Kurungot, S., Iancu, M., Badea, G., Boukherroub, R., and Szunerits, S. (2018). Sensitive electrochemical detection of cardiac troponin I in serum and saliva by nitrogen-doped porous reduced graphene oxide electrode. *Sensors and Actuators, B Chemicals* 262: 180–187.

55 Kumar, S., Kumar, S., Augustine, S., and Malhotra, B.D. (2017). Protein functionalized nanostructured zirconia based electrochemical immunosensor for cardiac troponin i detection. *Journal of Materials Research and Technology* 32 (15): 2966–2972.

56 Kazemi, S.H.K., Ghodsi, E., Abdollahi, S., and Nadri, S. (2016). Porous graphene oxide nanostructure as an excellent scaffold for label-free electrochemical biosensor: Detection of cardiac troponin I. *Materials Science and Engineering C* 69: 447–452.

57 Jo, H., Gu, H., Jeon, W., Youn, H., Her, J., Kim, S.K., Lee, J., Shin, J.H., and Ban, C. (2015). Electrochemical aptasensor of cardiac troponin i for the early diagnosis of acute myocardial infarction. *Analytical Chemistry* 87 (19): 9869–9875.

58 Tuteja, S.K., Kukkar, M., Suri, C.R., Paul, A.K., and Deep, A. (2015). One step in-situ synthesis of amine functionalized graphene for immunosensing of cardiac marker cTnI. *Biosensors & Bioelectronics* 66: 129–135.

59 Singal, S., Srivastava, A.K., Dhakate, S., and Biradar, A.M., Rajesh. (2015). Electroactive graphene-multi-walled carbon nanotube hybrid supported impedimetric immunosensor for the detection of human cardiac troponin-I. *RSC Advances* 5 (92): 74994–75003.

60 Chi, H., Han, Q., Chi, T., Xing, B., Ma, N., Wu, D., and Wei, Q. (2019). Manganese doped CdS sensitized graphene/Cu 2 MoS 4 composite for the photoelectrochemical immunoassay of cardiac troponin I. *Biosensors & Bioelectronics* 132 (December 2018): 1–7.

61 Rezaei, B., Shoushtari, A.M., Rabiee, M., Uzun, L., Mak, W.C., and Turner, A.P.F. (2018). An electrochemical immunosensor for cardiac Troponin I using electrospun carboxylated multi-walled carbon nanotube-whiskered nanofibres. *Talanta* 182 (October 2017): 178–186.

62 Yan, H., Tang, X., Zhu, X., Zeng, Y., Lu, X., Yin, Z., Lu, Y., Yang, Y., and Li, L. (2018). Sandwich-type electrochemical immunosensor for highly sensitive determination of cardiac troponin I using carboxyl-terminated ionic liquid and helical carbon nanotube composite as platform and ferrocenecarboxylic acid as signal label. *Sensors and Actuators, B Chemicals* 277 (July): 234–240.

63 Negahdary, M., Behjati-Ardakani, M., Sattarahmady, N., Yadegari, H., and Heli, H. (2017). Electrochemical aptasensing of human cardiac troponin I based on an array of gold nanodumbbells-Applied to early detection of myocardial infarction. *Sensors and Actuators, B Chemicals* 252: 62–71.

64 Negahdary, M. and Heli, H. (2019). An electrochemical troponin I peptisensor using a triangular icicle-like gold nanostructure. *Biochemical Engineering Journal* 151 (April): 107326.

65 Lopa, N.S., Rahman, M.M., Ahmed, F., Ryu, T., Sutradhar, S.C., Lei, J., Kim, J., Kim, D.H., Lee, Y.H., and Kim, W. (2019). Simple, low-cost, sensitive and label-free aptasensor for the detection of cardiac troponin I based on a gold nanoparticles modified titanium foil. *Biosensors & Bioelectronics* 126 (November 2018): 381–388.

66 Lee, T., Lee, Y., Park, S.Y., Hong, K., Kim, Y., Park, C., Chung, Y.H., Lee, M.H., and Min, J. (2019). Fabrication of electrochemical biosensor composed of multi-functional DNA structure/Au nanospike on micro-gap/PCB system for detecting troponin I in human serum. *Colloids Surfaces B Biointerfaces* 175 (December 2018): 343–350.

67 Grabowska, I., Sharma, N., Vasilescu, A., Iancu, M., Badea, G., Boukherroub, R., Ogale, S., and Szunerits, S. (2018). Electrochemical aptamer-based biosensors for the detection of cardiac biomarkers. *ACS Omega* 3 (9): 12010–12018.

68 Sandil, D., Srivastava, S., Malhotra, B.D., Sharma, S.C., and Puri, N.K. (2018). Biofunctionalized tungsten trioxide-reduced graphene oxide nanocomposites for sensitive electrochemical immunosensing of cardiac biomarker. *Journal of Alloys and Compounds* 763: 102–110.

69 Shen, Q., Liu, M., Lü, Y., Zhang, D., Cheng, Z., Liu, Y., Gao, H., and Jin, Z. (2019). Label-free electrochemical immunosensor based on a functionalized ionic liquid and helical carbon nanotubes for the determination of cardiac troponin I. *ACS Omega* 4 (7): 11888–11892.

70 Chen, Y., Mei, L.P., Feng, J.J., Yuan, P.X., Luo, X., and Wang, A.J. (2019). Simple one-pot aqueous synthesis of 3D superstructured PtCoCuPd alloyed tripods with hierarchical branches for ultrasensitive immunoassay of cardiac troponin I. *Biosensors & Bioelectronics* 145 (July): 111638.

71 Singh, N., Rai, P., Ali, M.A., Kumar, R., Sharma, A., Malhotra, B.D., and John, R. (2019). A hollow-nanosphere-based microfluidic biosensor for biomonitoring of cardiac troponin i. *Journal of Materials Chemistry B* 7 (24): 3826–3839.

72 Ma, Y., Shen, X.L., Wang, H.S., Tao, J., Huang, J.Z., Zeng, Q., and Wang, L.S. (2017). MIPs-graphene nanoplatelets-MWCNTs modified glassy carbon electrode for the determination of cardiac troponin I. *Analytical Biochemistry* 520: 9–15.

73 Yola, M.L. and Atar, N. (2019). Development of cardiac troponin-I biosensor based on boron nitride quantum dots including molecularly imprinted polymer. *Biosensors & Bioelectronics* 126 (November 2018): 418–424.

74 Sun, D., Luo, Z., Lu, J., Zhang, S., Che, T., Chen, Z., and Zhang, L. (2019). Electrochemical dual-aptamer-based biosensor for nonenzymatic detection of cardiac troponin I by nanohybrid electrocatalysts labeling combined with DNA nanotetrahedron structure. *Biosensors & Bioelectronics* 134 (March): 49–56.

75 Sun, D., Lin, X., Lu, J., Wei, P., Luo, Z., Lu, X., Chen, Z., and Zhang, L. (2019). DNA nanotetrahedron-assisted electrochemical aptasensor for cardiac troponin I detection based on the co-catalysis of hybrid nanozyme, natural enzyme and artificial DNAzyme. *Biosensors & Bioelectronics* 142 (May): 111578.

76 Qin, X., Dong, Y., Wang, M., Zhu, Z., Li, M., Chen, X., Yang, D., and Shao, Y. (2018). C-dots assisted synthesis of gold nanoparticles as labels to catalyze copper deposition for ultrasensitive electrochemical sensing of proteins. *Science China Chemistry* 61 (4): 476–482.

77 Zhang, T., Ma, N., Ali, A., Wei, Q., Wu, D., and Ren, X. (2018). Electrochemical ultrasensitive detection of cardiac troponin I using covalent organic frameworks for signal amplification. *Biosensors & Bioelectronics* 119 (July): 176–181.

78 Qian, X., Zhou, X., Ran, X., Ni, H., Li, Z., Qu, Q., Li, J., Du, G., and Yang, L. (2019). Facile and clean synthesis of dihydroxylatopillar[5]arene-stabilized gold nanoparticles integrated Pd/MnO 2 nanocomposites for robust and ultrasensitive detection of cardiac troponin I. *Biosensors & Bioelectronics* 130 (November 2018): 214–224.

79 Lv, H., Li, Y., Zhang, X., Li, X., Xu, Z., Chen, L., Li, D., and Dong, Y. (2019). Thionin functionalized signal amplification label derived dual-mode electrochemical immunoassay for sensitive detection of cardiac troponin I. *Biosensors & Bioelectronics* 133 (March): 72–78.

80 Gupta, R.K., Pandya, R., Sieffert, T., Meyyappan, M., and Koehne, J.E. (2016). Multiplexed electrochemical immunosensor for label-free detection of cardiac markers using a carbon nanofiber array chip. *Journal of Electroanalytical Chemistry* 773: 53–62.

81 Zhou, F., Lu, M., Wang, W., Bian, Z.P., Zhang, J.R., and Zhu, J.J. (2010). Electrochemical immunosensor for simultaneous detection of dual cardiac markers based on a poly(dimethylsiloxane)-gold nanoparticles composite microfluidic chip: A proof of principle. *Clinical Chemistry* 56 (11): 1701–1707.

82 Feng, L.N., Bian, Z.P., Peng, J., Jiang, F., Yang, G.H., Zhu, Y.D., Yang, D., Jiang, L.P., and Zhu, J.J. (2012). Ultrasensitive multianalyte electrochemical immunoassay based on metal ion functionalized titanium phosphate nanospheres. *Analytical Chemistry* 84 (18): 7810–7815.

83 Negahdary, M., Behjati-Ardakani, M., and Heli, H. (2019). An electrochemical troponin T aptasensor based on the use of a macroporous gold nanostructure. *Microchimica Acta* 186 (6).

84 Zanato, N., Talamini, L., Zapp, E., Brondani, D., and Vieira, I.C. (2017). Label-free Electrochemical Immunosensor for Cardiac Troponin T Based on Exfoliated Graphite Nanoplatelets Decorated with Gold Nanoparticles. *Electroanalysis* 29 (7): 1820–1827.

85 Karimi, M., Rabiee, M., Tahriri, M., Salarian, R., and Tayebi, L. (2019). A graphene based–biomimetic molecularly imprinted polyaniline sensor for ultrasensitive detection of human cardiac troponin T (cTnT). *Synthetic Metals* 256 (July): 116136.

86 Freitas, T.A., Mattos, A.B., Silva, B.V.M., and Dutra, R.F. (2014). amino-functionalization of carbon nanotubes by using a factorial design: Human cardiac troponin T immunosensing application. *BioMed Research International* 2014.

87 Kaur, G., Tomar, M., and Gupta, V. (2017). Nanostructured NiO-based reagentless biosensor for total cholesterol and low density lipoprotein detection. *Analytical and Bioanalytical Chemistry* 409 (8): 1995–2005.

88 Martín, M., Salazar, P., Álvarez, R., Palmero, A., López-Santos, C., González-Mora, J.L., and González-Elipe, A.R. (2017). Cholesterol biosensing with a polydopamine-modified nanostructured platinum electrode prepared by oblique angle physical vacuum deposition. *Sensors and Actuators, B Chemicals* 240: 37–45.

89 Shrestha, B.K., Ahmad, R., Shrestha, S., Park, C.H., and Kim, C.S. (2017). In situ synthesis of cylindrical spongy polypyrrole doped protonated graphitic carbon nitride for cholesterol sensing application. *Biosensors & Bioelectronics* 94 (March): 686–693.

90 Dervisevic, M., Çevik, E., Şenel, M., Nergiz, C., and Abasiyanik, M.F. (2016). Amperometric cholesterol biosensor based on reconstituted cholesterol oxidase on boronic acid functional conducting polymers. *Journal of Electroanalytical Chemistry* 776: 18–24.

91 Komathi, S., Muthuchamy, N., Lee, K.P., and Gopalan, A.I. (2016). Fabrication of a novel dual mode cholesterol biosensor using titanium dioxide nanowire bridged 3D graphene nanostacks. *Biosensors & Bioelectronics* 84: 64–71.

92 Lata, K., Dhull, V., and Hooda, V. (2016). Fabrication and optimization of ChE/ChO/HRP-AuNPs/c-MWCNTs based silver electrode for determining total cholesterol in Serum. *Biochemistry Research International* 2016.

93 Nandini, S., Nalini, S., Reddy, M.B.M., Suresh, G.S., Melo, J.S., Niranjana, P., Sanetuntikul, J., and Shanmugam, S. (2016). Synthesis of one-dimensional gold nanostructures and the electrochemical application of the nanohybrid containing functionalized graphene oxide for cholesterol biosensing. *Bioelectrochemistry* 110: 79–90.

94 Tang, S., Zhao, Q., and Tu, Y. (2016). A sensitive electrochemiluminescent cholesterol biosensor based on Au/hollowed-TiO2 nano-composite pre-functionalized electrode. *Sensors and Actuators, B Chemicals* 237: 416–422.

95 Tlı, G.A., Zeybek, D.K., and Pekyardlmcl, S. (2016). Fabrication of amperometric cholesterol biosensor based on SnO2nanoparticles and Nafion-modified carbon paste electrode. *Chemical Papers* 70 (4): i–xi.

96 Xu, Z.H., Cheng, X.D., Tan, J.H., and Gan, X. (2016). Fabrication of multiwalled carbon nanotube–polyaniline/platinum nanocomposite films toward improved performance for a cholesterol amperometric biosensor. *Biotechnology and Applied Biochemistry* 63 (6): 757–764.

97 Li, Z., Xie, C., Wang, J., Meng, A., and Zhang, F. (2015). Direct electrochemistry of cholesterol oxidase immobilized on chitosan-graphene and cholesterol sensing. *Sensors and Actuators, B Chemicals* 208: 505–511.

98 Sekretaryova, A.N., Beni, V., Eriksson, M., Karyakin, A.A., Turner, A.P.F., and Vagin, M.Y. (2014). Cholesterol self-powered biosensor. *Analytical Chemistry* 86 (19): 9540–9547.

99 Rahman, M.M., Li, X.B., Kim, J., Lim, B.O., Ahammad, A.J.S., and Lee, J.J. (2014). A cholesterol biosensor based on a bi-enzyme immobilized on conducting poly(thionine) film. *Sensors and Actuators, B Chemicals* 202: 536–542.

100 Dey, R.S. and Raj, C.R. (2014). Enzyme-integrated cholesterol biosensing scaffold based on in situ synthesized reduced graphene oxide and dendritic Pd nanostructure. *Biosensors & Bioelectronics* 62: 357–364.

101 Ruecha, N., Rangkupan, R., Rodthongkum, N., and Chailapakul, O. (2014). Novel paper-based cholesterol biosensor using graphene/polyvinylpyrrolidone/polyaniline nanocomposite. *Biosensors & Bioelectronics* 52: 13–19.

102 Wu, X., Chai, Y., Yuan, R., Zhong, X., and Zhang, J. (2014). Synthesis of multiwall carbon nanotubes-graphene oxide-thionine-Au nanocomposites for electrochemiluminescence detection of cholesterol. *Electrochimica Acta* 129: 441–449.

103 Dey, R.S. and Raj, C.R. (2013). Redox-functionalized graphene oxide architecture for the development of amperometric biosensing platform. *ACS Applied Materials & Interfaces* 5 (11): 4791–4798.

104 Zhu, L., Xu, L., Tan, L., Tan, H., Yang, S., and Yao, S. (2013). Direct electrochemistry of cholesterol oxidase immobilized on gold nanoparticles-decorated multiwalled carbon nanotubes and cholesterol sensing. *Talanta* 106: 192–199.

105 Tan, X., Zhang, L., Deng, X., Miao, L., Li, H., and Zheng, G. (2017). Redox active molybdophosphate produced by Cu3(PO4)2 nanospheres for enhancing enzyme-free electrochemical immunoassay of C-reactive protein. *New Journal of Chemistry* 41 (20): 11867–11871.

106 Wang, J., Guo, J., Zhang, J., Zhang, W., and Zhang, Y. (2017). RNA aptamer-based electrochemical aptasensor for C-reactive protein detection using functionalized silica microspheres as immunoprobes. *Biosensors & Bioelectronics* 95 (March): 100–105.

107 Lemos, A.J.G., Balvedi, R.P.A., Rodovalho, V.R., Resende, L.O., Castro, A.C.H., Cuadros-Orellana, S., Madurro, J.M., and Brito-Madurro, A.G. (2017). Immunosensor assembled on polymeric nanostructures for clinical diagnosis of C-reactive protein. *Microchemical Journal* 133: 572–576.

108 Zhang, X., Hu, R., Zhang, K., Bai, R., Li, D., and Yang, Y. (2016). An ultrasensitive label-free immunoassay for C-reactive protein detection in human serum based on electron transfer. *Analytical Methods : Advancing Methods and Applications* 8 (32): 6202–6207.

109 Yagati, A.K., Pyun, J.C., Min, J., and Cho, S. (2016). Label-free and direct detection of C-reactive protein using reduced graphene oxide-nanoparticle hybrid impedimetric sensor. *Bioelectrochemistry* 107: 37–44.

110 Kokkinos, C., Prodromidis, M., Economou, A., Petrou, P., and Kakabakos, S. (2015). Disposable integrated bismuth citrate-modified screen-printed immunosensor for ultrasensitive quantum dot-based electrochemical assay of C-reactive protein in human serum. *Analytica Chimica Acta* 886: 29–36.

111 Yuan, G., Yu, C., Xia, C., Gao, L., Xu, W., Li, W., and He, J. (2015). A simultaneous electrochemical multianalyte immunoassay of high sensitivity C-reactive protein and soluble CD40 ligand based on reduced graphene oxide-tetraethylene pentamine that directly adsorb metal ions as labels. *Biosensors & Bioelectronics* 72: 237–246.

112 Gupta, R.K., Periyakaruppan, A., Meyyappan, M., and Koehne, J.E. (2014). Label-free detection of C-reactive protein using a carbon nanofiber based biosensor. *Biosensors & Bioelectronics* 59: 112–119.

113 Esteban-Fernández De Ávila, B., Escamilla-Gómez, V., Campuzano, S., Pedrero, M., Salvador, J.P., Marco, M.P., and Pingarrón, J.M. (2013). Ultrasensitive amperometric magnetoimmunosensor for human C-reactive protein quantification in serum. *Sensors and Actuators, B Chemicals* 188: 212–220.

114 Bryan, T., Luo, X., Bueno, P.R., and Davis, J.J. (2013). An optimised electrochemical biosensor for the label-free detection of C-reactive protein in blood. *Biosensors & Bioelectronics* 39 (1): 94–98.

115 Ibupoto, Z.H., Jamal, N., Khun, K., and Willander, M. (2012). Development of a disposable potentiometric antibody immobilized ZnO nanotubes based sensor for the detection of C-reactive protein. *Sensors and Actuators, B Chemicals* 166–167: 809–814.

116 Li, Y., Tian, L., Liu, L., Khan, M.S., Zhao, G., Fan, D., Cao, W., and Wei, Q. (2018). Dual-responsive electrochemical immunosensor for detection of insulin based on dual-functional zinc silicate spheres-palladium nanoparticles. *Talanta* 179 (October 2017): 420–425.

117 Amouzadeh Tabrizi, M., Shamsipur, M., Saber, R., Sarkar, S., and Besharati, M. (2018). An electrochemical aptamer-based assay for femtomolar determination of insulin using a screen printed electrode modified with mesoporous carbon and 1,3,6,8-pyrenetetrasulfonate. *Microchimica Acta* 185 (1): 6–12.

118 Ensafi, A.A., Khoddami, E., and Rezaei, B. (2017). Aptamer@Au-o-phenylenediamine modified pencil graphite electrode: A new selective electrochemical impedance biosensor for the determination of insulin. *Colloids Surfaces B Biointerfaces* 159: 47–53.

119 Ma, H., Li, X., Yan, T., Li, Y., Liu, H., Zhang, Y., Wu, D., Du, B., and Wei, Q. (2016). Sensitive insulin detection based on electrogenerated chemiluminescence resonance energy transfer between Ru(bpy)32+ and Au Nanoparticle-Doped β-Cyclodextrin-Pb (II) Metal-Organic Framework. *ACS Applied Materials & Interfaces* 8 (16): 10121–10127.

120 Li, T., Liu, Z., Wang, L., and Guo, Y. (2016). Gold nanoparticles/Orange II functionalized graphene nanohybrid based electrochemical aptasensor for label-free determination of insulin. *RSC Advances* 6 (36): 30732–30738.

121 Singh, V. and Krishnan, S. (2015). Voltammetric immunosensor assembled on carbon-pyrenyl nanostructures for clinical diagnosis of type of diabetes. *Analytical Chemistry* 87 (5): 2648–2654.

122 Tertiş, M., Ciui, B., Suciu, M., Săndulescu, R., and Cristea, C. (2017). Label-free electrochemical aptasensor based on gold and polypyrrole nanoparticles for interleukin 6 detection. *Electrochimica Acta* 258: 1208–1218.

123 Sánchez-Tirado, E., Salvo, C., González-Cortés, A., Yáñez-Sedeño, P., Langa, F., and Pingarrón, J.M. (2017). Electrochemical immunosensor for simultaneous determination of interleukin-1 beta and tumor necrosis factor alpha in serum and saliva using dual screen printed electrodes modified with functionalized double-walled carbon nanotubes. *Analytica Chimica Acta* 959: 66–73.

124 Torrente-Rodríguez, R.M., Campuzano, S., Ruiz-Valdepeñas Montiel, V., Gamella, M., and Pingarrón, J.M. (2016). Electrochemical bioplatforms for the simultaneous determination of interleukin (IL)-8 mRNA and IL-8 protein oral cancer biomarkers in raw saliva. *Biosensors & Bioelectronics* 77: 543–548.

125 Sharma, R., Deacon, S.E., Nowak, D., George, S.E., Szymonik, M.P., Tang, A.A.S., Tomlinson, D.C., Davies, A.G., McPherson, M.J., and Wälti, C. (2016). Label-free electrochemical impedance biosensor to detect human interleukin-8 in serum with sub-pg/ml sensitivity. *Biosensors & Bioelectronics* 80: 607–613.

126 Wang, G., He, X., Chen, L., Zhu, Y., and Zhang, X. (2014). Ultrasensitive IL-6 electrochemical immunosensor based on Au nanoparticles-graphene-silica biointerface. *Colloids Surfaces B Biointerfaces* 116: 714–719.

127 Lou, Y., He, T., Jiang, F., Shi, J.J., and Zhu, J.J. (2014). A competitive electrochemical immunosensor for the detection of human interleukin-6 based on the electrically heated carbon electrode and silver nanoparticles functionalized labels. *Talanta* 122: 135–139.

128 Liu, P.Z., Hu, X.W., Mao, C.J., Niu, H.L., Song, J.M., Jin, B.K., and Zhang, S.Y. (2013). Electrochemiluminescence immunosensor based on graphene oxide nanosheets/polyaniline nanowires/CdSe quantum dots nanocomposites for ultrasensitive determination of human interleukin-6. *Electrochimica Acta* 113: 176–180.

129 Tang, C.K., Vaze, A., and Rusling, J.F. (2012). Fabrication of immunosensor microwell arrays from gold compact discs for detection of cancer biomarker proteins. *Lab on a Chip* 12 (2): 281–286.

130 Rodriguez-Silva, A.A., Movil-Cabrera, O., Oliveira Dos Anjos, C.T., and Staser, J.A. (2016). Supercapacitor-based biosensor for low density lipoprotein detection. *Journal of the Electrochemical Society* 163 (6): B256–B263.

131 Ali, M.A., Singh, C., Mondal, K., Srivastava, S., Sharma, A., and Malhotra, B.D. (2016). Mesoporous few-layer graphene platform for affinity biosensing application. *ACS Applied Materials & Interfaces* 8 (12): 7646–7656.

132 Ali, M.A., Srivastava, S., Agrawal, V.V., Willander, M., John, R., and Malhotra, B.D. (2016). A biofunctionalized quantum dot-nickel oxide nanorod based smart platform for lipid detection. *Journal of Materials Chemistry B* 4 (15): 2706–2714.

133 Kaur, G., Tomar, M., and Gupta, V. (2016). Realization of a label-free electrochemical immunosensor for detection of low density lipoprotein using NiO thin film. *Biosensors & Bioelectronics* 80: 294–299.

134 Ali, M.A., Solanki, P.R., Srivastava, S., Singh, S., Agrawal, V.V., John, R., and Malhotra, B.D. (2015). Protein functionalized carbon nanotubes-based smart lab-on-a-chip. *ACS Applied Materials & Interfaces* 7 (10): 5837–5846.

135 Ali, M.A., Singh, N., Srivastava, S., Agrawal, V.V., John, R., Onoda, M., and Malhotra, B.D. (2014). Chitosan-modified carbon nanotubes-based platform for low-density lipoprotein detection. *Appl. Biochem. Biotechnol.* 174 (3): 926–935.

136 Ali, M.A., Kamil Reza, K., Srivastava, S., Agrawal, V.V., John, R., and Malhotra, B.D. (2014). Lipid-lipid interactions in aminated reduced graphene oxide interface for biosensing application. *Langmuir* 30 (14): 4192–4201.

137 Pur, M.R.K., Hosseini, M., Faridbod, F., and Ganjali, M.R. (2017). Highly sensitive label-free electrochemiluminescence aptasensor for early detection of myoglobin, a biomarker for myocardial infarction. *Microchimica Acta* 184 (9): 3529–3537.

138 Ren, X., Zhang, Y., Sun, Y., and Gao, L. (2017). Development of electrochemical impedance immunosensor for sensitive determination of myoglobin. *International Journal of Electrochemical Science* 12 (8): 7765–7776.

139 Sun, L., Li, W., Wang, M., Ding, W., and Ji, Y. (2017). Development of an electrochemical impedance immunosensor for myoglobin determination. *International Journal of Electrochemical Science* 12 (7): 6170–6179.

140 Zhang, G., Liu, Z., Wang, L., and Guo, Y. (2016). Electrochemical aptasensor for myoglobin-specific recognition based on porphyrin functionalized graphene-conjugated gold nanocomposites. *Sensors (Switzerland)* 16 (11).

141 Taghdisi, S.M., Danesh, N.M., Ramezani, M., Emrani, A.S., and Abnous, K. (2016). A novel electrochemical aptasensor based on Y-shape structure of dual-aptamer-complementary strand conjugate for ultrasensitive detection of myoglobin. *Biosensors & Bioelectronics* 80: 532–537.

142 Singh, S., Tuteja, S.K., Sillu, D., Deep, A., and Suri, C.R. (2016). Gold nanoparticles-reduced graphene oxide based electrochemical immunosensor for the cardiac biomarker myoglobin. *Microchimica Acta* 183 (5): 1729–1738.

143 Khan, R., Pal, M., Kuzikov, A.V., Bulko, T., Suprun, E.V., and Shumyantseva, V.V. (2016). Impedimetric immunosensor for detection of cardiovascular disorder risk biomarker. *Materials Science and Engineering C* 68: 52–58.

144 Sun, C., Wang, D., Geng, Z., Gao, L., Zhang, M., Bian, H., Liu, F., Zhu, Y., Wu, H., and Xu, W. (2015). One-step green synthesis of a polypyrrole-Au nanocomposite and its application in myoglobin aptasensor. *Analytical Methods : Advancing Methods and Applications* 7 (12): 5262–5268.

145 Mishra, S.K., Srivastava, A.K., and Kumar, D., Rajesh. (2014). Bio-functionalized Pt nanoparticles based electrochemical impedance immunosensor for human cardiac myoglobin. *RSC Advances* 4 (41): 21267–21276.

146 Yagati, A.K., Lee, M.H., and Min, J. (2018). Electrochemical immunosensor for highly sensitive and quantitative detection of tumor necrosis factor-α in human serum. *Bioelectrochemistry* 122: 93–102.

147 Aydın, E.B., Aydın, M., and Sezgintürk, M.K. (2017). A highly sensitive immunosensor based on ITO thin films covered by a new semi-conductive conjugated polymer for the determination of TNFα in human saliva and serum samples. *Biosensors & Bioelectronics* 97 (June): 169–176.

148 Miao, P., Yang, D., Chen, X., Guo, Z., and Tang, Y. (2017). Voltammetric determination of tumor necrosis factor-α based on the use of an aptamer and magnetic nanoparticles loaded with gold nanoparticles. *Microchimica Acta* 184 (10): 3901–3907.

149 Arya, S.K. and Estrela, P. (2017). Electrochemical immunosensor for tumor necrosis factor-alpha detection in undiluted serum. *Methods* 116: 125–131.

150 Jiang, C., Alam, M.T., Silva, S.M., Taufik, S., Fan, S., and Gooding, J.J. (2016). Unique sensing interface that allows the development of an electrochemical immunosensor for the detection of tumor necrosis factor α in whole blood. *ACS Sensors* 1 (12): 1432–1438.

151 Yagati, A.K., Lee, G.Y., Ha, S., Chang, K.A., Pyun, J.C., and Cho, S. (2016). Impedimetric tumor necrosis factor-α sensor based on a reduced graphene oxide nanoparticle-modified electrode array. *Journal of Nanoscience and Nanotechnology* 16 (11): 11921–11927.

152 Mazloum-Ardakani, M. and Hosseinzadeh, L. (2015). Highly-sensitive label-free immunosensor for tumor necrosis factor α based on Ag@Pt core-shell nanoparticles supported on MWCNTs as an efficient electrocatalyst nanocomposite. *RSC Advances* 5 (87): 70781–70786.

153 Mazloum-Ardakani, M., Hosseinzadeh, L., and Khoshroo, A. (2015). Label-free electrochemical immunosensor for detection of tumor necrosis factor α based on fullerene-functionalized carbon nanotubes/ionic liquid. *Journal of Electroanalytical Chemistry* 757: 58–64.

154 Mazloum-Ardakani, M., Hosseinzadeh, L., and Khoshroo, A. (2015). Ultrasensitive electrochemical immunosensor for detection of tumor necrosis factor-α based on functionalized MWCNT-Gold nanoparticle/ionic liquid nanocomposite. *Electroanalysis* 27 (11): 2518–2526.

155 Kongsuphol, P., Ng, H.H., Pursey, J.P., Arya, S.K., Wong, C.C., Stulz, E., and Park, M.K. (2014). EIS-based biosensor for ultra-sensitive detection of TNF-α from non-diluted human serum. *Biosensors & Bioelectronics* 61: 274–279.

156 Mazloum-Ardakani, M., Hosseinzadeh, L., and Taleat, Z. (2014). Two kinds of electrochemical immunoassays for the tumor necrosis factor α in human serum using screen-printed graphite electrodes modified with poly(anthranilic acid). *Microchimica Acta* 181 (9–10): 917–924.

157 Hou, Y., Li, T., Huang, H., Quan, H., Miao, X., and Yang, M. (2013). Electrochemical immunosensor for the detection of tumor necrosis factor α based on hydrogel prepared from ferrocene modified amino acid. *Sensors and Actuators, B Chemicals* 182: 605–609.

158 Mondal, K., Ali, M.A., Singh, C., Sumana, G., Malhotra, B.D., and Sharma, A. (2017). Highly sensitive porous carbon and metal/carbon conducting nanofiber based enzymatic biosensors for triglyceride detection. *Sensors and Actuators, B Chemicals* 246: 202–214.

159 Narwal, V. and Pundir, C.S. (2017). An improved amperometric triglyceride biosensor based on co-immobilization of nanoparticles of lipase, glycerol kinase and glycerol 3-phosphate oxidase onto pencil graphite electrode. *Enzyme and Microbial Technology* 100: 11–16.

160 Zhu, M., Yang, Z., Cheng, Y., Sun, Y., Xing, J., Wei, J., Sun, J., Liu, H., and Song, X. (2017). Development of triglyceride biosensor based on the polydopamine-gold nanocomposite. *International Journal of Electrochemical Science* 12 (7): 6863–6873.

161 Pundir, C.S. and Aggarwal, V. (2017). Amperometric triglyceride bionanosensor based on nanoparticles of lipase, glycerol kinase, glycerol-3-phosphate oxidase. *Analytical Biochemistry* 517: 56–63.

162 Bhardwaj, S.K., Yadav, P., Ghosh, S., Basu, T., and Mahapatro, A.K. (2016). Biosensing test-bed using electrochemically deposited reduced graphene oxide. *ACS Applied Materials & Interfaces* 8 (37): 24350–24360.

163 Solanki, S., Pandey, C.M., Soni, A., Sumana, G., and Biradar, A.M. (2016). An amperometric bienzymatic biosensor for the triglyceride tributyrin using an indium tin oxide electrode coated with electrophoretically deposited chitosan-wrapped nanozirconia. *Microchimica Acta* 183 (1): 167–176.

164 Singh, C., Ali, M.A., and Sumana, G. (2016). Green synthesis of graphene based biomaterial using fenugreek seeds for lipid detection. *ACS Sustainable Chemistry & Engineering* 4 (3): 871–880.

165 Yücel, A., Özcan, H.M., and Saȷiroȷlu, A. (2016). A new multienzyme-type biosensor for triglyceride determination. *Prep. Biochem. Biotechnol.* 46 (1): 78–84.

166 Zhang, W., Tang, Y., Liu, J., Ma, Y., Jiang, L., Huang, W., Huo, F.W., and Tian, D. (2014). An electrochemical sensor for detecting triglyceride based on biomimetic polydopamine and gold nanocomposite. *Journal of Materials Chemistry B* 2 (48): 8490–8495.

167 Bravin, C. and Amendola, V. (2020). Wide range detection of C-Reactive protein with a homogeneous immunofluorimetric assay based on cooperative fluorescence quenching assisted by gold nanoparticles. *Biosensors & Bioelectronics* 169 (June): 112591.

168 Zheng, L., Li, M., Li, F., and Zhang, M. (2018). Paper-based chemiluminescence enzyme-linked immunosorbent assay enhanced by biotin-streptavidin system for high-sensitivity C-reactive protein detection. *Analytical Biochemistry* 559 (August): 86–90.

169 Çimen, D., Bereli, N., Günaydın, S., and Denizli, A. (2020). Detection of cardiac troponin-I by optic biosensors with immobilized anti-cardiac troponin-I monoclonal antibody. *Talanta* 219 (June): 121259.

170 Osman, B., Uzun, L., Beşirli, N., and Denizli, A. (2013). Microcontact imprinted surface plasmon resonance sensor for myoglobin detection. *Materials Science and Engineering C* 33 (7): 3609–3614.

4

Overview and Challenges of Wireless Communication and Power Transfer for Implanted Sensors

Mohamed Zied Chaari and Somaya Al-Maadeed

4.1 Introduction

Implanted sensors can measure the physiological and clinical parameters of interest, elaborate on them, and transmit information to healthcare staff through the internet to enable real-time decsion-making, as shown in Figure 4.1. Each sensor is an intelligent device, and the complete structural health supervision (SHM) system is a utilization of the internet of things (IoT) paradigm [1–4]. The bioinformatics data are sent to the cloud by internet link, allowing distributed systems and big data concepts to monitor and analyze them. Implementing the SHM system using the IoT model allows new technologies to facilitate the capability and reliability of progressive health supervising technology. Remotely following critical health bioinformatics helps patient in-home care and reduces the complexities of overseeing the healthcare of older people [5, 6], and is especially practical in COVID-19. If this advanced technology were implanted in the human body before, it would have helped us face the coronavirus pandemic, as the sensors measure the body temperature. If the temperature exceeds 39 °C, the doctor is informed directly. The patient then receives an instruction to stay at home until they have done a coronavirus test, and thus the spread of infection has been reduced.

New technology implant biosensors for supervising many biological parameters and improving wireless methods have led to progress in all-inclusive patient-focused technologies such as wireless body area networks (WBANs) [7] and body sensor networks (BSNs) for long-term healthcare [8, 9]. BSN is a short-range network consisting of an array of low-power sensors that can be inserted or attached to the body and work within a short-range. WBAN, on the other hand, offers several exciting new web-based applications for remote health monitoring, healthcare, and medicine, all of which benefit from the unrestricted freedom of movement provided by WBAN. The advantage of WBAN is that the patient does not have to stay in bed for long and can now leave the hospital and transmit medical data remotely. The essential component of these networks is an implantable chip. This research harness wireless energy transfer technologies to energize the chip implant sensors underneath the skin (invasive). Biosensors have several

Predicting Heart Failure: Invasive, Non-Invasive, Machine Learning, and Artificial Intelligence Based Methods, First Edition. Edited by Kishor Kumar Sadasivuni, Hassen M. Ouakad, Somaya Al-Maadeed, Huseyin C. Yalcin, and Issam Bait Bahadur.

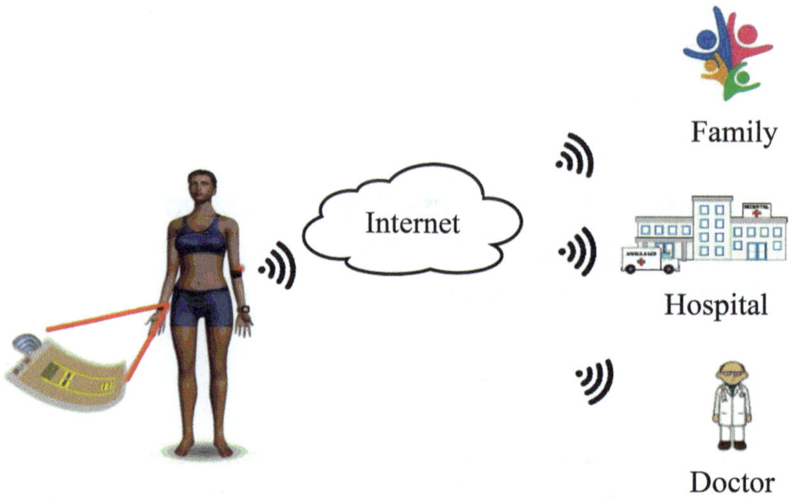

Figure 4.1 Implant sensor which can monitor physiological and clinical parameters.

advantages over amperometry sensors, including higher sensitivity, superior selectivity, and better stability. Another crucial benefit of the biosensor is that, if used correctly, it can offer a complete perfect diagnostic. If the cell volume of the biosensor is known and the varieties of benefits entirely electrolyze, the corresponding power-up is a final measure of quantity and concentration. Powering represents the fundamental challenge impeding the completion and medical use of implantable bioelectronic microdevices. Biosensors implanted in the body target vital areas to reach essential objectives in biomedicine and follow the patient's condition from a distance.

The realization of a new technique to collect and store radiofrequency energy in the dynamic and complex area underneath the skin is necessary to implement the biomedical microchip. So far, various techniques of transmitting energy wirelessly have been established, including ultrasonic guided waves, laser beam, electromagnetic induction, and transmission through radio frequency (RF). Including the listed alternatives, wireless energy transmission via RF signal is a highly advanced transmission technique. The uses of inductive charging are wide, but the narrow gap between coils (Rx, Tx) presents a challenge in the medical field. However, it is still a good solution in healthcare applications because skin depth is 3–5 mm. This method produces a heat process that interferes with the biological parameters of the human body. We cannot use all the techniques mentioned earlier in this section to penetrate human skin, for example laser might burn a patient's skin. In this chapter we will discuss the advanced techniques for developing the best technology to power-up the implantation of chips into the human body without intervention. Vital data checking is becoming an essential part of healthcare technologies. The chapter first explains the microchip insertion procedure. It then reviews wireless power transfer methods and gives some examples of applicative biomedical systems. This is followed by a discussion of the study of high-efficiency technology for charging wireless implant sensors, and then a conclusion.

4.2 Microchip Insertion Procedure

New improvements in biomedical chips and the latest CMOS techniques have led to invasive bioelectronics microchips for permanent human health monitoring. Microchips implanted in the human body allow doctors to continuously investigate a patient's medical vital data online, enabling savings of both money and time. In addition, the information acquired by the sensor from regular supervision helps the doctor and healthcare staff efficiently record a patient's medical history for analysis and emergencies. Figure 4.2 shows a complex implantable sensor system with various biosensors and the methods for entering the body. CMOS technologies offer many features, such as minor form elements and reliable processes, making them appropriate for implantable health applications.

Chips on this platform contain many sensors for oxygen, glucose, etc. The latest scientific study on implantable chip systems focuses on small form factors and lightweight features for ease of implementation and reasons of physical safety [10, 11]. Even though deep CMOS processes have substantially improved the overall sensor area, the power unit delivers a robust, comprehensive system.

The path to ultra-precise metering in CMOS technologies is not just limited to image sensors, wireless systems, microelectromechanical systems (MEMS), and radiofrequency systems. The implantable devices into the body demand low energy consumption and a small area fabricated by ultra-fine technology. Microchip sensor technology is very functional for biotechnology implementations in which fluorescence is frequently used for labeling, particularly for detecting neural activity or cells. These features are suitable for biomedical applications. CMOS technologies are thus entirely appropriate for an implantable microchip for biomedical fields and use in various applications. Increasing

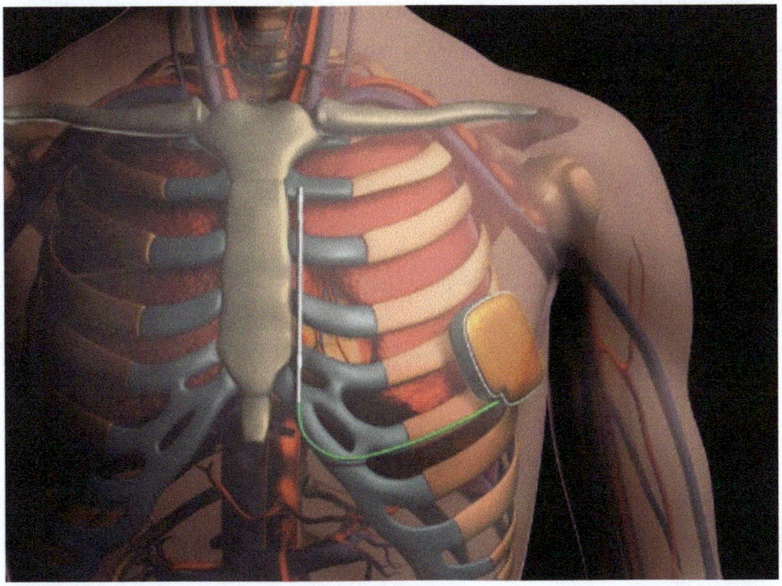

Figure 4.2 Implantable cardioverter defibrillators.

chip integration density has helped humans implant biosensors inside the human body to identify a problem in the human body before it occurs.

Removing the lithium battery as a permanent energizing source can potentially decrease the microchip size. In addition, the power unit (batteries) can cause a high risk of leakage, resulting in severe health risks to older people and necessitating regular replacement. A safe solution to this potential problem involves developing highly efficient wireless energy methods that can charge anytime and anywhere via the radio frequency coming from WiFi signals, television stations, etc. in our environment.

The power-collecting circuit includes one or more multiband antennae to collect any RF signals. The printed circuit board (PCB) is implanted in the body and connected to the biosensor battery. We can charge the microchip battery by collecting radio frequency energy in the environment. Unlike a battery-powered system, wireless battery charging minimizes periodic battery change [12–14]. Much research presents inductive correlation coupling [15] as a potential approach to wireless power charging. The non-surgical energy source is the best and most effective, along with developing a dedicated technology to transmit essential information during the charging method. The standard potentiostat comprises three electrodes: counter electrode, working electrode, and reference electrode. The difference potential between the reference electrodes and the working electrodes catalyzes the chemical reactivity. The counter electrode is related to the output signal provided to the processing unit. The implanted microsystem underneath the skin can wirelessly transmit data outside the human body to any device, such as a smartphone, laptop, or a programmable logic controller supervisory control and data acquisition (PLC SCADA) system, as shown in Figure 4.3. Peripheral integrated circuit (IC) biosensors or microsystems such as power supply units, sensors, and microcontroller unit (MCU) are integrated to make this schematic on a system on a chip (SoC) platform [16].

Healthcare sensors require certain rules to guarantee that they are chemically, physically, and biologically safe before being implantable in individuals. The necessary degree of regulation varies on the degree of risk associated with the sensor. Implantable biosensors, such as pacemakers, require stricter rules than non-invasive sensors. Therefore, when using health devices, it is essential to be aware of the regulations that pertain to a

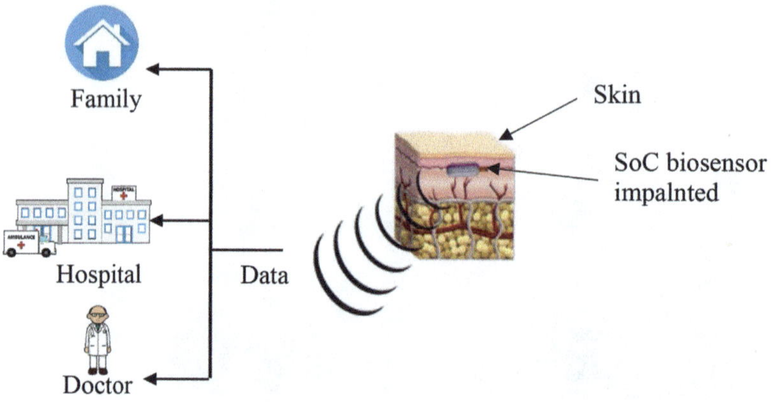

Figure 4.3 Implantable biosensor underneath the skin and the vital transmission data.

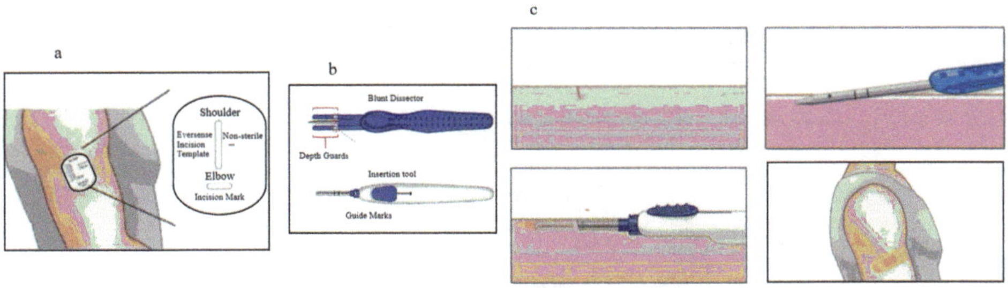

Figure 4.4 Biosensor sensor insertion procedure.

particular biochip and guarantee that the sensor is compliant. The bioelectronics microchip implant technique is demonstrated schematically in Figure 4.4.

According to World Health Organization regulations, only one implanted sensor is allowed in a patient. A health professional inserts the sensor in a short outpatient procedure [17]. First, the medical team makes a small incision, after which the bioelectronics sensor is inserted under the skin using a specialized biological chip. The incision is then closed using sterile tapes [18]. The chip implanted inside the body will not affect the body's organs because it does not contain any substances that present any danger for the body. A small chip inserted inside the body can detect many things such as blood pressure, sugar levels, heartbeat, and cancer and can subequently relay the results at precise times. It can lead to early detection of significant problems inside the body through physiological parameter measurements.

4.3 Wireless Power Transmission

Wireless electricity transfer technology transfers power from one place to another without physical support [19] and is therefore beneficial for transmitting electricity to sites and devices that are difficult to energize, such as implant sensors. In this subsection, we will highlight contemporary media for wireless power transmission. There are typically four technologies used for wireless energy transmission, depending on the physical energy grandeur sent [20, 21]:

- Microwave wireless power transfer
- Electromagnetic induction energy transfer
- Laser wireless power transmission
- Ultrasonic wireless power transmission.

4.3.1 Categories of Wireless Electricity Transmission

There are two main techniques of wireless electricity transmission: wireless power by induction and wireless power by radiation, as shown in Figure 4.5.

Many energy sources energize sensors, including dynamic and thermal power harvesters such as piezoelectric, RF harvesting, inductive link, and pyroelectric transducers.

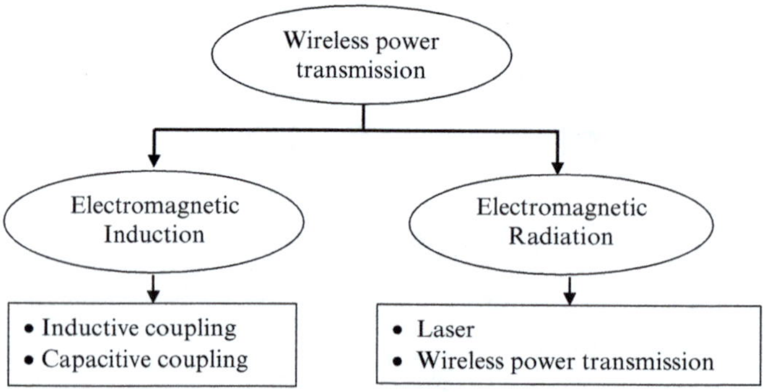

Figure 4.5 Different types of wireless energy transfer.

A summary is provided in Table 4.1, which shows their sizes, energy production, and related products [22, 23].

4.3.2 Microwave Wireless Power Transfer

Microwave power transmission (MPT) is a technique used to transfer electricity anywhere which is hard to reach (e.g. a microchip implant underneath the skin). The wireless energy transmission structure consists of three parts:

- Transmitter
- Traveling wave area (air, skin)
- RF/DC circuit (rectifying antenna).

Figure 4.6 shows the structure of a general wireless power transmission system.

The main requirement remains to efficiently convert direct current (DC) power into microwave energy and radiate the waves in a controlled, low-loss way. The wireless power transmission system needs to transmit enough power from RF radiation to the

Table 4.1 Comparison of different energy sources.

Method	Density	Advantage	Disadvantage
Microwave wireless power	5 W/cm^2	Long distance RF power transmitted to multiple receivers	Small amount of power
Electromagnetic induction	7–10 W/cm^2	Large amount of power	Depends on magnetic coupling Alignment required
Laser wireless power	2–4 W/cm^2	Long distance	Power can't transmit to multiple receivers Efficiency reduced by environment
Ultrasonic wireless power	1–3 W/cm^2	Long distance RF power transmitted to multiple receivers	Small amount of power Efficiency reduced by environment

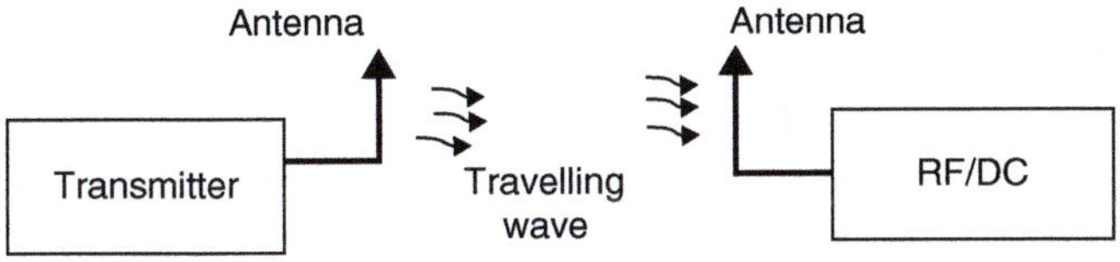

Figure 4.6 Block diagram of microwave wireless power transfer.

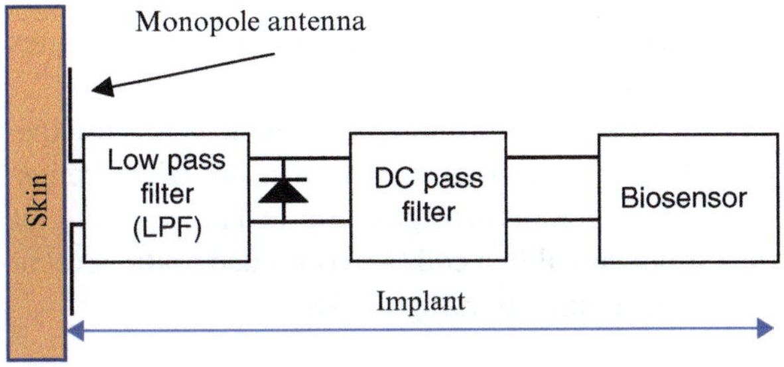

Figure 4.7 Rectenna (rectifying antenna). Based on Chaari and Al-Maadeed [24].

target place. All antennae types can be utilized for the microwave energy transmission and communication system, such as horn antennae, parabolic reflectors, patch antennae, Yagi-Uda, phased array antennae, cross-rhombic, etc. We regularly select a sizable parabolic antenna as a fixed point of the MPT technique to catch and collect maximum energy. As shown in Table 4.1, the amount of power that large parabolic antennae can capture is only about 5 W/cm^2. Therefore, we considered that the receiving antenna is part of the rectifying antenna (rectenna). The receiving RF energy then converts to DC, captured by the reception antenna, to DC using a rectenna design [24], as shown in Figure 4.7.

4.3.3 Electromagnetic Induction Energy Transfer

Electromagnetic inductive power transmission systems define techniques where inductive power is transferred from a transmission coil to a receiver coil using an alternating magnetic field [25, 26]. Various products utilize electromagnetic induction energy transmission, including mobile phones, trolleys, and cars. The concept of an inductive electricity transmission method is straightforward and integrable. The original design comprises an alternating current (AC) source, a transmission coil, a receiver coil, a rectenna, and the biosensor. The relation between the transmission and receiver coils creates electromagnetic energy. The main advantage of electromagnetic induction wireless power transmission is high efficiency at a low cost. The concept of an induction relation is simple, and highly efficient at small distances. The significant disadvantages of this technology are that the amount of energy transmitted is limited to the geometry of the coil, and the distance between the coils must not be multiples of a few millimeters. Professor Marin's method was to develop near-field communication between the inductive coil supplier and bulb light and utilize resonant objects linked through their magnetic

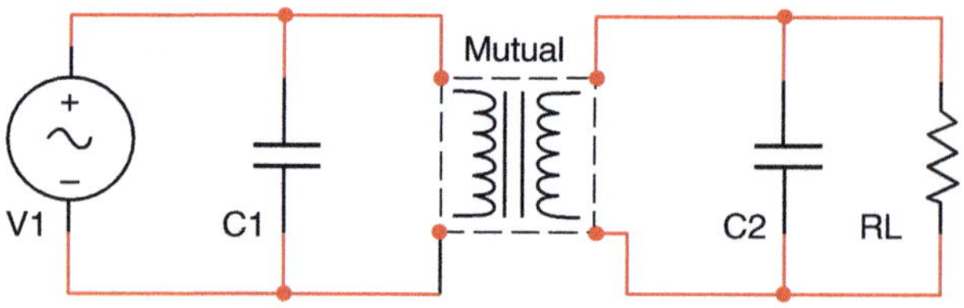

Figure 4.8 Inductive mutual coupling.

fields to attain mid-range energy transmission [27–29]. The linked resonance techniques can have a generally robust coupled regime of operation.

The transmitter coil (Tx) produces the desired electromagnetic field. The inductive coupling contains a loose-coupled transformer consisting of two coils. Part of the generated magnetic flux connects the receiver coil (Rx) corresponding to Faraday's law of electromagnetic induction. Thus, the output signal in a coil (Rx) is related to the level of change of magnetic flux in the receiver coil, as shown in Figure 4.8.

4.3.4 Laser Wireless Power Transmission

A laser is the best technique for transmitting electricity for a space energy beaming experiment. Investigation into the available laser technologies is presented [30, 31]. Laser energy transfer is performed by first converting DC into light using a laser source. These waves are transmitted wirelessly by laser light and then received and converted back into electricity, as shown in Figure 4.9. Historically, the main disadvantages with this technology were low efficiency of between 12 and 20% and safety concerns. However, the European Aeronautic Defense and Space Company (EDAS) successfully powered-up a robot with laser wireless power transfer.

We cannot use laser energy as a wireless charging solution for the implanted microchip, because the laser beam can pose a risk to the patient's skin.

4.3.5 Ultrasonic Wireless Power Transfer

This section discusses wireless ultrasound energy transmission to miniature medical implants in the human body [32–34]. The ultrasound produces vibrations or sound waves with the help of piezoelectric transducers. The ultrasonic frequency outside the audible scale is greater than 20 kHz [35] and, thus, the ultrasonic technique provides better penetration depths and shorter wavelengths. It can also transmit electromagnetic energy through hard-to-reach materials and neither the ultrasound method nor

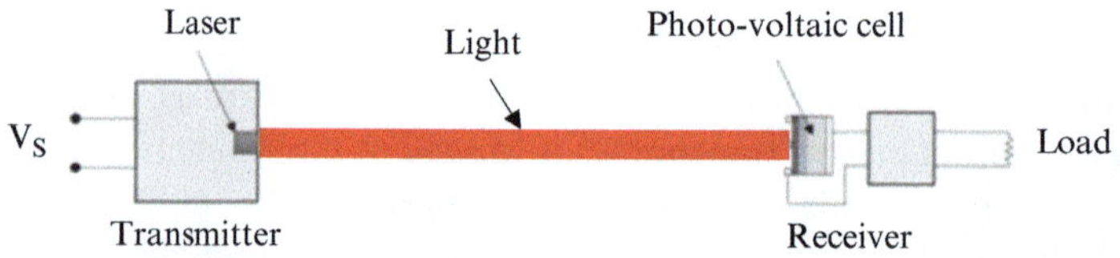

Figure 4.9 A schematic description of typical wireless power transfer using a laser beam.

electromagnetic interference harms human tissues. The ultrasound device comprises an external apparatus and a slide implanted underneath the skin with piezoelectric transducers on both sides and separated by tissue, as shown in Figure 4.10. This technology depends on the generation and propagation of sound via the tissues. Transmission of energy through tissue requires an external transducer (Transmitter (Tx)) placed on the tissue surface and counteracting the ultrasonic frequency to the biosensor chip directly under the skin (Receiver (Rx)). The power source activates a piezoelectric transducer that converts electricity into ultrasound waves. These ultrasound waves channel energy through the tissue toward a receiver implanted inside the body. The transducer's receiver transforms ultrasonic strength into electricity. The low-loss rectifier network rectifies and filters the output voltage of power-up the biosensor chip and charging battery.

An incorrect choice of the transmission frequency can adversely affect the skin attenuation and sizes of the emitter and receiver transducers (Tx and Rx) and Rayleigh distance. Therefore, the maximum power that a transducer can provide complete at its resonant frequency (f_r) depends on the transducer's material and size:

$$f_r = \frac{C}{2d} \tag{4.1}$$

where:

C = acoustic velocity
d = transducer thickness.

According to this equation, increasing (f_r) minimizes the transducer volume and boosts the Rayleigh range at the cost of boost tissue absorption.

Having presented the classification for wireless electricity, we will focus on inductive and radio frequency harvesting technology to charge the subcutaneous SoC implant. This work designs and realizes an inductive wireless charging system using mutual

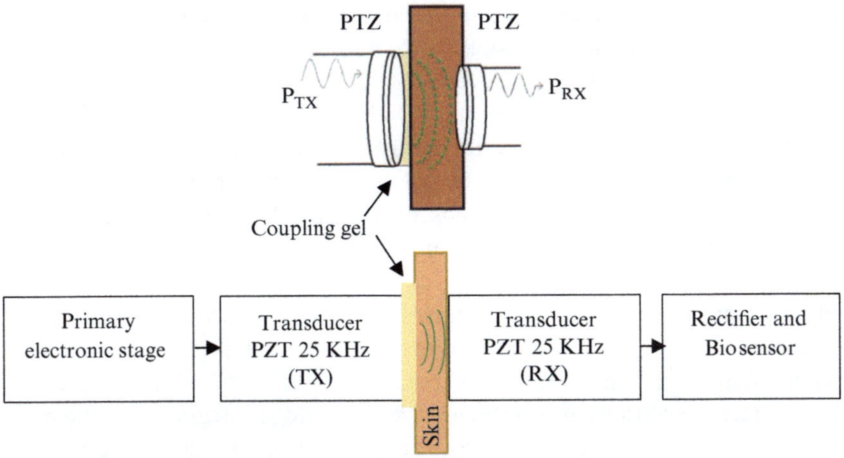

Figure 4.10 Ultrasound wireless power transfer.

inductive radiation. An inductive link between two coils operates the SoC, despite the tissue thickness of 3-5 mm (tissue width). Although this technique has a short space, the inductive distance range can be boosted using a high-power class E amplifier to enhance the magnetic resonance.

According to the following equation, the efficiency of ultrasonic wireless power (η) usually relies on transducer losses, the amount of energy used by the receiver transducer, acoustic impedance matching, the efficiency of the coupling gel, losses due to rectifier losses, and skin absorption:

$$\eta = \left| \frac{P_{out}}{P_{in}} \right| \tag{4.2}$$

The proposed circuit considers all of the above technical parameters to provide adequate power to operate the applied biosensor in the patient. The real success of the implanted chips varies according to how safely they work without any harmful effect on the skin.

4.4 The High-Efficiency Technique to Wirelessly Power Up Implanted Sensors

Currently, there are many technologies to power-up and transfer data between the implanted biosensor and the external reader unit. We will present and discuss two solutions here: magnetic resonant coupling and ambient RF energy harvesting for power energizing and for data transmission in any implant biosensor.

4.4.1 Inductive Wireless Electricity Transfer and Data Transmission through a Common Inductive Coupling

In this technique, inductive energy transmission depends on electromagnetic resonant coupling. The scale of this technique very short, no more than a few millimeters, which presents a significant limitation to its feasible implementation. However, the analytical model of an inductive link structure can develop through coupled-mode theory (CMT). We utilize the CMT approach to propose multicoil inductive links, increasing the power transfer efficiency considerably at large coupling distances, skin absorption losses, and RF-DC rectifier losses. The multicoil inductive link has been studied from a circuit perspective for power transmission to energize biosensors. A block diagram of the wireless electricity and biomedical data transmission through a shared connection, is given in Figure 4.11.

The system presented in Figure 4.11 comprises two parts: the external reader unit (inductive transmitter) is the primary part, and the biosensor chip part (SoC) is the second part. The inductive connection bridges the primary and biosensor chip sides, which is essential for wireless electricity transmission. The full-bridge integrated on the chip delivers enough power to the biosensor through the inductive coupling. A rectifier is employed on the harvester to convert the inductive flux into electricity. The

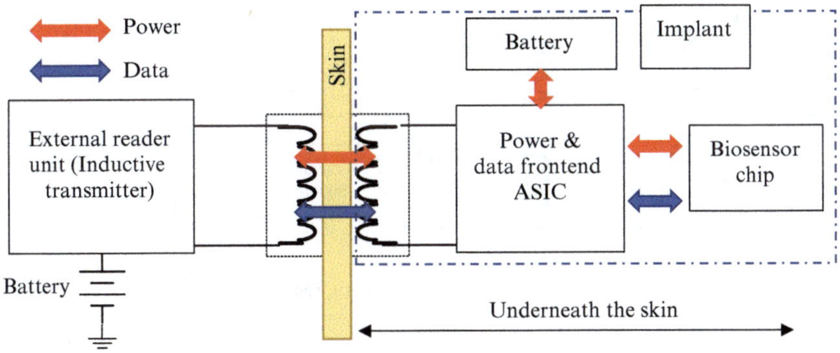

Figure 4.11 Block diagram of the biosensor implant system with a wireless data and inductive wireless power link.

recommended communication transmit data is implemented on both sides and magnetically coupled with the resonant power tank by the ferrite-core coupled inductors. The transmission data has two process methods: the transmitter and receiver methods controlled by electronic switch commutation. A signal amplifier employs an information source to broadcast data in the primary part. An impedance matching network connects to receive the data carrier from the transmitter circuit at the receiver circuit, and the information is demodulated and read by an MCU data acquisition. Thus, this design can work in two conditions: forward data and backward data conditions, as shown in Figure 4.12. The primary circuit works on power-up in forwarding information conditions, and the biosensor chip works on the receiver circuit. In backward information conditions, the external reader unit works on transmission data mode. The sensor is working on the transmitter circuit.

A magnetic resonant link utilizes similar concepts as inductive coupling but with resonance to boost the flux transfer scale with high efficiency. This technique provides a higher-quality factor and a lower strength loss proportional to the energy of the flux oscillator. The quality factor is a primary factor that explains the character of a rectangular wave oscillation and characterizes a resonator's bandwidth comparative to the resonant frequency center. Firstly, we fabricate two coils (Rx, Tx); for each, we wrap five turns of

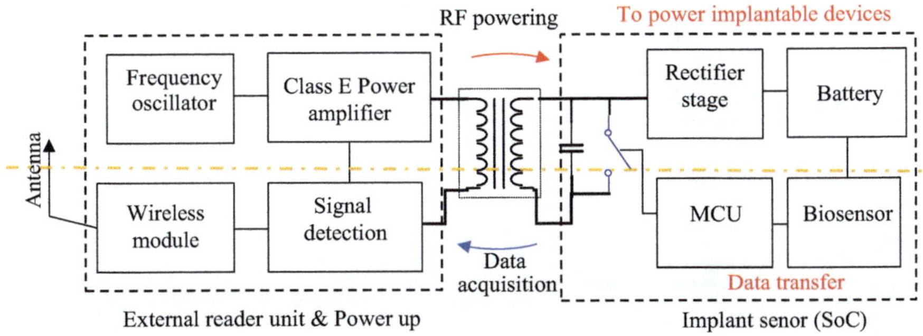

Figure 4.12 Simple block diagram of inductive wireless electricity and data transmission circuit.

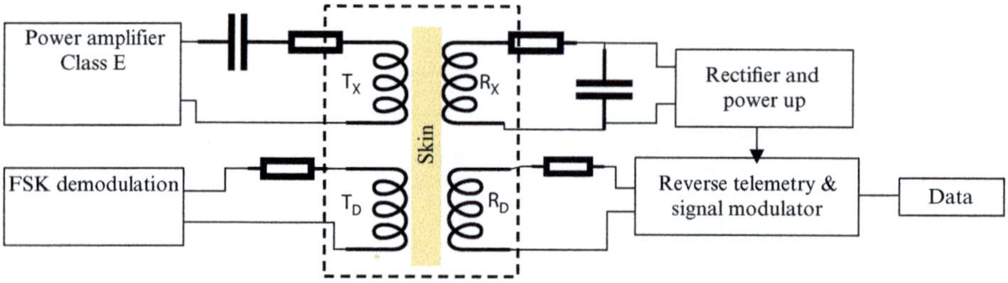

Figure 4.13 Schematic of bidirectional data transfer and magnetic resonant coupling.

tinned copper wires around a 5 mm diameter. Every loop has an internal inductance (L) and resistance (R), and the two coils are fine-tuned at the same frequency (50 kHz). Next, a rectangular oscillator signal is coupled to the transmitter coil via the power amplifier class E, linked with resonant inductively to a biosensor. The power transmission coil (Tx), adjusted to the resonant frequency, receives the power via the flux generated by the coil (Rx). The data coil (T_d), adjusted to the resonant frequency, receives the data via the magnetic field generated by the transmitter data coil (R_D), as shown in Figure 4.13.

The method offered in this work is separated into two parts: the wireless power-up device (external reader unit), as shown in Figure 4.14, and the implant microsystem (biosensor). Each of these presents its own challenges.

4.4.2 External Reader Unit

The external reader unit consists of a power amplifier class E for powering-up the implanted chip and a high-frequency demodulation block for data acquisition from the chip underneath the skin.

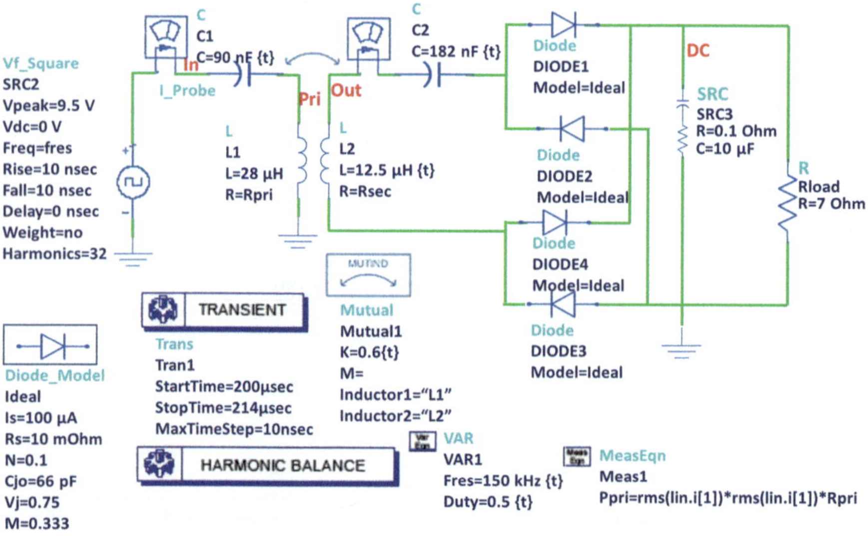

Figure 4.14 Simplified ADS schematic of resonant link.

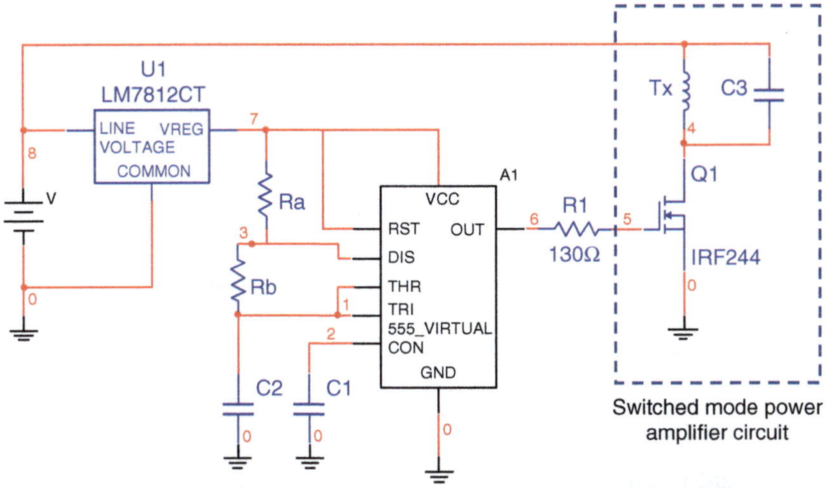

Figure 4.15 Schematic circuit of transmitting section.

Many shapes can be used for constructing a rectangular-wave oscillator. In this application, we utilize the oscillator NE555 [36, 37]. Our purpose is to establish the frequency oscillation of 50 kHz and duty cycle of 50%. The output signal is insufficient to power-up the biosensor because of the range of 3–5 mm; we will add a power amplifier stage in the oscillator's output.

For a biosensor to be operational, it needs to receive enough energy. The power collected from the square wave oscillator is insufficient to energize the biosensor wirelessly due to the coil losses, the inductive impedance matching losses, skin absorption losses, and RF-DC rectifier losses. Many techniques can be used to experiment with this work to increase the electricity transferred. For example, we can use a power amplifier to boost the output power of electromagnetic radiation. Nevertheless, it should stabilize high power and prevent the device temperature from going over safe levels. We utilize a power MOSFET transistor to drive a transmitter coil (Tx). The power transistor operates from a rectangular oscillator with a frequency of around 50 kHz.

The external reader unit is powered-up with 12 V DC to control the source coil via the switched-mode power amplifier (Figure 4.15). Thus, when the output power signal increases, the wirelessly electricity transmission level also increases. The amount of power required to operate the biosensor is within 2 W.

4.4.2.1 High-Frequency Demodulation

When the biosensor chip transmits the information, the signal is accepted by the receiver (VR) and handled by the demodulation circuit. The demodulator module consists of an RF envelope detector, a low-pass filter (LPF), an RF amplifier, and a comparator, as shown in Figure 4.16. The data carrier is first dispatched into a one-stage high-pass filter (HPF) to remove the power carrier, whose cut-off frequency equals 1.2 MHz and then to the envelope detector for detection of the data [38–41]. The RC LPF is usually used for reducing high-frequency interference [42, 43]. Next, the amplifier gets a reference input power. The last component of the demodulation module is the comparator. The decoded

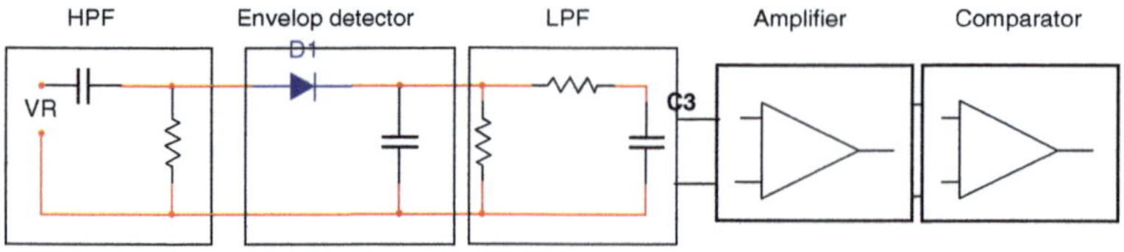

Figure 4.16 Block diagram of the demodulation module.

information is dispatched to the MCU with reference voltages, matching the conventional series transmission interface. Due to this modulation module technique, we minimize data transfer loss during the high-frequency demodulation technique.

4.4.3 Microchip Implant

The microchip implant underneath the skin consists of a receiver circuit section and data transmission via an induction link.

The receiver circuit consists of two blocks: a rectifier circuit and a data transmitter circuit through the magnetic field but with a frequency range greater than the frequency of the RF power circuit. The coil antenna is made using a wire-wound component on a PCB board. The implanted chip underneath the skin comprises the receiver coil connected to the bridge rectifier and the ultra-capacitor to harvest maximum electricity, as shown in Figure 4.17. To keep a constant output signal, a voltage regulator is used.

The full-wave rectifier is a prominent part of the electronic circuit that transforms the inductive flux signal to stable output voltage, as shown in Figure 4.18. The process is known as rectification. The DC voltage harvested changes according to the RF strength level. We make a simulation with two different input power; the first RF input, 34 dBm, and the output voltage, 9.219 V. The second input RF power is 45 dBm and gives us an output voltage of 20.742 V. This means that if the RF strength is very high, the output is elevated.

4.4.4 Data Transmission through a Common Inductive Connection

The proposed information transfer method, presented in Figure 4.19, is implemented on both sides and magnetically linked with the resonant power tank by the coupled inductances. The frequency of the inductive power is established at 50 kHz, and the information carrier frequency fixes at 1.2 MHz [44, 45]. Thus, the frequency of the bioinformatics carrier must be at least an order of magnitude higher than that of an energy transmission wave in this design. The voltage drop of the power frequency on the information

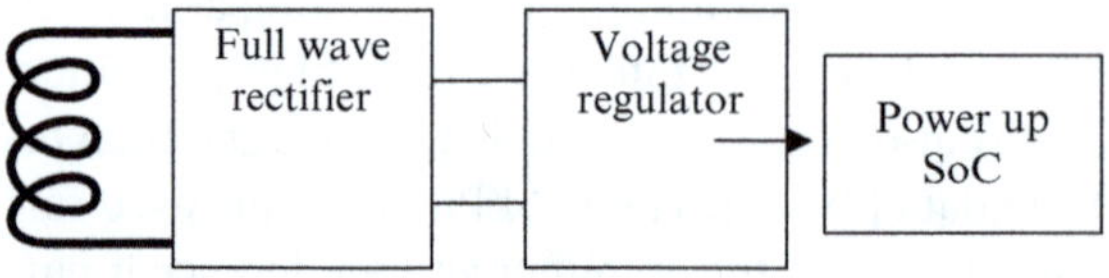

Figure 4.17 Block diagram of the inductive wireless rectifier circuit.

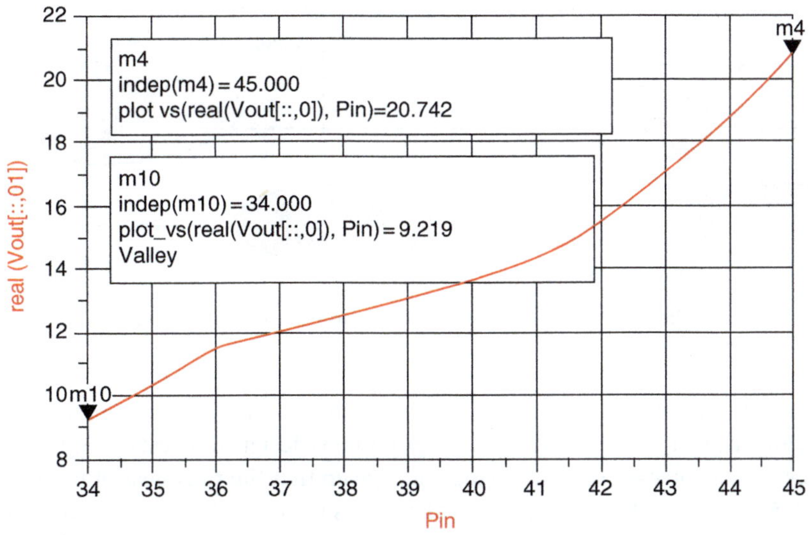

Figure 4.18 Output voltage.

transmission is relatively small, only in this situation, so the data would not substantially reduce energy transmission efficiency [46]. The reduced noise of data transmission from the power transmitted considerably suppresses the demodulation circuit design and guarantees bioinformatics transmission without loss.

4.4.5 Discussion and Results

The electromagnetic radiation technique is a safe method of wireless energy transfer, depending on being near a magnetic field. However, the power received from the oscillator is not enough to energize the implant SoC chip.

Transferred power wirelessly from a gap of 5 mm (width of the skin) depends on the efficiency of the Tx coil and the Rx coil, the alignment required to power-up the biosensor. However, more work and study are needed to increase the electromagnetic radiation area so that the subcutaneous implant can harvest electricity anywhere in the external reader unit.

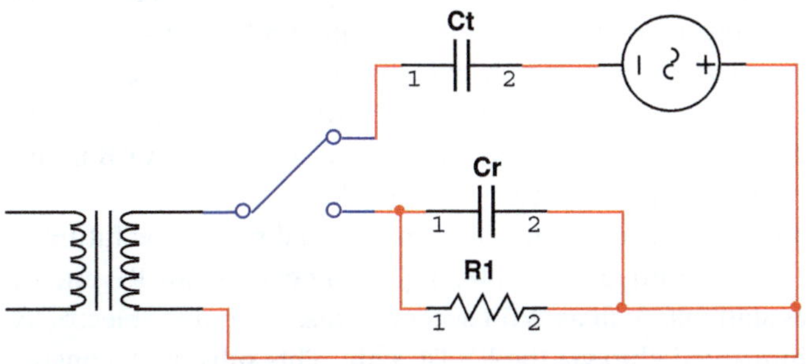

Figure 4.19 Block diagram of the data transfer structure.

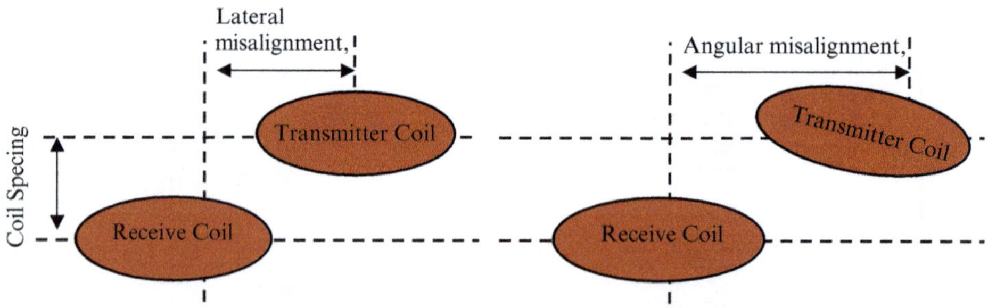

Figure 4.20 Inductive coupling between two coils with lateral misalignment and angular misalignment.

The main goal is to show that the biosensor wirelessly charges outside the human body without damaging the skin. In addition, the configuration is designed to test energy coupling efficiency with a constant separation distance (given that the thickness of human skin is about 3–5 mm). The efficiency of this technique is related to the coupling of two coils with angular misalignment and lateral misalignment, as shown in Figure 4.20.

The performance of the inductive link depends on three parameters: diameter of coils, number of turns, and spacing and alignment. The inductive coupling method presented in section 4.1 has its advantages as well as drawbacks. The technique that is highly available for these drawbacks is wireless energy transmission. On the other hand, ambient RF harvesting is manageable enabling powering-up of the implant devices independent of the individual's trajectory [47], is always available around us, and presents a higher efficiency than all the power sources cited in Table 4.1. Section 4.5 will investigate ambient RF energy harvesting techniques that require no external power-up, the power-up energy coming from any RF source.

We have successfully studied the method of powering-up and communicating the implant sensor simultaneously.

4.5 Study and Realization of Ambient RF Energy Harvesting for Invasive Charging

We concentrate in this section on RF energy pollution. We utilize the RF strength produced from commercial RF broadcasting stations like Global System for Mobile (GSM), television, WiFi, or radar to power-up the SoC chip implant underneath the skin. Recently, wireless telecommunication has shown extraordinary improvement. As a result, there is an increasing number of radio stations in the urban atmosphere, such as GSM mobile base stations and WiFi access points. This density variation in dBm/cm^2 depends on the frequency scale and time, as shown in Figure 4.21.

In this context, the idea of RF energy recycling offers an essential role in the future of microchips for implantation in the human body [48, 49]. Many can obtain RF energy from many radio frequencies stations, such as WiFi access points, to produce electricity and effectively operate the implanted chip via the RF-DC chip. This subsystem consists of two sections: the microwave energy harvester and the RF-DC converter. RF energy

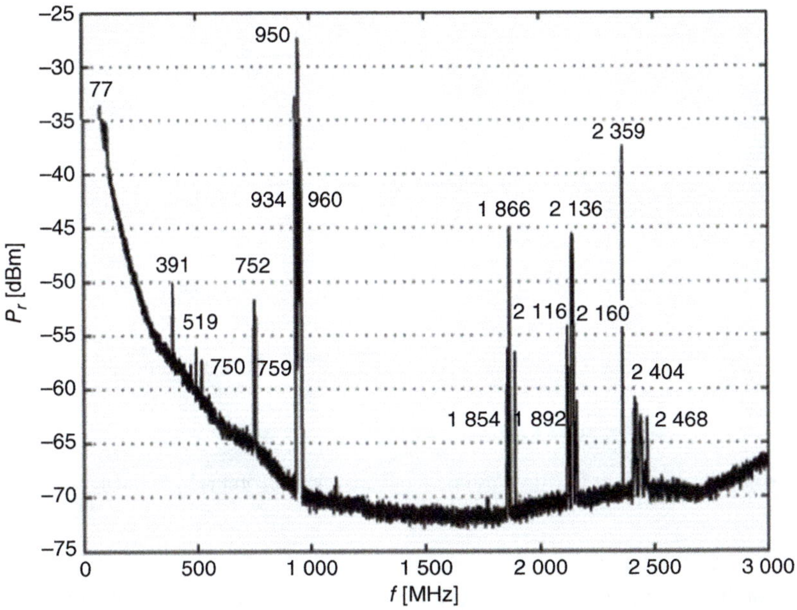

Figure 4.21 Average ambient RF power.

harvesting depends on the strength of the RF level, the type of patch antenna, and the efficiency of the RF-DC circuit installed on the SoC platform. The microwave energy harvested is usually on the milliwatt scale, which is a severe hurdle that limits the popularity of WiFi energy harvesting.

The penetration depth of RF microwaves into the physical skin is a function of different frequencies, which shows that lower microwave frequencies ranging from 1 to 4 GHz have much better dermal penetration than high-frequency radiation above 4 GHz, as shown in Figure 4.22. In biological samples, it is a function of frequency. According to Thiele and Elsner's *Oxidants and Antioxidants in Skin Biology* [52, see also 50, 51, 53, 54], the penetration depth of the most common microwave frequency of 9 GHz is less than 1 mm due to the high-water content of biological samples. According to the same study, the WiFi strength signal can infiltrate human skin up to 7 mm.

This research presents a novel solution to power up implant chips independent of a person's trajectory and position. The WiFi microwave energy, with a frequency range of 2.4 GHz, has an enormous capacity to penetrate a patient's skin and power-up the implanted chip underneath the tissue. We evaluate the efficiency and the application, as shown in Figure 4.23.

This powering technique can be a very exciting solution to the problem of wirelessly charging the implanted SoC chip where other energy sources, like laser or wind energy, are not feasible. The DC power (P_{dc})*it* relies on the accessible RF energy (P_{RF}) and on the efficiency of RF-DC circuits:

$$P_{dc} = \eta_{RF/DC} . P_{RF} \tag{4.3}$$

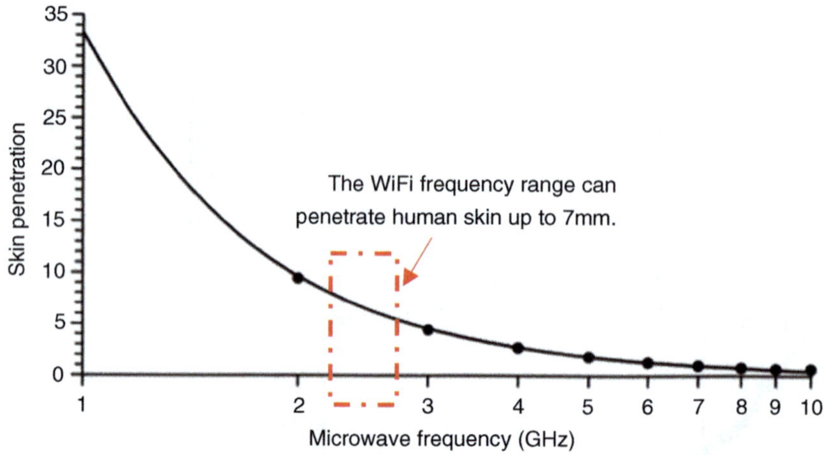

Figure 4.22 The penetration depth of microwaves into biological skin according to frequency.

Efficiency $\left(\eta_{RF/DC}\right)$ is defined as in (1), where (P_{dc}) is the output DC power and (P_{RF}) is the input RF power. The voltage sensitivity γ is given by (1), where V_{out} is the output DC voltage.

$$\gamma = \frac{P_{dc}}{V_{out}} \tag{4.4}$$

The attractive structures of the fractal antenna array, such as planar shape, ruggedness, and low cost, have been of considerable importance in implementing SoC chips under the skin to recover power microwaves primarily accessible around us. However, the advantage of using a fractal antenna array is that it receives WiFi frequency with high efficiency. Therefore, we can accumulate and recycle a lot of microwave energy around the human body with this solution.

4.5.1 Antenna Design and Simulation

The WiFi technique comprises the IEEE 802.16d standard for nomadic customers utilizing a 2.3–2.4 GHz frequency band and IEEE 802.16e. For this reason, the fractal

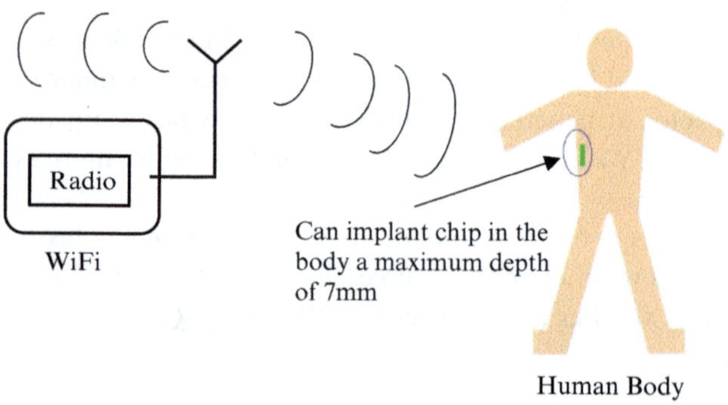

Figure 4.23 Typical WiFi energy harvesting to power-up implant chip.

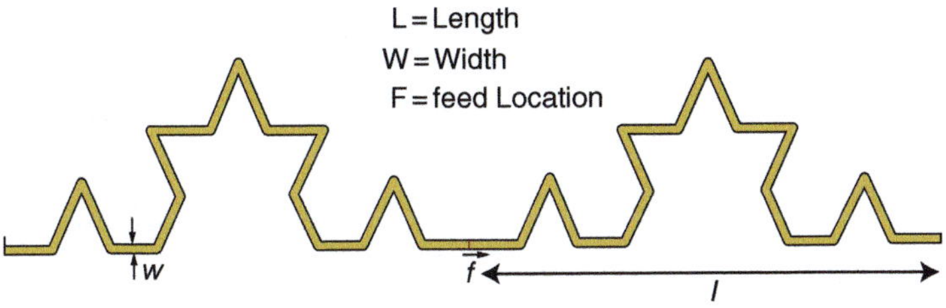

Figure 4.24 Fractal antenna.

antenna array provides an alternative to broadband planar patch antennae in applications. The main advantage of fractal antennae is that they are compact, which is essential for small and complex circuits, as shown in Figure 4.24. Moreover, these fractals antennae are used in multiband and wideband applications like GSM, Universal Mobile Telecommunications Service (UMTS), WiFi, and Bluetooth.

Microwave strength acquired from the atmosphere is mainly in milliwatts, which is a severe obstacle that restricts the attractiveness of WiFi energy harvest technology. Therefore, we create an array of fractal Koch antennae. The fractal antenna bandwidth and gain requirements are expected to meet the needs of several products. The area is 120 mm long and 80 mm wide. The geometry of the array of fractal Koch antennae, is shown in Figure 4.25. Typically, the fractal patch antenna necessitates 100 MHz of bandwidth at a 2.3–2.5 GHz frequency range. The fractal patch antenna is designed and simulated with a MATLAB antenna designer. After simulation, we can determine the following parameters' values: S-parameter, radiation pattern 3D, directivity.

S-parameter: We achieve a perfect return loss, –16.23 dB, at the working frequency of 2.45 GHz, as shown in Figure 4.26. Therefore, this antenna's bandwidth is about

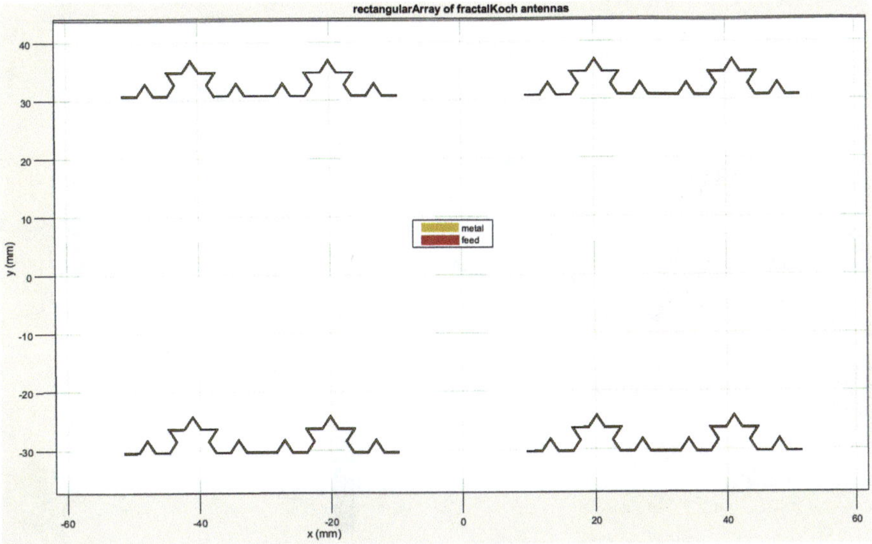

Figure 4.25 Array of fractal Koch antennae patch.

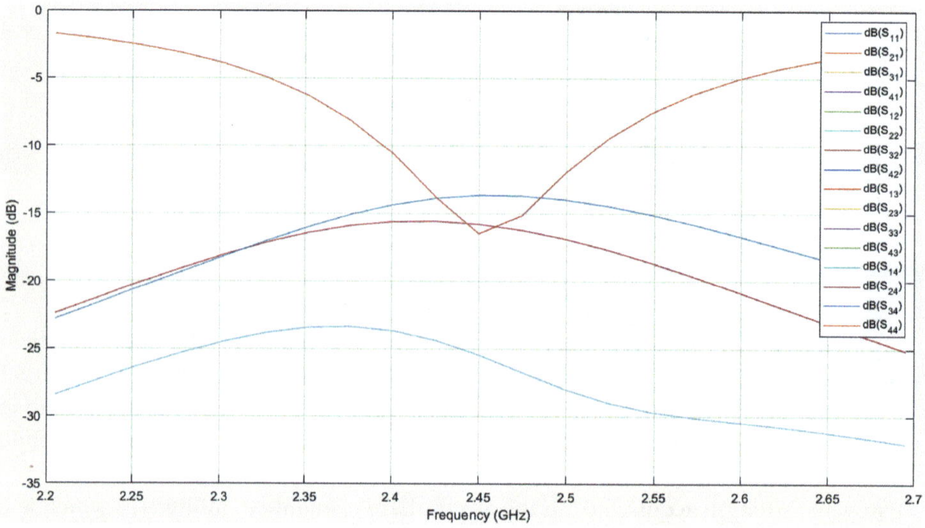

Figure 4.26 S-parameter.

550 MHz (18.26%), and the voltage standing wave ratio (VSWR) within 1.10 at 2.45 GHz.

Radiation pattern 3D: According to the 3D radiation pattern plots, we can consider that the fractal antenna is very directive and has a high-efficiency maximum gain of around 7.06 dBi, as shown in Figure 4.27.

Directivity: The fractal antenna array directivity gain at 2.45 GHz is −7.05 dB, as shown in Figure 4.28.

A fractal antenna's essential characteristics are its input impedance and its radiation pattern, both being frequency-dependent amounts. These quantities can obtain for

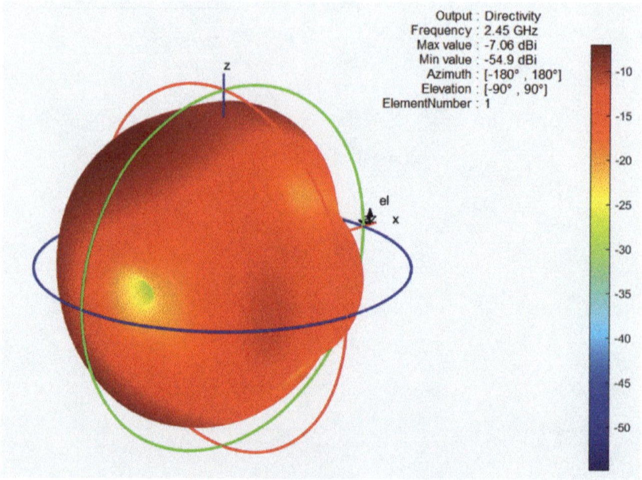

Figure 4.27 3D radiation pattern plots.

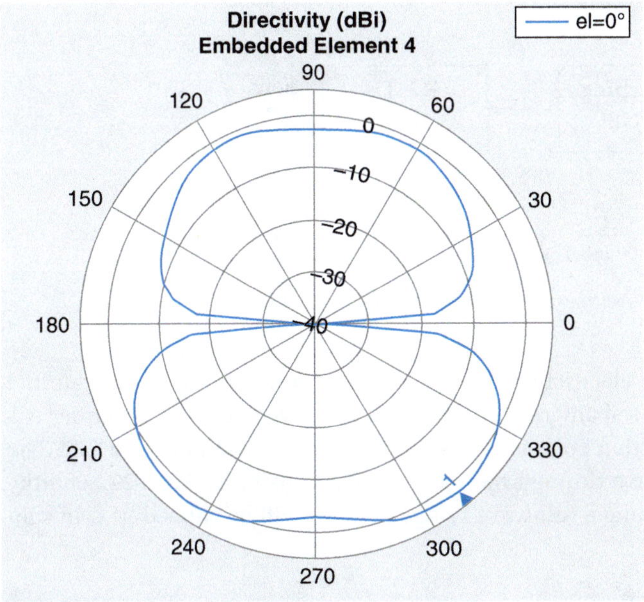

Figure 4.28 Directivity of the proposed antenna.

lossless antennae from the array impedance or scattering matrix, thus escaping numerical integration. The simulation reaches an active impedance (R = 48.3 Ω and Z = 10 Ω), as shown in Figure 4.29.

The subcutaneous antenna harvests electromagnetic energy from any WiFi access point. This radio frequency input signal is transmitted to the RF-DC circuit to convert

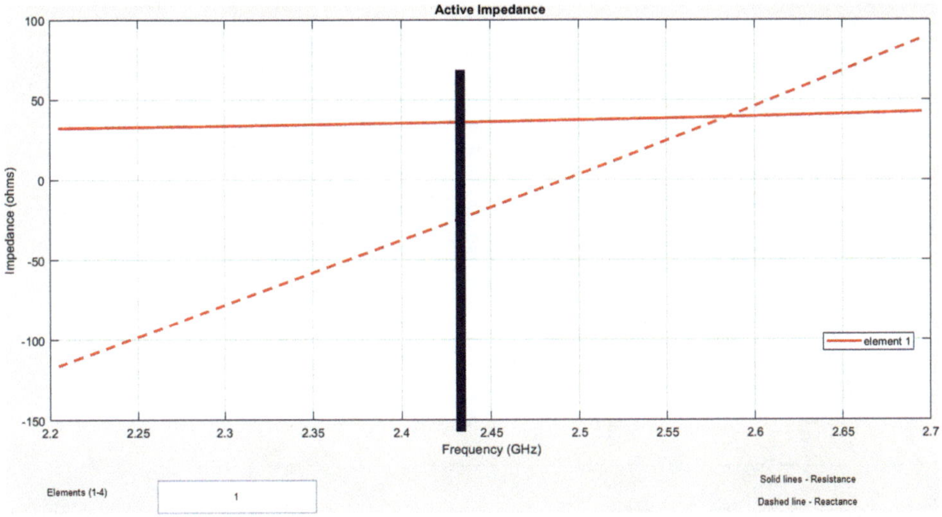

Figure 4.29 Active impedance.

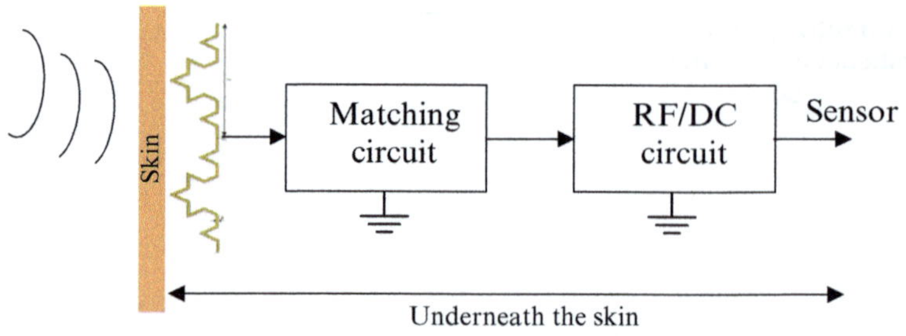

Figure 4.30 Block diagram of powering-up the implanted chip.

electromagnetic energy into electricity, with which we can continuously operate the implanted chip and do not need any medical intervention to recharge. The rectifier is a Schottky diode that aligns with dipoles by a low-pass filter, as shown in Figure 4.30. The receiver signal is then effective through the rectifier circuit using HSMS2822 Schottky diodes. Selecting and evaluating a full-wave bridge rectifier will be studied next in subsection 4.5.2.

4.5.2 Design a Full-Wave Bridge Rectenna

The RF-DC rectifier design uses a full-wave bridge rectenna. The rectifier's input impedance (Z_{in} = 50 Ω) is constructed to maximize the electricity transmission and boost the signal reflected from the sensor. As indicated in subsection 4.5.1, the fractal antenna design operates at 2.45 GHz with an output impedance of 50 Ω [55]. Figure 4.31 presents the schematic configuration of the rectifier circuit.

The power-up pump configuration used in this circuit is the modified Dickson power-up pump. This circuit has been used extensively in other RF energy harvesting projects and closely resembles the form of the Cockcroft–Walton voltage multiplier.

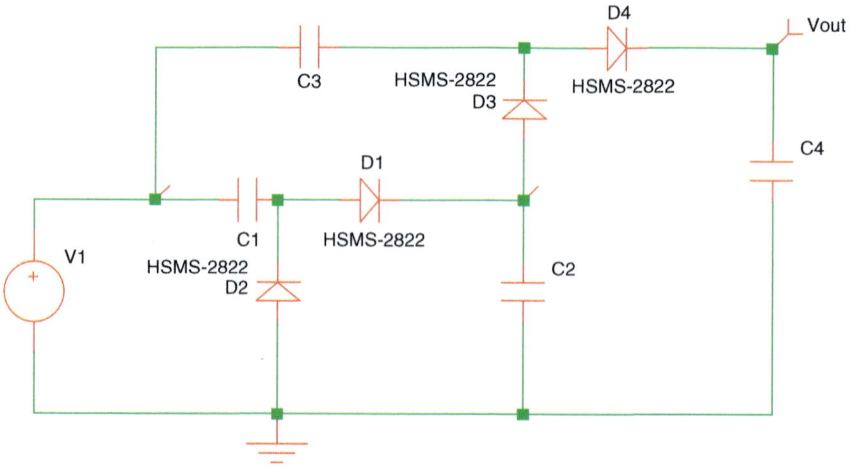

Figure 4.31 Power-up pump circuit.

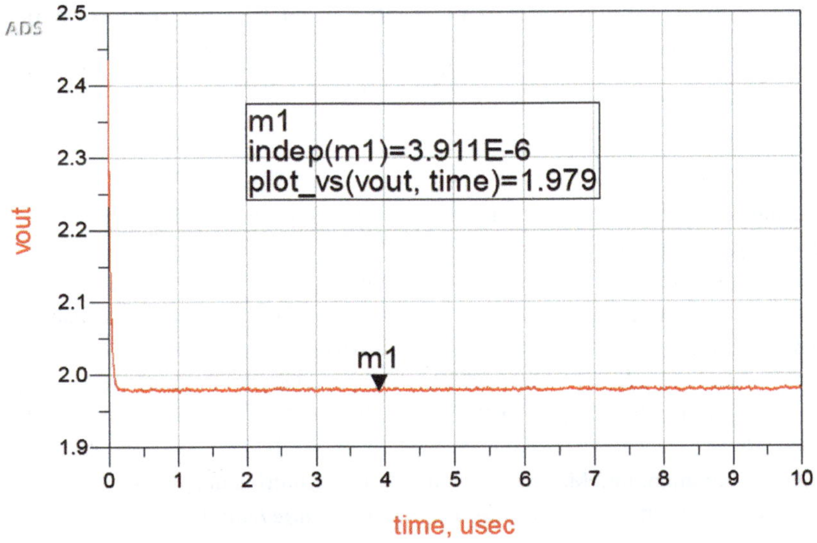

Figure 4.32 Charge pump stage voltage.

The output voltage of the simulation result of the RF-DC full-wave bridge circuit utilizing a Schottky diode is (1.979 V), as shown in Figure 4.32.

4.6 Conclusion

The method of charging chips implanted inside the human body were simulated for radio frequency energy and verified experimentally in this work. Ambient RF harvesting is clean and controllable, and the implanted slices operate independently of patient movement, anytime, anywhere. Conversely, inductive radio transmission produces heat at the implant position, interfering with the body's physiological activity.

In this chapter, we examined how an implanted SoC chip can be charged wirelessly. We demonstrated the possibility of using inductive flux and RF harvesting signals to activate any microchips implanted inside the body. We tested this research, and we prove that the S-band (WiFi) is a suitable power for charging the SoC chip. The fractal harvester antenna has a reflection coefficient of S11 of −16.23 dB. Therefore, the maximum gain direction of this antenna is −7.06 dBm. We chose Schottky diode HSMS2822 and fractal combiner antenna dimensions tested and approved for the full-wave bridge rectifier topology.

Each harvester circuit can supply 1.92 V, and this energy is sufficient to operate the sensor implanted under the skin wirelessly. In this study, we agreed that we could wirelessly improve the configuration of implant chips and can unlock a new solution for using radiation in our lives as a source of energy to activate sensors implanted inside a human. This technology is essential for many applications both in civilian life and in military sectors.

In future, we will study how to obtain energy to run the implanted chips from human temperature, arm movement, breathing devices, leg movement, or any human movements made while working or during any activity that can be converted into energy to charge implanted chips.

References

1 RFID, IoT, and AIDC News: Implanted RFID chips in humans being taken to whole new levels. *Supply Chain Digest*, August 2016.

2 Mani, V., Beduk, T., Khushaim, W., Ceylan, A.E., Timur, S., Wolfbeis, O.S., and Salama, K.N. (2021). Electrochemical sensors targeting salivary biomarkers: A comprehensive review. *TrAC Trends in Analytical Chemistry* 135: 116164.

3 Lamonaca, F., Sciammarella, P.F., Scuro, C., Carnì, D., and Olivito, R. (2018). *Internet of Things for Structural Health Monitoring*. 2018 Workshop on Metrology for Industry 4.0 and IoT, 95–100.

4 Sonmezoglu, S., Fineman, J.R., Maltepe, E. et al. (2021).Monitoring deep-tissue oxygenation with a millimeter-scale ultrasonic implant. *Nature Biotechnology* 39: 855–864.

5 Mohamed, M. and Chaudhry, B. (2021) Preliminary investigations on subcutaneous implantable microchip health and security risks, 612–618. In: Russo D., Ahram T., Karwowski W., Di Bucchianico G., Taiar R. (eds) Intelligent Human Systems Integration 2021. IHSI 2021. Advances in Intelligent Systems and Computing, vol 1322. Springer, Cham.

6 Mohamed, M. (2021) Modeling of subcutaneous implantable microchip intention of use, 842–847.

7 Manickavasagam, B., Balakrishnan, A., and Sudhakara, P. (2019) Review of wireless body area networks (WBANs), pp. 645–656. International Conference on Communications and Cyber Physical Engineering 2018. doi: 10.1007/978-981-13-0212-1_66.

8 Wali, S. and Al Salam, M. (2020). Review of wireless body sensor networks. *International Journal of Engineering and Technology (IJET)* 9: 863–870.

9 Yilmaz, A. and Ppp, Ppp. (2021) Wireless body sensor networks. https://www.researchgate.net/publication/342339094_Wireless_Body_Sensor_Networks

10 Annema, A.-J., Nauta, B., Van Langevelde, R., and Tuinhout, H. (2005). Analog circuits in ultra-deep-submicron CMOS. *IEEE Journal of Solid-state Circuits* 40 (1): 132–143.

11 Datta, B. On-chip thermal sensing in deep sub-micron Cmos. Masters thesis, Feb. 2014, University of Massachusetts Amherst, 127.

12 Owens, B.B. (ed.) (1986). *Batteries for Implantable Biomedical Devices*. Boston, MA: Springer US.

13 Algora, C. and Peña, R. (2009). Recharging the battery of implantable biomedical devices by light. *Artificial Organs* 33 (10): 855–860.

14 Staff, E. (2020). Assessing lithium-ion battery life for implantable medical devices. *Embedded.com*.

15 Inductive coupling - an overview. *ScienceDirect Topics*. https://www.sciencedirect.com/topics/engineering/inductive-coupling

16 System-on-chip - an overview. *ScienceDirect Topics*. https://www.sciencedirect.com/topics/engineering/system-on-chip

17 Deiss, D., Szadkowska, A., Gordon, D., Mallipedhi, A., Schütz-Fuhrmann, I., Aguilera, E., Ringsell, C., Block, C., and Irace, C. (2019). Clinical practice recommendations on the routine use of Eversense, the first long-term implantable continuous glucose monitoring system. *Diabetes Technology & Therapeutics* 21.

18 Christiansen, M., Klaff, L., Brazg, R., Chang, A., Levy, C., Lam, D., Denham, D., Atiee, G., Bode, B., Walters, S., Kelley, L., and Bailey, T. (2018). A prospective multicenter evaluation of the accuracy of a novel implanted continuous glucose sensor: PRECISE II. *Diabetes Technology & Therapeutics* 20.

19 Chaari, M.Z. Design and production of a system for wirelessly charging the batteries of a robot. US20130147430A1, filed Jun. 13, 2013.

20 Chaari, M.Z. (2018). *Design and Production of a System for Wireless Charging the Battery the Wireless Power Transmission Device*. Scholars Press.

21 Chaari, M.Z. and Al-Maadeed, S.A. (2019). Spiral antenna mounted on the t-shirt to harvested RF energy. *2019 1st International Conference on Electrical, Control and Instrumentation Engineering (ICECIE)* 1–6. doi: 10.1109/ICECIE47765.2019.897475.

22 Kumari, N. and Rakotondrabe, M. (2020). Development, presentation and tests of a hybrid thermal vibrational energy harvester based on lead free piezoelectric material. *2020 IEEE 2nd International Conference on Electronics, Control, Optimization and Computer Science (ICECOCS)* 1–6. doi: 10.1109/ICECOCS50124.2020.9314542.

23 Zhang, Y., Phuong, P.T.T., Roake, E., Khanbareh, H., Wang, Y., Dunn, S., and Bowen, C. (2020). Thermal energy harvesting using pyroelectric-electrochemical coupling in ferroelectric materials. *Joule* 4 (2): 301–309.

24 Chaari, M.Z. and Al-Maadeed, S. (2020). Wireless power transmission for the internet of things (IoT). *IEEE International Conference on Informatics, IoT, and Enabling Technologies (ICIoT)* 549–554. doi: 10.1109/ICIoT48696.2020.9089547.

25 Jang, S.G., Kim, J., Lee, J., Kim, J.S., Hwan Kim, D., and Park, S.M. (2020). Wireless power transfer based implantable neurostimulator. *2020 IEEE Wireless Power Transfer Conference (WPTC)* 365–368. doi: 10.1109/WPTC48563.2020.9295553.

26 Lee, C.C., Ouyang, H., and Che, G. (2020). Development of new wireless charging system with improved energy efficiency for electric vehicles. *IECON 2020 The 46th Annual Conference of the IEEE Industrial Electronics Society* 3617–3621. doi: 10.1109/IECON43393.2020.9255192.

27 Joannopoulos, J.D., Karalis, A., and Soljacic, M. (2020). Wireless non-radiative energy transfer. https://scholar.google.com/citations?view_op=view_citation&hl=en&user=jpqAJIMAAAAJ&cstart=20&pagesize=80&sortby=pubdate&citation_for_view=jpqAJIMAAAAJ:71d7Y1FijdoC.

28 Cheng, C., Li, X., Xu, G., Lu, Y., Low, S.S., Liu, G., Zhu, L., Li, C., and Liu, Q. (2021). Battery-free, wireless, and flexible electrochemical patch for in situ analysis of sweat cortisol via near field communication. *Biosensors & Bioelectronics* 172: 112782.

29 Olenik, S., Lee, H.S., and Güder, F. (2021). The future of near-field communication-based wireless sensing. *Nature Reviews Materials* 6 (4): 286–288.

30 Lee, S., Lim, N., Choi, W., Lee, Y., Baek, J., and Park, J. (2020). Study on battery charging converter for MPPT control of laser wireless power transmission system. *Electronics* 9 (10): 1745.

31 Kim, S.-M. and Park, H. (2020). Optimization of optical wireless power transfer using near-infrared laser diodes. *Chinese Optics Letters* 18 (4): 042603.

32 Taalla, R.V., Arefin, M.S., Kaynak, A., and Kouzani, A.Z. (2019). A review on miniaturized ultrasonic wireless power transfer to implantable medical devices. *IEEE Access* 7: 2092–2106.

33 Radice, J.J., Tseng, V.F.-G., Drummond, T., Diamond, D., Schieuer, N., and Bedair, S. (2020). Multiphysics modeling of ultrasonic elastic wave attenuation for wireless power transfer including viscoelasticity and acoustic emission. *Mechanics Research Communications* 115: 103600.

34 Guida, R., Demirors, E., Dave, N., and Melodia, T. (2020). Underwater ultrasonic wireless power transfer: A battery-less platform for the internet of underwater things. *IEEE Transactions on Mobile Computing* 1–1. doi: 10.1109/TMC.2020.3029679.

35 Kural, A., Pullin, R., Featherston, C., Paget, C., and Holford, K. (2011). Wireless power transmission using ultrasonic guided waves. *Journal of Physics: Conference Series* 305: 012088.

36 Besharati, B., Lak, A., Ghaffari, H., Karimi, H., and Fattahzadeh, M. (2021). Development of a model to estimate moisture contents based on physical properties and capacitance of seeds. *Sensors and Actuators A: Physical* 318: 112513.

37 Orovwode, H., Matthew, S., Agbetuyi, A.F., Adoghe, U.A., and Amuta, E. (2021). Development of a starter with protective systems for a three-phase induction motor. *Journal of Engineering* 2021: 1–8.

38 Estes, N. and Chisum, J. (2021). A 10MHz-1GHz mitigated shunt capacitance hybrid LNA for use in a Ka-band envelope detector baseband output. *2019 United States National Committee of URSI National Radio Science Meeting (USNC-URSI NRSM)* 226–227. doi: 10.23919/USNC-URSINRSM51531.2021.9336482.

39 Gazivoda, M., Oletic, D., and Bilas, V. (2020). Characterization and comparison of envelope detectors for wake-up sensor interfaces at audio frequencies. *2020 IEEE International Instrumentation and Measurement Technology Conference (I2MTC)* 1–6. doi: 10.1109/I2MTC43012.2020.9128810.

40 Delshadpour, S. and Geng, M. (2020). A PLL based FSK demodulator with auxiliary path. *2020 IEEE 11th Latin American Symposium on Circuits & Systems (LASCAS)* 1–4. doi: 10.1109/LASCAS45839.2020.9069002.

41 Zahiruddin, S., Srinivasulu, A., and Sarada, M. (2020). A novel FSK generator using a second generation current controlled conveyor. *Nanoscience & Nanotechnology-Asia* 10 (6): 902–908.

42 Li, L., Xu, Y., Zhang, Z., Yin, J., Chen, W., and Han, Z. (2019). A prediction-based charging policy and interference mitigation approach in the wireless powered internet of things. *IEEE Journal on Selected Areas in Communications* 37 (2): 439–451.

43 Mathur, P. and Raman, S. (2020). Electromagnetic interference (EMI): Measurement and reduction techniques. *Journal of Electronic Materials* 49 (5): 2975–2998.

44 Patiño, A.G. and Menon, C. (2021). Inductive textile sensor design and validation for a wearable monitoring device. *Sensors* 21 (1): 225.

45 Kassanos, P., Rosa, B.G., Keshavarz, M., and Yang, G.-Z. (2021). Power and data communication in wearable and implantable devices. In: *Wearable Sensors* (ed. E. Sazonov), 279–309. Elsevier.

46 Wu, J., Zhao, C., Lin, Z., Du, J., Hu, Y., and He, X. (2015). Wireless power and data transfer via a common inductive link using frequency division multiplexing. *IEEE Transactions on Industrial Electronics* 62 (12): 7810–7820.

47 Clerckx, B., Zhang, R., Schober, R., Ng, D.W.K., Kim, D.I., and Poor, H.V. (2019). Fundamentals of wireless information and power transfer: From RF energy harvester models to signal and system designs. *IEEE Journal on Selected Areas in Communications* 37 (1): 4–33.

48 Grossi, M. (2021). Energy harvesting strategies for wireless sensor networks and mobile devices: A review. *Electronics* 10 (6): 661.

49 Moghaddam, N.A. and Maleki, A. (2019). *RF Energy Harvesting System and Circuits for Charging of Wireless Devices Using Spectrum Sensing*. IntechOpen.

50 Cleary, S.F. (1983). Microwave radiation effects on humans. *BioScience* 33 (4): 269–273.

51 Elston, D.M. (2020). Occupational skin disease among health care workers during the coronavirus (COVID-19) epidemic. *Journal of the American Academy of Dermatology* 82 (5): 1085–1086.

52 Thiele, J. and Elsner, P. (eds.) (2001). *Oxidants and Antioxidants in Cutaneous Biology*. Basel; New York: Karger.

53 Bajakke, P.A., Malik, V.R., Mugali, P., and Deshpande, A.S. (2021). Microwave processing of engineering materials. In: *Coatings: Materials, Processes, Characterization and Optimization* (ed. K. Kumar, B.S. Babu, and J.P. Davim), 31–55. Cham: Springer.

54 Amin, B., Shahzad, A., Crocco, L., Wang, M., O'Halloran, M., González-Suárez, A., and Elahi, M.A. (2021). A feasibility study on microwave imaging of bone for osteoporosis monitoring. *Medical & Biological Engineering & Computing* 59 (4): 925–936.

55 Khan, D., Oh, S.J., Shehzad, K., Basim, M., Verma, D., Pu, Y.G., Lee, M., Hwang, K.C., Yang, Y., and Lee, K. (2020). An efficient reconfigurable RF-DC converter with wide input power range for RF energy harvesting. *IEEE Access* 8: 79310–79318.

5

Minimally Invasive and Non-Invasive Sensor Technologies for Predicting Heart Failure

An Overview

Huseyin Enes Salman, Mahmoud Khatib A. A. Al-Ruweidi, Hassen M. Ouakad, and Huseyin C. Yalcin

5.1 Introduction

Heart failure (HF) is one of most prevalent clinical syndromes, in which the heart muscles are not capable of providing adequate blood flow to the circulatory system. The symptoms of HF are reported as ankle swelling, dyspnea, and fatigue due to elevated jugular venous pressure, pulmonary crackles, and peripheral edema [1–3]. The estimated number of patients suffering from HF worldwide is reported as 26 million [4]. Frequent hospitalization and poor life quality are serious risks for HF patients. It has been reported that only about 10% of patients with chronic HF survive 10 years after diagnosis [5, 6]. HF is a chronic and progressive disease and, therefore, HF patients have high rehospitalization rates and emergency visits. About 25% of HF patients are readmitted within a month and at least half of these readmissions are due to HF related symptoms [7]. These facts demonstrate the high economic burden and hospital workload for HF treatment.

Hospitalization is required for HF patients in case of congestion, which is the excessive accumulation of body fluid [8]. Congestion is mainly related to water and sodium retention in the body, leading to high left ventricular end-diastolic pressure [9, 10]. The symptoms of congestion can be listed as dyspnea, rales, and edema [11]. The most-used therapy for congestion is to intravenously inject diuretics to minimize the fluid accumulation in the body [8]. The diuretics help kidneys to excrete more sodium into the urine, and the excessive sodium results in more water absorption from the blood, which reduces the amount of fluid in the body.

The current gold standard for HF diagnosis is to measure intracardiac filling pressures using implantable pressure sensors via cardiac catheterization [12]. However, the invasive nature of cardiac catheterization prevents its routine usage for HF patients [10]. In addition, the cost of the implantable pressure sensors is more than US$ 20,000, which is not affordable for millions of HF patients [7]. This demonstrates the need for an inexpensive, non-invasive, easy-to-apply, and accurate method for HF diagnosis.

Predicting Heart Failure: Invasive, Non-Invasive, Machine Learning, and Artificial Intelligence Based Methods, First Edition. Edited by Kishor Kumar Sadasivuni, Hassen M. Ouakad, Somaya Al-Maadeed, Huseyin C. Yalcin, and Issam Bait Bahadur.

In the literature, alternative non-invasive modalities are suggested to monitor HF patients and diagnose the critical HF stages which require hospitalization. This way, unnecessary hospitalizations can be prevented by remotely monitoring the patient using non-invasive and minimally invasive sensors [3]. The efficiency of remote monitoring is still open to debate, but many studies have indicated a reduced rehospitalization rate and increased life quality for patients with external monitoring [3]. For this purpose, external devices or wearables with embedded non-invasive sensors are employed. By retrieving data from the non-invasive sensors, the health status of an HF patient is followed, and clinical therapy is offered in emergency cases, which are identified by evaluating the abnormal changes in measured data. This method is also known as home monitoring or remote patient monitoring [3].

In this chapter, we explain the non-invasive and minimally invasive sensor technologies and techniques employed for HF diagnosis. We also summarize landmark studies and clinical trials which prove the potential of non-invasive monitoring of HF patients.

5.2 Methods

The methods for identifying worsening HF can be listed as body weight measurements, electrocardiography (ECG), bioimpedance monitoring, activity tracking, implanted pressure sensors, lung ultrasound monitoring, measurements with sound and Doppler sensors, seismocardiography, ballistocardiography, photoplethysmography, and measurement of natriuretic peptides levels in circulating blood. These methods are explained in detail in this chapter.

5.2.1 Body Weight Measurement

The state of worsening HF is characterized by excessive reduction in circulatory volume and body water retention [3, 13]. Depending on the change in water balance in the body, a sudden increase in weight is observed in an emergency case. If the increase rate in body weight is higher than 2 kg/48 hours, it can be evaluated as a deterioration due to the impending HF decompensation [3].

Many remote monitoring studies used body weight measurements as a rehospitalization indicator for HF patients [14–24]. Weight measurements can be easily performed on a daily basis using weight scales or shoe-integrated pressure sensors. However, pressure sensors used in shoes can lead to inaccuracy in long-term monitoring [25] as there are several factors reducing the accuracy of measurements, such as different levels of activity in daily life and individual-dependent posture and gait disturbances. Alternatively, weight measurements can be performed daily by patients using bathroom scales as a part of HF self-management [26, 27].

5.2.2 Electrocardiographic (ECG) Measurement

ECG measurement is a widely used non-invasive method for HF diagnosis [28, 29]. The method is based on measuring the electrical activity of the heart using electrodes placed on the chest skin [30]. The electrodes identify voltage differences resulting from heart muscle depolarization and repolarization during the heartbeat [31]. In 12-lead ECG measurements, 10 electrodes are placed on limbs and the chest. The electric potential of the heart is measured by taking capitalizing on the different angles between the heart and electrodes

Measurements are generally recorded for 10 seconds so that the electrical depolarization is monitored during the entire cardiac cycle [32, 33]. The main components of ECG signals are P-wave, QRS complex, and T-wave.

Several ECG parameters are utilized for predicting HF and also its worsening in HF patients [3]. The most-used ECG parameters are reduced heart rate variability [34], increased heart rate [35], increase in QRS/T angle [36], atrial and ventricular tachyarrhythmias [37, 38], increased ECG left ventricle mass index [28, 39], QT prolongation [40], increased QRS duration [41, 42], and left ventricle strain [20, 43, 44]. Reduced heart rate variability can be determined using Holter monitoring by evaluating the time differences in heart rate between day and night [34]. The heart rate variability can be determined by examining the standard deviation of sequential 5-minute R-R interval means. If the ECG left ventricle mass exceeds 70 ± 9 g/m^2 in men and 61 ± 8 g/m^2 in women [28, 39], or the corrected QR duration is longer than 450 ms in men and 460 ms in women [40], there is a potential risk factor for the presence of HF. QRS durations higher than 100 ms [41, 42, 45], T-wave inversions, and ST segment depression [20] are also evaluated as indications of HF.

5.2.3 Bioimpedance Monitoring

Bioimpedance analysis is a non-invasive method for assessing the body composition and fluid overload [46]. Impedance is an electrical parameter defining the resistance to the electrical current flow. In bioimpedance monitoring, a high-frequency and low-amplitude electrical current is used in the body to measure the bioimpedances [47]. Body tissues and fluids have different resistances which change the flow behavior of the electrical current. In an HF decompensation scenario, fluid retention leads to pulmonary congestion, and this fluid overload in the lungs influences the bioimpedance of the thoracic area. The blood and fluids have lower resistance to electrical current flow compared to thoracic tissues and air. This means that bioimpedance decreases with increasing fluid content. Therefore, there is an inverse correlation between the bioimpedance and the amount of fluid [48–50]. Healthy and relatively dry lungs are expected to have higher impedances than lungs with pulmonary edema that develop as a result of HF [51]. The bioimpedance monitoring is important for HF patients, because the thoracic impedance changes start in advance of the observation of serious symptoms and hospitalization.

The traditional non-invasive bioimpedance analysis, also known as transthoracic impedance cardiography, is performed using four or six electrodes placed on the skin for measuring the changes in thorax resistance. Low-amplitude constant electrical current is sent from one of the electrodes and measured by the other electrodes, enabling the voltage difference and impedance through the thorax to be determined [47].

Biompedance levels show variability for each patient due to individual-dependent characteristics such as fat and muscle percentage in the body composition, amount of body hair, and skin condition [10]. For this reason, defining the exact values of critical impedances for HF emergency conditions is challenging. Therefore, individualized analysis is employed for each patient for tracking the relative increases in bioimpedance levels [10]. By remotely performing bioimpedance measurements at every hour or every day, clinicians can track the relative behavior of impedances and have the opportunity to take therapeutic action in case of a sudden and sharp decrease in thoracic impedance.

As a recent application of bioimpedance monitoring, remote dielectric sensing technology (ReDS) utilizes the changes in lung fluid status and dielectric properties of thoracic tissues for predicting the HF state [52–54]. In this application, a wearable vest is used with two sensors placed on the anterior and posterior sides. Low-power electromagnetic signals are emitted and received by the implemented sensors after passing through the thoracic tissues [55]. There is no need for direct skin contact to perform the measurements, and therefore the method can be applied over light clothing. The electromagnetic signals are mostly affected by the fluid content of the thoracic tissues in the path [55], and the predicted fluid balance in the lungs can be used for identification of congestion in case of HF decompensation [53].

5.2.4 Pedometers and Activity Trackers

One of the common symptoms of HF is the restricted exercise ability that prevents people performing daily tasks. Regular physical activity is recommended for HF patients to improve their functional capacity [56–58]. Walking is a safe and efficient form of physical activity, and pedometers are used for counting the number of steps [56]. In this way, the activity levels of patients can be remotely monitored using biosensing products integrated into accessories and clothing [3].

Pedometers and activity trackers are portable electronic devices which measure the distance traveled by the patient using a global positioning system (GPS) receiver. Since the step size of each individual varies, a calibration is required for determining the accurate number of steps. There are also pedometers including inertial microelectromechanical system (MEMS) sensors for detecting the number of steps utilizing the body accelerations in three spatial dimensions [58–60]. Using these portable devices, clinicians can track the total physical activity of HF patients, and in case of severe reduction in physical activity, patients can be called for medical care. This also helps HF patients in tracking their own physical data and taking preventive precautions before being face with more serious HF symptoms.

5.2.5 Implanted Pressure Sensors

The concept of sensors-based device monitoring is a prime prospect for improving the outcomes of any long-lasting HF disease supervision [61]. With the rapid increase of cardiac implantable sensors in HF patients, some HF monitoring strategies have taken broader advantage of such chips [61]. Certainly, the usage of implantable sensors has several advantages over other HF monitoring standards (such as in-clinic monitoring, where the patient acts as the sensor during the live physical contact), which are mainly limited by several factors including subjectivity, variable patient ability, and poor sensitivity to symptoms during a premature HF diagnosis process [61]. In addition, implantable sensors have several advantages, including live continuous monitoring, autonomous assessment based on subjective measurements, and the ability to provide a timely profile about a particular patient with relative ease in analyzing its medical status.

One of the chief methods in identifying deteriorating HF can be implantable devices such as pressure sensors [62]. It is worth mentioning that the early detection of signs of any clinical condition deterioration permits rapid medical preventive intervention to optimize and identify an HF status. Consequently, it is not only healthcare specialists who can take advantage of a decrease in medical treatments and monotonous checks, but also patients who can profit from effective supervision of their HF status. Indeed, over the past decade, and with the increasing recognition of the value of monitoring HF, there has been an exponential growth in the insertion of devices for cardiovascular therapy [62]. Employing implantable pressure sensors in cardiovascular therapy-based devices represents an exceptional prospect for constant tending of a patient's clinical HF status through real-time measuring of physical activity and cardiac rhythms/events, as well as sensing any health malfunction by monitoring different cardiac pressures.

A key factor in diagnosing an HF is an elevation of the ventricular filling pressures and, therefore, much of the focus of HF disease monitoring has centered on achieving the lowest ventricular filling pressures possible with medical and device-based therapy. Consequently, the opportunity for continuous monitoring of cardiac pressure via implantable sensors has been shown to be an attractive opportunity. Early effort [63] established the safety and practicability of long-term cardiac pressure-based sensors monitoring and also recognized an outstanding connection between the implantable heart pressure sensors measurements and the HF attack. From this perspective, coupling a pressure transducer to a heart ventricle lead of a pacemaker or defibrillator provides the simplest form of continuous cardiac pressure monitoring. Through implanted pressure sensors, three major classes of arterial pressures can be remotely supervised to mirror a patient's HF status: (i) the right ventricular (RV) pressure, (ii) the left ventricular (LV) pressure, and (iii) the pulmonary arterial (PA) pressure.

Indeed, a patient's RV pressure can be monitored using a piezoelectric-based chip merged at the tip of a pacemaker lead in the RV outflow area [64]. Then, the arterial diastolic pressures can be estimated by taking the value of the RV pressure at the peak time (first rate of change of the pressure with respect to the time) [65]. A particular study on a RV pressure-guided treatment group [66] showed a decrease in HF hospitalization and a reduction of about 20% in the need for intravenous diuretics. A subsequent analysis on the same group showed an approximately 20% reduction in HF events. Furthermore, high RV pressure was correlated to an augmented risk of ventricular tachyarrhythmias [67, 68].

The left atrial (LA) pressure sensor is composed of a sensor lead positioned at the interventricular septum and attached to a coil antenna for telemetry of sensor signals from the LA. In a severe HF patient trial [69], the use of LA pressure monitoring resulted in a fall in LA pressure and proved the stability, safety, and efficacy (potential risk of pulmonary embolism) of LA pressure sensors.

Various studies, including that of Abraham et al. [39], have proved that an increase in the intracardiac and the PA pressures comes before the commencement of an HF dissociation. A pressure transducer, such as the CardioMEMS HF sensor [70, 71], can be arranged in any branch of the pulmonary artery. Such a sensor allows monitoring of the PA pressure to improve the outcomes of HF patients. The trial by Smeets et al. [10] showed that daily measurement of PA pressures in addition to ordinary care led to an approximate 40% reduction in HF-related hospitalization and improved quality of life scores compared with the control group, while the duration of an in-patient stay was significantly shortened from 4 almost to 2 days.

The CardioMEMS HF sensor [39, 72, 73] is the first clinically proven HF monitoring system confirmed to significantly decrease HF hospital admissions and improve quality of life [39]. Additionally, it has been clinically demonstrated to reduce hospital admissions by about 60% over an average of 1 year [72]. This HF system, almost batteryless, revealed many benefits, including the use of sensor information without the patient needing to visit the clinic or hospital as the system regularly communicates the measurements wirelessly to the respective care person/doctor.

In summary, remote wireless pressure sensors-based systems are valuable apparatuses that can support several HF clinics by keeping the respective patients regulated, out of the medical health centers, and a relatively stable quality of life [74]. As cardiac pressure sensors-based monitoring systems become automated in terms of data collection, smarter and smaller remote nursing will evolve into an essential piece of HF patients' health evaluation, especially with the recently developed emphasis on virtual visits in light of the COVID-19 pandemic [74].

5.2.6 Lung Ultrasound

Lung ultrasound (LUS) is an accurate non-invasive method that can be used for quantification of extravascular lung water (EVLW) in patients with known or suspected HF [75]. It is a safe, efficient, and reliable method [76].

The concept of LUS in critical care and cardiovascular medicine is perhaps seen as new idea emerging over the past few decades, but its origin dates back to much further – to 1946 [77]. It was neglected for a long time [78] due to the belief that lungs are an inadequate medium for ultrasound waves because of high air content [79]. The discovery of B-lines artifacts and utilizing their presence and summation as an indicator for HF made LUS significant in cardiology. The study of ultrasound includes three essential modes that form soft tissue imaging: (i) amplitude mode (A-mode), (ii) motion mode (M-mode), (iii) brightness mode (B-mode) [80]. In this section, we are limiting discussion to the third mode only.

The LUS for HF applications relies mostly on B-lines artifacts detection. The presence of multiple and diffuse B-lines is correlated with the presence of EVLW [81, 82]. In a typical B-mode, the ultrasound pulses construct a 2D image [83]. In a normally aerated lung, ultrasound images will show A-lines consisting of regularly spaced horizontal lines and reverberation artifacts between two bordering surfaces, which are the probe/body surface and the pleura/air in alveoli [84]. An image for a lung that contains A-line artifacts is usually called dry lung. The presence of B-lines begins to take shape upon the presence of fluids in the interstitial or interalveolar spaces due to the reverberation phenomenon, which is currently understood to mean that when an ultrasound wave is trapped between materials that possess different acoustic impedance, a reverberation artifact will occur [85]. The increase of lung tissue density causes a change from the dominant A-line to diffuse B-lines in what is known as sliding [86]. B-lines, previously known as comet tails or lung cosmists, are defined as discrete laser-like vertical lines that arise from the bottom of screen and move synchronously with lung sliding [81, 87]. Lung B-lines are not exclusive to HF symptoms, and can be seen in many other conditions such as pulmonary edema [88], pneumonia [89], systemic sclerosis [90], acute lung injury [91], and other respiratory diseases [92].

There are multiple factors that affect the quality and quantity of B-lines appearances in LUS images, such as the position of the patients, the equipment utilized, clip-length, probe selection, the experience of the practitioner, and the number of zones [93]. The current settings to examine designated thoracic zones can be as low as two up to 36 zones. The optimum recommendation is eight zones.

The visualization of B-lines is possible with cardiac, convex, or linear probes [94]. There are two main scanning approaches in LUS, but either way the probe has to be placed in intercostal spaces. The first approach is the longitudinal scan, while the second is the transverse (oblique) scan. The ribs and their shadows are a part of the image in the longitudinal scan. On the other hand, the transversal approach allows the practitioner to visualize a wider view of the pleural lines uninterrupted by rib shadows [95]. The most important reference point is the pleural line with its lung sliding as it would be impossible to obtain any information about lung aeration without clearly visualizing it. Patients should be positioned either sitting upright, semi-recumbent or supine. In addition, patients should maintain the same position if serial examinations are being performed as the B-lines appearances in the imaging are greatly influenced by the patient's position [96, 97]. The length of the imaging clip is optimally 6 seconds, if the patient is breathing normally [98].

In HF diagnosis and monitoring, the B-lines should be diffuse, bilateral, and multiple. Diffuse means that the lines should be adjacent in two areas, bilateral means that they should be visible in the left and right hemithorax, and multiple means that they should be in abundance [95]. There are many quantification systems that have been developed to classify and assess B-lines numbers in order to identify the level of risk that at patient is at during and after hospital discharge. The methods can be categorized as: (i) score methods and (ii) count-based methods. Score methods often rely on a minimum number of B-lines in one intercostal space, labeling it as a positive zone and adding up the number of positive zones. In addition, lines can be counted one by one, or upon confluence, or as percentage, cumulatively known as count-based methods [99]. These quantification systems can be important in predicting mortality and hospitalization of worsening HF, and are a prognostic marker for HF as shown by many studies [100–108].

There are many protocols for LUS for diagnosis and prognosis monitoring of HF. The most famous protocols being used are: (i) bedside lung ultrasound in emergency (BLUE) [109], (ii) fluid administration limited by lung sonography (FALLS-protocol) [110], (iii) cardiac arrest ultrasound exam (C.A.U.S.E.) [84], (iv) lung and cardiac ultrasound (LuCUS) [111].

LUS is a powerful and sensitive technique for the prediction and prognosis monitoring of HF. It is easy-to-apply, widely available, and has a short learning curve [112]. Although

LUS is a powerful tool for pulmonary and cardiology imaging, there are some limitations, including the dependence on the skill of the practitioner, the quality and the setting of the hardware [113], and the lack of specificity as B-lines can be present in many other conditions. Nevertheless, the future is open for LUS to be further developed and specific with the integration of new algorithms and reliability on deep learning methods [114].

5.2.7 Sound Sensors

The flow of blood in and out of the heart and the movement of the structures responsible for controlling this flow allow the heart to make sounds [115]. There are four types of heart sounds: (i) primary heart sounds in healthy adults, including the first heart sound (S1) and the second heart sound (S2) [115–118], (ii) extra heart sounds including gallop rhythms of the third heart sound (S3) and fourth heart sound (S4) [119–123], (iii) heart murmurs, which are present in congenital abnormalities [124–128], (iv) other abnormal sounds such as adventitious sounds, click [129, 130], rubs [131], snaps [132], knocks [133], and plops [134–136].

Before the invention of the stethoscope in 1816 by Laënnec, listening to the sounds of heart was not possible without physicians applying their ears to the chest of the patient [137]. Stethoscopes enabled listening to and interpreting heart sounds for diagnosis. The contribution of scientists and introduction of physical concepts and technological additions have allowed us to arrive at sound sensors for the classification of heart sounds.

The normal sounds in healthy adults are S1 and S2 [138]. The presence of other sounds could be an indicator for cardiovascular problems. For instance, the presence of S3 sound could be an indicator for pathological problems such as anemia, thyrotoxicosis, mitral regurgitation, hypertrophic cardiomyopathy, aortic and tricuspid regurgitation, and LV dysfunction [135]. The S4 sound can result from hypertension, aortic stenosis and regurgitation, severe mitral regurgitation, cardiomyopathy, and ischemic heart disease [139]. The ability to distinguish the different heart sounds is uniform across all practitioners, especially as it is difficult to distinguish some sounds, like the S3 sound, which is crucial for HF diagnosis. Therefore, it became important to move toward the automatic classification of heart sound signals in order to achieve better diagnosis, through signals detected with, for example, stethoscopes, electret microphones or piezoelectric acoustic sensors [140–142].

Over the past few decades, multiple sensors have emerged for better detection of heart sounds based on phonocardiography and echocardiography. The sensors focus on improving signal processing and noise reduction. In 2004, Reed et al. developed a model for the production of heart sounds through a prototype based on wavelet decomposition of sounds and a neural network-based classifier that could detect abnormal heart sounds, which was very useful in predicting HF [143]. In another work, a chest-worn accelerometer with high sensitivity for cardiorespiratory sound was based on an asymmetrical gapped cantilever, which is composed of a bottom mechanical layer and a top piezoelectric layer separated by a gap with a built-in amplifier to amplify the output of the voltage sensor [144]. Mubarak et al. published their work centered on improving the quality of phonocardiogram (PCG) signals and the removal of noisy and corrupted signals, which allowed them to accurately identify and localize S1 and S2 sounds based on homomorphic filtering using support vector machine [145]. Gupta et al. utilized commercially available Audicor (Inovise Medical, Oregon, USA) devices that use 10 second PCG to detect S3 sounds. They used a proprietary algorithm and the S3 intensity is graded on a scale of 0–10. S3 sound is considered present when its intensity is greater than 5. They were able to reproduce the data upon replacing the old sensors with new pairs of sensors [146]. In their work, Chen et al. used a deep neural network (DNN) to recognize S1 and S2 sounds based only on acoustic characters through converting signals first into a sequence of Mel-frequency cepstral coefficients (MFCCs).

The K-means algorithm is applied to cluster MFCC features into two groups to refine their representation and discriminative capability. The refined features are then fed to a DNN classifier to perform S1 and S2 recognition [147]. In a non-invasive pilot study on HF patients with audible S3, Siejeko et al. studied the feasibility of heart sound measurements from an accelerometer within an implantable cardioverter defibrillator (ICD) pulse generator. In their findings S1, S2, and S3 vibrations were detected in all accelerometer locations including 16 subjects. However, S3 was not audible because when the signal bandwidth was increased, a substantial portion of S2 was infrasonic (below 20 Hz). In their conclusions they found that heart sounds, including S3 amplitude and heart sound time intervals, can be measured using pulse generator embedded circuitry at implant sites without special-purpose leads [148].

5.2.8 Seismocardiography

Seismocardiography (SCG) is a non-invasive method based on measuring the vibration on the chest in response to the movement of heart and blood in the arterial tree [149]. Vibration measurements can be performed using a MEMS-based 3-axis accelerometer placed on the chest, particularly around the mid-sternum [7, 150]. Since SCG measurements are not confounded by body fluid, there is no need to use multiple sensors. The waveforms of SCG signals consist of parts that correspond to the opening and closure states of the aortic valve, and the ejection of blood from the left ventricle to the aorta. The hypothesis of SCG studies depends on the similarity of signals for HF patients before and after physical exercise [7], because HF patients have less reserve to increase cardiac performance during exercise. In other words, SCG signals of HF patients are similar during exercise and rest conditions. On the other hand, healthy individuals have relatively altered signal amplitudes during exercise and rest. By comparing the recorded signals during rest and exercise, the HF severity of the patient can be predicted in a non-invasive way. Recorded time signals are converted into frequency domain for detailed investigation. During exercise, high-frequency components in SCG waves are more visible in healthy individuals compared with the SCG signals of HF patients [7].

5.2.9 Ballistocardiography

Ballistocardiography (BCG) is a non-invasive technique that examines the movements which occur as a result of the ejection of blood during the cardiac cycle [151]. BCG measures the response of the whole body in terms of displacement, velocity, or acceleration to the mechanical forces generated by the movement of blood in heart chambers and in arteries, particularly in the aorta, and the movement of the heart muscles.

BCG signals can be determined using a modified weighing scale capable of measuring the response at the bottom of the foot. There is a phase difference between the peaks of ECG and BCG signals due to wave propagation through the body. There are also secondary peaks in the BCG wave which are not observed in ECG signals. In the classic BCG, early peak H occurs due to the heart contraction in systole and main IJK complex is observed due to the ventricular ejection and aortic flow [151, 152]. After BCG had been studied extensively between 1955 and 1980, the method was almost extinct by 2010, mainly due to the lack of standardized measurement techniques and lack of understanding of the signal source [151]. However, BCG research has increased again in recent years, thanks to the advancements in sensing technologies such as static-charge-sensitive sensors and piezoelectric films [153–155]. These sensing technologies simplify the non-invasive measurements of BCG signals using weighing scale implemented or bed/chair implemented sensor applications that are capable of measuring BCG signals during standing or sitting [156, 157]. BCG signals vary depending on the cardiovascular health status of the individual [158, 159]. The peak amplitudes of BCG signals are significantly lower for HF patients compared with the rest or exercise states of healthy individuals [158].

5.2.10 Photoplethysmography

Photoplethysmogram (PPG) is an optical signal used for the quantification of blood volume changes during the heartbeat [158]. PPG signal is generally measured to monitor the oxygen saturation using a pulse oximeter [160]. The scatter of light is different for oxygenated and deoxygenated blood and the amount of oxygen can be predicted using this difference [161]. A pulse oximeter is generally used on the finger [161, 162]; a beam of light is emitted toward one side of the finger and the level of collected light is measured on the other side. As a result, the scattered light intensity provides a measure to determine the level of oxygen saturation in the body [163]. The baseline oxygen saturation decreases progressively due to inadequate cardiovascular performance of HF patients, and HF worsening may be suspected when the baseline oxygen saturation is less than 93% [164].

5.2.11 Monitoring Natriuretic Peptides Levels

B-type natriuretic peptide (BNP) and amino-terminal pro-B-type natriuretic peptide (NT-proBNP) are biomarkers of HF, and they can be used for the assessment of HF severity [165–167]. BNP is a cardiac hormone which is released from the myocytes (heart muscle cells) in response to increased wall stress [168]. For the measurements of BNP levels, minimally invasive finger-stick self-testing can be used [3].

In the case of HF, ventricular stress increases, leading to higher levels of BNP and NT-proBNP release. It has been reported that the cut-off levels for HF diagnosis are 100 pg/mL of BNP [168] or 300 pg/mL of NT-proBNP [169]. Natriuretic peptide levels less than these cut-off values are not considered to indicate HF. There are several factors which influence the level of BNP and NT-proBNP; therefore, in addition to BNP measurements, other supporting diagnostic tools should be employed for accurate HF diagnosis [2]. In case of acute coronary syndrome, renal insufficiency, RV dysfunction, atrial fibrillation, and advanced aging, higher levels of BNP are observed than the expected levels [167]. On the other hand, obesity, flash pulmonary edema, and end-stage cardiomyopathy lead to lower levels of BNP than those expected [167]. For individuals under 50 years old, presence of HF can be considered when the BNP level is higher than 400 pg/mL or NT-proBNP is higher than 450 pg/mL. For the groups between 50 and 75 years of age and older than 75 years of age, these threshold levels become 900 pg/mL and 1800 pg/mL, respectively [167]. It is reported that impending HF deterioration can be predicted using daily home BNP measurements [170, 171]. McDonald et al. (2018) used an averaged filter to reduce the variations in daily BNP measurements and provide better assessment of weekly changes for predicting emerging HF failure [170].

5.3 Clinical Trials on Remote Monitoring Using Non-Invasive Sensors

The non-invasive modalities discussed in this chapter are used for remote monitoring of HF patients. Many remote monitoring trials investigated different population groups and employed different monitoring techniques. Several researchers performed meta-analysis by combining randomized control trials (RCTs).

Klersy et al. (2009) conducted a meta-analysis, using 20 RCTs and 12 cohort studies, to identify the effect of remote patient monitoring (RPM) on the outcome of HF patients [172]. The RCTs included 6258 patients and had a 6-month follow-up period. The RCTs showed that RPM results in a significant reduction in the number of deaths (relative risk: 0.83, 95% confidence interval: 0.73 to 0.95, $p = 0.006$) and hospitalizations (relative risk: 0.93, 95% confidence interval: 0.87 to 0.99, $p = 0.030$), indicating that RPM has a clinical protective effect compared with usual care [172]. Inglis et al. (2010) performed a similar meta-analysis and reported that RPM decreased the number of deaths (2710 subjects were included, relative risk: 0.66), all-cause hospitalizations (2343 subjects were included, relative risk: 0.91), and HF-related hospitalizations (1570 subjects were included, relative risk: 0.79) [42].

The meta-analysis of Yun et al. (2018) reported that RPM reduced all-case mortality (relative risk: 0.81) and HF-related mortality (relative risk: 0.81), but no significant change is reported for all-cause hospitalizations and HF-related hospitalizations [173]. Chaudhry et al.'s (2010) study was a randomized controlled clinical trial of RPM by means of measuring weight and collecting daily information about the symptoms [14]. They stated that there was no effect of remote monitoring system on the number of deaths and hospitalizations. The possible reason for this ineffectiveness might be related to using only weight as the indicator. The most commonly used parameter for remote monitoring is weight because of its simplicity [51]; however, it is not sufficient alone to capture the warning of impending HF decompensation [19]. Large-scale trials that use only one remote monitoring parameter tend to generate neutral results and show limited positive effect of remote monitoring. Similarly, if thoracic impedance is used as the only remote monitoring parameter, large trials result in low sensitivity and specificity [174, 175]. It can be concluded that including several monitoring parameters is critical to improve the effectiveness of RPM [51]. The findings of Pekmezaris et al. (2018) support this fact as, by utilizing blood pressure measurement and a pulse oximeter in addition to the weight scale, lower hospitalization rates are achieved [22].

In several trials which employ multiple monitoring parameters, thoracic impedance, heart rate, heart rate variability, and physical activity are used synchronously [176, 177]. In the study of Anand et al. (2012), an algorithm was developed to predict impending acute HF decompensation [178]. A total of 543 patients were monitored over three months using a device with multiple sensors measuring heart rate, respiratory rate, body impedance, and physical activity. It is reported that the algorithm predicted HF events with 63% sensitivity, 92% specificity, and a false positive rate of 0.9 per patient-year.

In Table 5.1, remote patient monitoring studies are listed by indicating the subject numbers and the non-invasive sensing parameters used.

5.4 Discussion

HF is a chronic cardiovascular disease which results in frequent hospitalizations, increasing the economic burden in healthcare systems and negatively affecting the hospital workload. Many rehospitalizations are unnecessary or can be avoided by employing remote monitoring of HF patients.

Hemodynamic effects of HF decompensation begin about 30 days before hospitalization [185]. In current practice, in-hospital invasive techniques are applied for assessing the HF state by measuring ventricular pressure levels. However, filling ventricle pressures can be determined using a catheter and cannot be applied frequently because of their invasive nature. An accurate and low-cost non-invasive modality is an important requirement for the recognition of HF decompensation. The signs of HF decompensation can be sensed in the form of intrathoracic impedance alterations measured by non-invasive tools up to 15 days before hospitalization. Systematic use of non-invasive techniques allows remote monitoring of the patient's condition. With the development in sensor technologies and data science, lightweight and wearable sensors can be designed and the measurements taken can be remotely monitored by clinicians.

The exact role and effectiveness of remote monitoring remains unclear [3, 24, 182]. Although several RPM studies have reported reduced mortality rates and HF-related hospitalizations, large-scale trials tend to give neutral results for mortality and hospitalizations [19]. In future, it is necessary to elucidate the effect of remote monitoring modalities for HF prediction on large-scale RCTs. We have seen that using only one monitoring parameter is not sufficient to reduce hospitalization and mortality rates, and multiparameter methods with optimized algorithms are recommended for the increased benefit and for improving the life quality of patients [22].

The use of weight scales is common among RPM trials, but the increase in weight provides an imprecise estimation because weight can change due to many factors other than HF decompensation [186]. A relative increase in thoracic bioimpedance provides better prediction of HF-related congestion [3]. ECG is among the under-investigated techniques for HF remote monitoring [182]. There is an effort to perform ambulatory ECG measurements with

Table 5.1 Summary of trials employing non-invasive remote measurements for monitoring HF patients.

Author	Number of Patients	Measured Parameters	Results
Cleland et al. (2005) [179]	426	Body weight, ECG signal, blood pressure	Decreased all-cause mortality
Klersy et al. (2009) [172]	8612	ECG signal	Decreased all-cause mortality and HF-related hospitalization
Chaudry et al. (2010) [14]	1653	Body weight	No positive effect
Ferrante et al. (2010) [15]	1518	Body weight, blood pressure	Decreased all-cause mortality and HF-related hospitalization
Koehler et al. (2011) [16]	710	Body weight, ECG signal, blood pressure, pulse oximeter	No positive effect
Anand et al. (2012) [178]	543	Bioimpedance monitoring	HF decompensation is predicted using an algorithm
Angermann et al. (2012) [18]	1007	Body weight, ECG signal, blood pressure	Decreased mortality
Lyngå et al. (2012) [180]	344	Body weight	No positive effect
Dovancescu et al. (2015) [181]	180	Bioimpedance monitoring	Decreased hospitalization
Kotb et al. (2015) [182]	193	ECG signal	Decreased all-cause mortality and HF-related hospitalization
Inglis et al. (2015) [20]	9332	Body weight, ECG signal, blood pressure	Decreased all-cause mortality and HF-related hospitalization
Ong et al. (2016) [19]	1437	Body weight, ECG signal, pressure signal	No positive effect
Lin et al. (2017) [21]	11,758	Body weight, ECG signal, blood pressure	Decreased all-cause mortality and HF-related hospitalization
Koehler et al. (2018) [17]	1571	Body weight, ECG signal, blood pressure, pulse oximeter	Decreased all-cause mortality and HF-related hospital admission
Nouryan et al. (2018) [183]	89	Body weight, blood pressure, pulse oximeter	Decreased all-cause hospitalization
Ware et al. (2018) [23]	98	Body weight, blood pressure	Increased life quality
Gingele et al. (2019) [184]	382	ECG signal, pulse oximeter	No positive effect
Zhu et al. (2020) [24]	10,981	Body weight, ECG signal, blood pressure, pulse oximeter	Decreased all-cause mortality and hospitalization

the use of smartphone applications and miniaturized devices; on the other hand, large-scale randomized trials are necessary to prove ECG reliability in home monitoring systems [28, 187–189]. In the study of Kotb et al. (2015), it is stated that ECG analysis plays a prominent role in lowering all-cause mortality and hospitalization, and in improving quality of life [182]. The highest HF prediction performance is observed for RPM trials including multiple monitoring parameters. Through these, early warnings of HF may be better recognized using efficient algorithms that analyze various sensor measurements [190].

Another aspect of non-invasive remote monitoring is the adherence of HF patients in order to improve the efficiency of proposed trials. It is stated that most HF patients are older than 65 years [191]. Proposed RPM systems should be portable and easy-to-use for increased adherence. Ware et al. (2019) conducted a study to evaluate patient adherence to a remote monitoring program [192]. It is reported that the highest patient adherence is observed in older patients, while participation of younger patients decreased over time, indicating that older patients adapted better to remote monitoring system [3, 192]. There are several recommended systems for increasing patient adherence, such as the toilet-seat based cardiovascular monitoring system and the clothing-integrated sensor system, which do not require any effort from the patient to develop the habit of monitoring themselves [158, 189].

Non-invasive measurements are cheap and easy-to-apply. As a result, these modalities can be used in large number of patients. Beyond the effectiveness of the methods, these measurements encourage patients to make lifestyle changes and increase their sensitivity to healthcare, thereby increasing the life quality of HF patients. Two important questions for non-invasive RPM are which type of HF patients should benefit from remote monitoring and at with what frequency should the measurements be performed. Measurements on a daily basis are recommended for increasing the efficiency of monitoring systems, as relative changes in the measured data provide important clues about upcoming HF decompensation. The viable method for remote data analysis systems is that large numbers of patients with low HF severity should be encouraged to become involved in RPM with non-invasive measurements, and a smaller group of patients with severe HF should be directed to invasive measurement techniques.

5.5 Conclusion

In this chapter, we explained non-invasive and minimally invasive measurement techniques and summarized the results of emerging RPM systems to predict impending HF decompensation. The use of remote monitoring techniques employing non-invasive sensors helps to reduce all-cause mortality, HF-related mortality, and rehospitalization. With the advances in sensor technologies, these measurements can be performed by patients at home using smart devices and wearables. The data obtained can be monitored remotely by the clinicians, providing the opportunity to take precautions before serious symptoms are encountered. This also helps reduce the workload of hospitals and the economic burden of HF treatment in healthcare systems. The positive results of clinical trials with large numbers of patients show the high potential of non-invasive sensors for diagnosing HF.

Acknowledgments

This study was funded by Qatar National Research Fund (QNRF), National Priority Research Program (NPRP13S-0108-200024) and Qatar University International Research Collaboration Co-Fund (IRCC) program (IRCC-2020-002). Dr. Ouakad is grateful for the support of the Research Grant provided by the Deanship of Research at Sultan Qaboos University (SQU) through grant number CL/SQU-QU/ENG/20/01.

References

1 Ponikowski, P., Voors, A.A., Anker, S.D., Bueno, H., Cleland, J.G.F., Coats, A.J.S., Falk, V., González-Juanatey, J.R., Harjola, V.P., Jankowska, E.A., et al. (2016). 2016 ESC Guidelines for the diagnosis and treatment of acute and chronic heart failure: The Task Force for the diagnosis and treatment of acute and chronic heart failure of the European Society of Cardiology (ESC)Developed with the special contribution of the Heart Failure Association (HFA) of the ESC. *European Heart Journal* 37: 2129–2200. doi:10.1093/eurheartj/ehw128.

2 Yancy Clyde, W., Jessup, M., Bozkurt, B., Butler, J., Casey Donald, E., Colvin Monica, M., Drazner Mark, H., Filippatos Gerasimos, S., Fonarow Gregg, C., Givertz Michael, M., et al. (2017). 2017 ACC/AHA/HFSA focused update of the 2013 ACCF/AHA guideline for the management of heart failure. *Journal of the American College of Cardiology* 70: 776–803. doi:10.1016/j.jacc.2017.04.025.

3 Faragli, A., Abawi, D., Quinn, C., Cvetkovic, M., Schlabs, T., Tahirovic, E., Düngen, H.D., Pieske, B., Kelle, S., Edelmann, F., et al. (2020). The role of non-invasive devices for the telemonitoring of heart failure patients. *Heart Failure Reviews*. doi:10.1007/s10741-020-09963-7.

4 Savarese, G. and Lund, L.H. (2017). Global public health burden of heart failure. *Cardiac Failure Review (CFR)* 3: 7–11. doi:10.15420/cfr.2016:25:2.

5 Cowie, M.R., Wood, D.A., Coats, A.J.S., Thompson, S.G., Suresh, V., Poole-Wilson, P.A., and Sutton, G.C. (2000). Survival of patients with a new diagnosis of heart failure: A population based study. *Heart* 83: 505. doi:10.1136/heart.83.5.505.

6. Mosterd, A., Cost, B., Hoes, A.W., De Bruijne, M.C., Deckers, J.W., Hofman, A., and Grobbee, D.E. (2001). The prognosis of heart failure in the general population. The Rotterdam study. *European Heart Journal* 22: 1318–1327. doi:10.1053/euhj.2000.2533.

7 Inan Omer, T., Baran Pouyan, M., Javaid Abdul, Q., Dowling, S., Etemadi, M., Dorier, A., Heller, J.A., Bicen, A.O., Roy, S., De Marco, T., et al. (2018). Novel wearable seismocardiography and machine learning algorithms can assess clinical status of heart failure patients. *Circulation. Heart Failure* 11: e004313. doi:10.1161/CIRCHEARTFAILURE.117.004313.

8 Gheorghiade, M., Follath, F., Ponikowski, P., Barsuk, J.H., Blair, J.E.A., Cleland, J.G., Dickstein, K., Drazner, M.H., Fonarow, G.C., Jaarsma, T., et al. (2010). Assessing and grading congestion in acute heart failure: A scientific statement from the Acute Heart Failure Committee of the Heart Failure Association of the European Society of

Cardiology and endorsed by the European Society of Intensive Care Medicine. *European Journal of Heart Failure* 12: 423–433. https://doi.org/10.1093/eurjhf/hfq045.

9 Adams, K.F., Fonarow, G.C., Emerman, C.L., LeJemtel, T.H., Costanzo, M.R., Abraham, W.T., Berkowitz, R.L., Galvao, M., and Horton, D.P. (2005). Characteristics and outcomes of patients hospitalized for heart failure in the United States: Rationale, design, and preliminary observations from the first 100,000 cases in the Acute Decompensated Heart Failure National Registry (ADHERE). *American Heart Journal* 149: 209–216. https://doi.org/10.1016/j.ahj.2004.08.005.

10 Smeets, C.J.P., Lee, S., Groenendaal, W., Squillace, G., Vranken, J., De Cannière, H., Van Hoof, C., Grieten, L., Mullens, W., Nijst, P., et al. (2020). The added value of in-hospital tracking of the efficacy of decongestion therapy and prognostic value of a wearable thoracic impedance sensor in acutely decompensated heart failure with volume overload: Prospective cohort study. *JMIR Cardio* 4: e12141.

11 Selvaraj, S., Claggett, B., Pozzi, A., McMurray John, J.V., Jhund Pardeep, S., Packer, M., Desai Akshay, S., Lewis Eldrin, F., Vaduganathan, M., Lefkowitz Martin, P., et al. (2019). Prognostic implications of congestion on physical examination among contemporary patients with heart failure and reduced ejection fraction. *Circulation* 140: 1369–1379. doi:10.1161/CIRCULATIONAHA.119.039920.

12 Le Jemtel, T.H. and Alt, E.U. (2006). Are hemodynamic goals viable in tailoring heart failure therapy? Hemodynamic goals are outdated. *Circulation* 113: 1027–1032. Discussion 1033.

13 Gronda, E., Vanoli, E., Sacchi, S., Grassi, G., Ambrosio, G., and Napoli, C. (2020). Risk of heart failure progression in patients with reduced ejection fraction: Mechanisms and therapeutic options. *Heart Failure Reviews* 25: 295–303. doi:10.1007/s10741-019-09823-z.

14 Chaudhry, S.I., Mattera, J.A., Curtis, J.P., Spertus, J.A., Herrin, J., Lin, Z., Phillips, C.O., Hodshon, B.V., Cooper, L.S., and Krumholz, H.M. (2010). Telemonitoring in patients with heart failure. *New England Journal of Medicine* 363: 2301–2309. doi:10.1056/NEJMoa1010029.

15 Ferrante, D., Varini, S., Macchia, A., Soifer, S., Badra, R., Nul, D., Grancelli, H., and Doval, H. (2010). Long-term results after a telephone intervention in chronic heart failure. *Journal of the American College of Cardiology* 56 (372–378): doi:10.1016/j.jacc.2010.03.049.

16 Koehler, F., Winkler, S., Schieber, M., Sechtem, U., Stangl, K., Böhm, M., Boll, H., Baumann, G., Honold, M., Koehler, K., et al. (2011). Impact of remote telemedical management on mortality and hospitalizations in ambulatory patients with chronic heart failure. *Circulation* 123: 1873–1880. doi:10.1161/CIRCULATIONAHA.111.018473.

17 Koehler, F., Koehler, K., Deckwart, O., Prescher, S., Wegscheider, K., Winkler, S., Vettorazzi, E., Polze, A., Stangl, K., Hartmann, O., et al. (2018). Telemedical interventional management in heart failure II (TIM-HF2), a randomised, controlled trial investigating the impact of telemedicine on unplanned cardiovascular hospitalisations and mortality in heart failure patients: Study design and description of the intervention. *European Journal of Heart Failure* 20: 1485–1493. https://doi.org/10.1002/ejhf.1300.

18 Angermann Christiane, E., Störk, S., Gelbrich, G., Faller, H., Jahns, R., Frantz, S., Loeffler, M., and Ertl, G. (2012). Mode of action and effects of standardized collaborative disease management on mortality and morbidity in patients with systolic heart failure. *Circulation. Heart Failure* 5: 25–35. doi:10.1161/CIRCHEARTFAILURE.111.962969.

19 Ong, M.K., Romano, P.S., Edgington, S., Aronow, H.U., Auerbach, A.D., Black, J.T., De Marco, T., Escarce, J.J., Evangelista, L.S., Hanna, B., et al. (2016). Effectiveness of remote patient monitoring after discharge of hospitalized patients with heart failure: The better effectiveness after transition–heart failure (BEAT-HF) randomized clinical trial. *JAMA Internal Medicine* 176: 310–318. doi:10.1001/jamainternmed.2015.7712.

20 Inglis, S.C., Clark, R.A., Dierckx, R., Prieto-Merino, D., and Cleland, J.G.F. (2015). Structured telephone support or non-invasive telemonitoring for patients with heart failure. *Cochrane Database of Systematic Reviews*. doi:10.1002/14651858.CD007228.pub3.

21 Lin, M.-H., Yuan, W.-L., Huang, T.-C., Zhang, H.-F., Mai, J.-T., and Wang, J.-F. (2017). Clinical effectiveness of telemedicine for chronic heart failure: A systematic review and meta-analysis. *Journal of Investigative Medicine* 65: 899. doi:10.1136/jim-2016-000199.

22 Pekmezaris, R., Nouryan, C.N., Schwartz, R., Castillo, S., Makaryus, A.N., Ahern, D., Akerman, M.B., Lesser, M.L., Bauer, L., Murray, L., et al. (2018). A randomized controlled trial comparing telehealth self-management to standard outpatient management in underserved black and hispanic patients living with heart failure. *Telemedicine and e-Health* 25: 917–925. doi:10.1089/tmj.2018.0219.

23 Ware, P., Ross, H.J., Cafazzo, J.A., Laporte, A., Gordon, K., and Seto, E. (2018). Evaluating the implementation of a mobile phone–based telemonitoring program: Longitudinal study guided by the consolidated framework for implementation research. *JMIR Mhealth Uhealth* 6: e10768. doi:10.2196/10768.

24 Zhu, Y., Gu, X., and Xu, C. (2020). Effectiveness of telemedicine systems for adults with heart failure: A meta-analysis of randomized controlled trials. *Heart Failure Reviews* 25: 231–243. doi:10.1007/s10741-019-09801-5.

25 Elian, A., Sada, N., Elfadel, I., Saeed, M., and Shabra, A. (2016). A preliminary evaluation of continuous, shoe-integrated weight measurements for heart failure patients. *Proceedings of 2016 38th Annual International Conference of the IEEE Engineering in Medicine and Biology Society (EMBC), 16-20 Aug* 4768–4771. doi: 10.1109/EMBC.2016.7591793

26 Evangelista, L.S. and Shinnick, M.A. (2008). What do we know about adherence and self-care? *The Journal of Cardiovascular Nursing* 23: 250–257. doi:10.1097/01.JCN.0000317428.98844.4d.

27 Sohn, A., Speier, W., Lan, E., Aoki, K., Fonarow, G.C., Ong, M.K., and Arnold, C.W. (2020). Integrating remote monitoring into heart failure patients' care regimen: A pilot study. *PLOS ONE* 15: e0242210. doi:10.1371/journal.pone.0242210.

28 Kennedy, H.L. (2013). The evolution of ambulatory ECG monitoring. *Progress in Cardiovascular Diseases* 56: 127–132. https://doi.org/10.1016/j.pcad.2013.08.005.

29 Bhurane, A.A., Sharma, M., San-Tan, R., and Acharya, U.R. (2019). An efficient detection of congestive heart failure using frequency localized filter banks for the diagnosis with ECG signals. *Cognitive Systems Research* 55: 82–94. https://doi.org/10.1016/j.cogsys.2018.12.017.

30 Sovilj, S., Magjarević, R., Lovell, N.H., and Dokos, S. (2013). A simplified 3D model of whole heart electrical activity and 12-lead ECG generation. *Computational and Mathematical Methods in Medicine* 2013: 134208. doi:10.1155/2013/134208.

31 Ramsey, M., Barr, R.C., and Spach, M.S. (1977). Comparison of measured torso potentials with those simulated from epicardial potentials for ventricular depolarization and repolarization in the intact dog. *Circulation Research* 41: 660–672. doi:10.1161/01.res.41.5.660.

32 Gajda, R. (2020). Is continuous ECG recording on heart rate monitors the most expected function by endurance athletes, coaches, and doctors? *Diagnostics (Basel, Switzerland)* 10. doi: 10.3390/diagnostics10110867.

33 Lim, Y.G., Kim, K.K., and Park, K.S. (2007). ECG recording on a bed during sleep without direct skin-contact. *IEEE Transactions on Biomedical Engineering* 54: 718–725. doi:10.1109/TBME.2006.889194.

34 Potpara, T.S., Polovina, M.M., Licina, M.M., Marinkovic, J.M., and Lip, G.Y.H. (2013). Predictors and prognostic implications of incident heart failure following the first diagnosis of atrial fibrillation in patients with structurally normal hearts: The belgrade atrial fibrillation study. *European Journal of Heart Failure* 15: 415–424. https://doi.org/10.1093/eurjhf/hft004.

35 Lang, N.N., Wong, C.M., Dalzell, J.R., Jansz, S., Leslie, S.J., and Gardner, R.S. (2014). The ease of use and reproducibility of the Alere™ heart check system: A comparison of patient and healthcare professional measurement of BNP. *Biomarkers in Medicine* 8: 791–796. doi:10.2217/bmm.14.48.

36 Maisel, A.S., Shah, K.S., Barnard, D., Jaski, B., Frivold, G., Marais, J., Azer, M., Miyamoto, M.I., Lombardo, D., Kelsay, D., et al. (2016). How B-type natriuretic peptide (BNP) and body weight changes vary in heart failure with preserved ejection fraction compared with reduced ejection fraction: Secondary results of the HABIT (HF assessment with BNP in the home) trial. *Journal of Cardiac Failure* 22: 283–293. https://doi.org/10.1016/j.cardfail.2015.09.014.

37 Rice, M.J. and Coursin, D.B. (2016). Glucose meters: Here today, gone tomorrow? *Critical Care Medicine* 44.

38 Schwamm Lee, H., Chumbler, N., Brown, E., Fonarow Gregg, C., Berube, D., Nystrom, K., Suter, R., Zavala, M., Polsky, D., Radhakrishnan, K., et al. (2017). Recommendations for the implementation of telehealth in cardiovascular and stroke care: A policy statement from the American Heart Association. *Circulation* 135: e24–e44. doi:10.1161/CIR.0000000000000475.

39 Abraham, W.T., Adamson, P.B., Bourge, R.C., Aaron, M.F., Costanzo, M.R., Stevenson, L.W., Strickland, W., Neelagaru, S., Raval, N., Krueger, S., et al. (2011). Wireless pulmonary artery haemodynamic monitoring in chronic heart failure: A randomised controlled trial. *The Lancet* 377: 658–666. https://doi.org/10.1016/S0140-6736(11)60101-3.

40 Anker, S.D., Koehler, F., and Abraham, W.T. (2011). Telemedicine and remote management of patients with heart failure. *The Lancet* 378: 731–739. https://doi.org/10.1016/S0140-6736(11)61229-4.

41 Dickinson, M.G., Allen, L.A., Albert, N.A., DiSalvo, T., Ewald, G.A., Vest, A.R., Whellan, D.J., Zile, M.R., and Givertz, M.M. (2018). Remote monitoring of patients with heart failure: A white paper from the heart failure society of America Scientific Statements Committee. *Journal of Cardiac Failure* 24: 682–694. https://doi.org/10.1016/j.cardfail.2018.08.011.

42 Inglis, S.C., Clark, R.A., McAlister, F.A., Ball, J., Lewinter, C., Cullington, D., Stewart, S., and Cleland, J.G. (2010). Structured telephone support or telemonitoring programmes for patients with chronic heart failure. *The Cochrane Database of Systematic Reviews*. doi:10.1002/14651858.CD007228.pub2.

43 Aronson, D., Mittleman, M.A., and Burger, A.J. (2004). Measures of heart period variability as predictors of mortality in hospitalized patients with decompensated congestive heart failure. *The American Journal of Cardiology* 93: 59–63. https://doi.org/10.1016/j.amjcard.2003.09.013.

44 Inglis, S.C., Clark, R.A., McAlister, F.A., Stewart, S., and Cleland, J.G.F. (2011). Which components of heart failure programmes are effective? A systematic review and meta-analysis of the outcomes of structured telephone support or telemonitoring as the primary component of chronic heart failure management in 8323 patients: Abridged Cochrane Review. *European Journal of Heart Failure* 13: 1028–1040. https://doi.org/10.1093/eurjhf/hfr039.

45 Norland, K., Sveinbjornsson, G., Thorolfsdottir, R.B., Davidsson, O.B., Tragante, V., Rajamani, S., Helgadottir, A., Gretarsdottir, S., Van Setten, J., Asselbergs, F.W., et al. (2019). Sequence variants with large effects on cardiac electrophysiology and disease. *Nature Communications* 10: 4803. doi:10.1038/s41467-019-12682-9.

46 Abbas, S.R., Zhu, F., and Levin, N.W. (2015). Bioimpedance can solve problems of fluid overload. *Journal of Renal Nutrition* 25: 234–237. https://doi.org/10.1053/j.jrn.2014.10.014.

47 Folan, L. and Funk, M. (2008). Measurement of thoracic fluid content in heart failure: The role of impedance cardiography. *AACN Advanced Critical Care* 19: 47–55. doi:10.4037/15597768-2008-1007.

48 Whellan, D.J., Droogan, C.J., Fitzpatrick, J., Adams, S., McCarey, M.M., Andrel, J., Mather, P., Rubin, S., Bonita, R., and Keith, S. (2012). Change in intrathoracic impedance measures during acute decompensated heart failure admission: Results from the diagnostic data for discharge in heart failure patients (3D-HF) pilot study. *Journal of Cardiac Failure* 18: 107–112. https://doi.org/10.1016/j.cardfail.2011.10.017.

49 Lee, S., Squillace, G., Smeets, C., Vandecasteele, M., Grieten, L., Francisco, R.D., and Hoof, C.V. (2015). Congestive heart failure patient monitoring using wearable bio-impedance sensor technology. *In Proceedings of 2015 37th Annual International Conference of the IEEE Engineering in Medicine and Biology Society (EMBC)* 25–29 Aug: 438–441. doi: 10.1109/EMBC.2015.7318393.

50 Cuba-Gyllensten, I., Gastelurrutia, P., Riistama, J., Aarts, R., Nuñez, J., Lupon, J., and Bayes-Genis, A. (2014). A novel wearable vest for tracking pulmonary congestion in acutely decompensated heart failure. *International Journal of Cardiology* 177: 199–201. doi:10.1016/j.ijcard.2014.09.041.

51 Ali, O., Hajduczok, A.G., and Boehmer, J.P. (2020). Remote physiologic monitoring for heart failure. *Current Cardiology Reports* 22: 68. doi:10.1007/s11886-020-01309-x.

52 Amir, O., Ben-Gal, T., Weinstein, J.M., Schliamser, J., Burkhoff, D., Abbo, A., and Abraham, W.T. (2017). Evaluation of remote dielectric sensing (ReDS) technology-guided therapy for decreasing heart failure re-hospitalizations. *International Journal of Cardiology* 240: 279–284. https://doi.org/10.1016/j.ijcard.2017.02.120.

53 Murphy, N., Shanks, M., and Alderman, P. (2019). Management of heart failure with outpatient technology. *The Journal for Nurse Practitioners* 15: 12–18. https://doi.org/10.1016/j.nurpra.2018.07.004.

54 Chouvarda, I., Philip, N.Y., Natsiavas, P., Kilintzis, V., Sobnath, D., Kayyali, R., Henriques, J., Paiva, R.P., Raptopoulos, A., Chételat, O., et al. (2014). WELCOME — Innovative integrated care platform using wearable sensing and smart cloud computing for COPD patients with comorbidities. *Proceedings of 2014 36th Annual International Conference of the IEEE Engineering in Medicine and Biology Society* 26–30 Aug: 3180–3183. doi:10.1109/EMBC.2014.6944298.

55 Amir, O., Rappaport, D., Zafrir, B., and Abraham, W.T. (2013). A novel approach to monitoring pulmonary congestion in heart failure: Initial animal and clinical experiences using remote dielectric sensing technology. *Congestive Heart Failure* 19: 149–155. https://doi.org/10.1111/chf.12021.

56 Vetrovsky, T., Siranec, M., Parenica, J., Griva, M., Stastny, J., Precek, J., Pelouch, R., Bunc, V., Linhart, A., and Belohlavek, J. (2017). Effect of a 6-month pedometer-based walking intervention on functional capacity in patients with chronic heart failure with reduced (HFrEF) and with preserved (HFpEF) ejection fraction: Study protocol for two multicenter randomized controlled trials. *Journal of Translational Medicine* 15: 153. doi:10.1186/s12967-017-1257-x.

57 Chang, V.M., Dallas, M.I., Lampley, T.M., and Milner, K.A. (2015). Effects of pedometer use in veterans with chronic heart failure. *The Journal for Nurse Practitioners* 11: 819–823. https://doi.org/10.1016/j.nurpra.2015.04.027.

58 Tumkur, K. and Subbiah, S. (2012). Modeling human walking for step detection and stride determination by 3-axis accelerometer readings in pedometer. *Proceedings of 2012 Fourth International Conference on Computational Intelligence, Modelling and Simulation* 25–27 Sept: 199–204. doi:10.1109/CIMSim.2012.65

59 Zhao, N. Full-featured pedometer design realized with 3-axis digital accelerometer.

60 Sai, R., Bapanapalle, S., Praveen, K., and Sunil, M. (2016). Pedometer and calorie calculator for fitness tracking using MEMS digital accelerometer. *2016 International Conference on Inventive Computation Technologies (ICICT)* 1: 1–6.

61 Merchant Faisal, M., Dec, G.W., and Singh Jagmeet, P. (2010). Implantable sensors for heart failure. *Circulation. Arrhythmia and Electrophysiology* 3: 657–667. doi:10.1161/CIRCEP.110.959502.

62 Shasha Liu, P. and Tse, H.-F. (2013). Implantable sensors for heart failure monitoring. *Journal of Arrhythmia* 29: 314–319. https://doi.org/10.1016/j.joa.2013.06.003.

63 Magalski, A., Adamson, P., Gadler, F., Böehm, M., Steinhaus, D., Reynolds, D., Vlach, K., Linde, C., Cremers, B., Sparks, B., et al. (2002). Continuous ambulatory right heart pressure measurements with an implantable hemodynamic monitor: A multicenter,

12-month follow-up study of patients with chronic heart failure. *Journal of Cardiac Failure* 8: 63–70. https://doi.org/10.1054/jcaf.2002.32373.

64 Steinhaus David, M., Lemery, R., Bresnahan Dennis, R., Handlin, L., Bennett, T., Moore, A., Cardinal, D., Foley, L., and Levine, R. (1996). Initial experience with an implantable hemodynamic monitor. *Circulation* 93: 745–752. doi:10.1161/01.CIR.93.4.745.

65 Reynolds, D.W., Bartelt, N., Taepke, R., and Bennett, T.D. (1995). Measurement of pulmonary artery diastolic pressure from the right ventricle. *Journal of the American College of Cardiology* 25: 1176–1182. https://doi.org/10.1016/0735-1097(94)00510-W.

66 Bourge Robert, C., Abraham William, T., Adamson Philip, B., Aaron Mark, F., Aranda Juan, M., Magalski, A., Zile Michael, R., Smith Andrew, L., Smart Frank, W., O'Shaughnessy Mark, A., et al. (2008). Randomized controlled trial of an implantable continuous hemodynamic monitor in patients with advanced heart failure. *Journal of the American College of Cardiology* 51: 1073–1079. doi:10.1016/j.jacc.2007.10.061.

67 Reiter Michael, J., Stromberg Kurt, D., Whitman Teresa, A., Adamson Philip, B., Benditt David, G., and Gold Michael, R. (2013). Influence of intracardiac pressure on spontaneous ventricular arrhythmias in patients with systolic heart failure. *Circulation. Arrhythmia and Electrophysiology* 6: 272–278. doi:10.1161/CIRCEP.113.000223.

68 Adamson, P.B., Gold, M.R., Bennett, T., Bourge, R.C., Stevenson, L.W., Trupp, R., Stromberg, K., Wilkoff, B.L., Costanzo, M.R., Luby, A., et al. (2011). Continuous hemodynamic monitoring in patients with mild to moderate heart failure: Results of the reducing decompensation events utilizing intracardiac pressures in patients with chronic heart failure (REDUCEhf) trial. *Congestive Heart Failure* 17: 248–254. https://doi.org/10.1111/j.1751-7133.2011.00247.x.

69 Ritzema, J., Troughton, R., Melton, I., Crozier, I., Doughty, R., Krum, H., Walton, A., Adamson, P., Kar, S., Shah Prediman, K., et al. (2010). Physician-directed patient self-management of left atrial pressure in advanced chronic heart failure. *Circulation* 121: 1086–1095. doi:10.1161/CIRCULATIONAHA.108.800490.

70 Shavelle, D. and Jermyn, R. (2016). The CardioMEMS heart failure sensor: A procedural guide for implanting physicians. *The Journal of Invasive Cardiology* 28: 273–279.

71 Volterrani, M., Spoletini, I., Angermann, C., Rosano, G., and Coats, A.J. (2019). Implantable devices for heart failure monitoring: The CardioMEMS™ system. *European Heart Journal Supplements* 21: M50–M53. doi:10.1093/eurheartj/suz265.

72 Shavelle, D.M., Desai, A.S., Abraham, W.T., Bourge, R.C., Raval, N., Rathman, L.D., Heywood, J.T., Jermyn, R.A., Pelzel, J., Jonsson, O.T., et al. (2020). Lower rates of heart failure and all-cause hospitalizations during pulmonary artery pressure-guided therapy for ambulatory heart failure: One-year outcomes from the CardioMEMS post-approval study. *Circulation. Heart Failure* 13: e006863. doi:10.1161/circheartfailure.119.006863.

73 Abraham, J., McCann, P.J., Guglin, M.E., Bhimaraj, A., Benjamin, T.-A.S., Robinson, M.R., Jonsson, O.T., Feitell, S.C., Bhatt, K.A., Bennett, M.K., et al. (2020). Management of the patient with heart failure and an implantable pulmonary artery hemodynamic sensor. *Current Cardiovascular Risk Reports* 14: 12. doi:10.1007/s12170-020-00646-4.

74 Lander, M.M., Aldweib, N., and Abraham, W.T. (2021). Wireless hemodynamic monitoring in patients with heart failure. *Current Heart Failure Reports* 18: 12–22. doi:10.1007/s11897-020-00498-4.

75 Pellicori, P., Platz, E., Dauw, J., Ter Maaten, J.M., Martens, P., Pivetta, E., Cleland, J.G.F., McMurray, J.J.V., Mullens, W., Solomon, S.D., et al. (2020). Ultrasound imaging of congestion in heart failure: Examinations beyond the heart. *European Journal of Heart Failure* n/a. https://doi.org/10.1002/ejhf.2032.

76 Mayo, P.H., Beaulieu, Y., Doelken, P., Feller-Kopman, D., Harrod, C., Kaplan, A., Oropello, J., Vieillard-Baron, A., Axler, O., Lichtenstein, D., et al. (2009). American College of Chest Physicians/La Société de Réanimation de Langue Française Statement on Competence in Critical Care Ultrasonography. *Chest* 135: 1050–1060. https://doi.org/10.1378/chest.08-2305.

77 Denier, A. (1946). Les ultrasons: Leurs applications au diagnostic: Ultra-Sonoscopie et a la therapeutique Ultra-Sonoscopie. *Journal Radiology Electrocardiology* 27: 281–283.

78 Desai, S.R. and Hansell, D.M. (1997). Lung imaging in the adult respiratory distress syndrome: Current practice and new insights. *Intensive Care Medicine* 23: 7–15. http://dx.doi.org/10.1007/s001340050284.

79 Lichtenstein, D., Mézière, G., Biderman, P., Gepner, A., and Barré, O. (1997). The Comet-tail Artifact. *American Journal of Respiratory and Critical Care Medicine* 156: 1640–1646. doi:10.1164/ajrccm.156.5.96-07096.

80 Carovac, A., Smajlovic, F., and Junuzovic, D. (2011). Application of ultrasound in medicine. *Acta Informatica Medica : AIM : Journal of the Society for Medical Informatics of Bosnia & Herzegovina : Casopis Drustva Za Medicinsku Informatiku BiH* 19: 168–171. doi:10.5455/aim.2011.19.168-171.

81 Dietrich, C.F., Mathis, G., Blaivas, M., Volpicelli, G., Seibel, A., Wastl, D., Atkinson, N.S.S., Cui, X.-W., Fan, M., and Yi, D. (2016). Lung B-line artefacts and their use. *Journal of Thoracic Disease* 8: 1356–1365. doi:10.21037/jtd.2016.04.55.

82 Jambrik, Z., Monti, S., Coppola, V., Agricola, E., Mottola, G., Miniati, M., and Picano, E. (2004). Usefulness of ultrasound lung comets as a nonradiologic sign of extravascular lung water. *The American Journal of Cardiology* 93: 1265–1270. https://doi.org/10.1016/j.amjcard.2004.02.012.

83 Demi, M., Prediletto, R., Soldati, G., and Demi, L. (2020). Physical mechanisms providing clinical information from ultrasound lung images: Hypotheses and early confirmations. *IEEE Transactions on Ultrasonics, Ferroelectrics, and Frequency Control* 67: 612–623. doi:10.1109/TUFFC.2019.2949597.

84 Francisco Neto, M.J., Rahal Junior, A., Vieira, F.A.C., Silva, P.S.D.D., and Funari, M.B.D.G. (2016). Advances in lung ultrasound. *Einstein (São Paulo)* 14: 443–448.

85 Bakhru, R.N. and Schweickert, W.D. (2013). Intensive care ultrasound: I. Physics, equipment, and image quality. *Annals of the American Thoracic Society* 10: 540–548. doi:10.1513/AnnalsATS.201306-191OT.

86 Bouhemad, B., Mojoli, F., Nowobilski, N., Hussain, A., Rouquette, I., Guinot, P.-G., and Mongodi, S. (2020). Use of combined cardiac and lung ultrasound to predict weaning failure in elderly, high-risk cardiac patients: A pilot study. *Intensive Care Medicine* 46: 475–484. doi:10.1007/s00134-019-05902-9.

87 Volpicelli, G., Elbarbary, M., Blaivas, M., Lichtenstein, D.A., Mathis, G., Kirkpatrick, A.W., Melniker, L., Gargani, L., Noble, V.E., Via, G., et al. (2012). International evidence-based recommendations for point-of-care lung ultrasound. *Intensive Care Medicine* 38: 577–591. doi:10.1007/s00134-012-2513-4.

88 Lichtenstein, D. and Mezière, G. (1998). A lung ultrasound sign allowing bedside distinction between pulmonary edema and COPD: The comet-tail artifact. *Intensive Care Medicine* 24: 1331–1334. doi:10.1007/s001340050771.

89 Caiulo, V.A., Gargani, L., Caiulo, S., Fisicaro, A., Moramarco, F., Latini, G., Picano, E., and Mele, G. (2013). Lung ultrasound characteristics of community-acquired pneumonia in hospitalized children. *Pediatric Pulmonology* 48: 280–287. https://doi.org/10.1002/ppul.22585.

90 Gargani, L., Bruni, C., Romei, C., Frumento, P., Moreo, A., Agoston, G., Guiducci, S., Bellando-Randone, S., Lepri, G., Belloli, L., et al. (2020). Prognostic value of lung ultrasound B-lines in systemic sclerosis. *Chest* 158: 1515–1525. doi:10.1016/j.chest.2020.03.075.

91 Jambrik, Z., Gargani, L., Adamicza, Á., Kaszaki, J., Varga, A., Forster, T., Boros, M., and Picano, E. (2010). B-lines quantify the lung water content: A lung ultrasound versus lung gravimetry study in acute lung injury. *Ultrasound in Medicine & Biology* 36: 2004–2010. https://doi.org/10.1016/j.ultrasmedbio.2010.09.003.

92 Pierce, C.W. (2020). Clarifying the role of lung ultrasonography in COVID-19 respiratory disease. *Canadian Medical Association Journal* 192: E436. doi:10.1503/cmaj.75311.

93 Saraogi, A. (2015). Lung ultrasound: Present and future. *Lung India : Official Organ of Indian Chest Society* 32: 250–257. doi:10.4103/0970-2113.156245.

94 Picano, E. and Pellikka, P.A. (2016). Ultrasound of extravascular lung water: A new standard for pulmonary congestion. *European Heart Journal* 37: 2097–2104. doi:10.1093/eurheartj/ehw164.

95. Vannan, M. (2019). Imaging the failing heart, an issue of heart failure clinics, ebook. *Elsevier Health Sciences* 15.

96 Bikdeli, B., Madhavan Mahesh, V., Jimenez, D., Chuich, T., Dreyfus, I., Driggin, E., Nigoghossian Caroline, D., Ageno, W., Madjid, M., Guo, Y., et al. (2020). COVID-19 and thrombotic or thromboembolic disease: Implications for prevention, antithrombotic therapy, and follow-up. *Journal of the American College of Cardiology* 75: 2950–2973. doi:10.1016/j.jacc.2020.04.031.

97 Frasure, S.E., Matilsky, D.K., Siadecki, S.D., Platz, E., Saul, T., and Lewiss, R.E. (2015). Impact of patient positioning on lung ultrasound findings in acute heart failure. *European Heart Journal. Acute Cardiovascular Care* 4: 326–332. doi:10.1177/2048872614551505.

98 Platz, E., Campbell Ross, T., Claggett, B., Lewis Eldrin, F., Groarke John, D., Docherty Kieran, F., Lee Matthew, M.Y., Merz Allison, A., Silverman, M., Swamy, V., et al. (2019). Lung ultrasound in acute heart failure. *JACC. Heart Failure* 7: 849–858. doi:10.1016/j.jchf.2019.07.008.

99 Platz, E., Lattanzi, A., Agbo, C., Takeuchi, M., Resnic, F.S., Solomon, S.D., and Desai, A.S. (2012). Utility of lung ultrasound in predicting pulmonary and cardiac pressures. *European Journal of Heart Failure* 14: 1276–1284. https://doi.org/10.1093/eurjhf/hfs144.

100 Coiro, S., Rossignol, P., Ambrosio, G., Carluccio, E., Alunni, G., Murrone, A., Tritto, I., Zannad, F., and Girerd, N. (2015). Prognostic value of residual pulmonary congestion at discharge assessed by lung ultrasound imaging in heart failure. *European Journal of Heart Failure* 17: 1172–1181. https://doi.org/10.1002/ejhf.344.

101 Gargani, L., Pang, P.S., Frassi, F., Miglioranza, M.H., Dini, F.L., Landi, P., and Picano, E. (2015). Persistent pulmonary congestion before discharge predicts rehospitalization in heart failure: A lung ultrasound study. *Cardiovascular Ultrasound* 13: 40. doi:10.1186/s12947-015-0033-4.

102. Bidaut, A., Hubert, A., Charton, M., Paven, E., Leclercq, C., Galli, E., and Donal, E. (2021). One year prognostic value of B-lines in dyspnoeic patients. *ESC Heart Failure* n/a. https://doi.org/10.1002/ehf2.12739.

103 Chouihed, T., Coiro, S., Zannad, F., and Girerd, N. (2016). Lung ultrasound: A diagnostic and prognostic tool at every step in the pathway of care for acute heart failure. *The American Journal of Emergency Medicine* 34: 656–657. doi:10.1016/j.ajem.2015.12.030.

104 Russell, F.M., Ehrman, R.R., Ferre, R., Gargani, L., Noble, V., Rupp, J., Collins, S.P., Hunter, B., Lane, K.A., Levy, P., et al. (2019). Design and rationale of the B-lines lung ultrasound guided emergency department management of acute heart failure (BLUSHED-AHF) pilot trial. *Heart & Lung* 48: 186–192. https://doi.org/10.1016/j.hrtlng.2018.10.027.

105 Kobayashi, M., Watanabe, M., Coiro, S., Bercker, M., Paku, Y., Iwasaki, Y., Chikamori, T., Yamashina, A., Duarte, K., Ferreira, J.P., et al. (2019). Mid-term prognostic impact of residual pulmonary congestion assessed by radiographic scoring in patients admitted for worsening heart failure. *International Journal of Cardiology* 289: 91–98. https://doi.org/10.1016/j.ijcard.2019.01.091.

106 Pivetta, E., Goffi, A., Nazerian, P., Castagno, D., Tozzetti, C., Tizzani, P., Tizzani, M., Porrino, G., Ferreri, E., Busso, V., et al. (2019). Lung ultrasound integrated with clinical assessment for the diagnosis of acute decompensated heart failure in the emergency department: A randomized controlled trial. *European Journal of Heart Failure* 21: 754–766. https://doi.org/10.1002/ejhf.1379.

107 Platz, E., Merz, A.A., Jhund, P.S., Vazir, A., Campbell, R., and McMurray, J.J. (2017). Dynamic changes and prognostic value of pulmonary congestion by lung ultrasound in acute and chronic heart failure: A systematic review. *European Journal of Heart Failure* 19: 1154–1163. https://doi.org/10.1002/ejhf.839.

108 Cogliati, C., Casazza, G., Ceriani, E., Torzillo, D., Furlotti, S., Bossi, I., Vago, T., Costantino, G., and Montano, N. (2016). Lung ultrasound and short-term prognosis in heart failure patients. *International Journal of Cardiology* 218: 104–108. https://doi.org/10.1016/j.ijcard.2016.05.010.

109 Lichtenstein, D.A. and Mezière, G.A. (2008). Relevance of lung ultrasound in the diagnosis of acute respiratory failure*: The BLUE protocol. *Chest* 134: 117–125. https://doi.org/10.1378/chest.07-2800.

110 Lichtenstein, D. (2012). Fluid administration limited by lung sonography: The place of lung ultrasound in assessment of acute circulatory failure (the FALLS-protocol). *Expert Review of Respiratory Medicine* 6: 155–162. doi:10.1586/ers.12.13.

111 Dehbozorgi, A., Eslami Nejad, S., Mousavi-roknabadi, R.S., Sharifi, M., Tafakori, A., and Jalli, R. (2019). Lung and cardiac ultrasound (LuCUS) protocol in diagnosing acute heart failure in patients with acute dyspnea. *The American Journal of Emergency Medicine* 37: 2055–2060. https://doi.org/10.1016/j.ajem.2019.02.040.

112 Gargani, L. (2015). Prognosis in heart failure: Look at the lungs. *European Journal of Heart Failure* 17: 1086–1088. https://doi.org/10.1002/ejhf.423.

113 Raheja, R., Brahmavar, M., Joshi, D., and Raman, D. (2019). Application of lung ultrasound in critical care setting: A review. *Cureus* 11: e5233–e5233. doi:10.7759/cureus.5233.

114 Baloescu, C., Toporek, G., Kim, S., McNamara, K., Liu, R., Shaw, M.M., McNamara, R.L., Raju, B.I., and Moore, C.L. (2020). Automated lung ultrasound B-line assessment using a deep learning algorithm. *IEEE Transactions on Ultrasonics, Ferroelectrics, and Frequency Control* 67: 2312–2320. doi:10.1109/tuffc.2020.3002249.

115 Luisada, A.A. (1964). The areas of auscultation and the two main heart sounds. *Medical Times* 92: 8–11.

116 Curtiss, E.I., Matthews, R.G., and Shaver, J.A. (1975). Mechanism of normal splitting of the second heart sound. *Circulation* 51: 157–164.

117 Counihan, T., Lee Messer, A., Rappaport Maurice, B., and Sprague Howard, B. (1951). The initial vibrations of the first heart sound. *Circulation* 3: 730–732. doi:10.1161/01.CIR.3.5.730.

118 Luisada, A.A., Alimurung, M.M., and Lewis, L. (1951). Mechanisms of production of the first heart sound. *American Journal of Physiology-Legacy Content* 168: 226–233.

119 Tavel, M.E. (1974). The fourth heart sound-a premature requiem? *Circulation* 49: 4–6.

120 Reid, K. (1969). Origin of the third heart sound. *British Medical Journal* 3: 597.

121 Timmis, A.J. (1987). The third heart sound. *British Medical Journal (Clinical Research Ed.)* 294: 326.

122 Ewing, G.J. A new approach to the analysis of the third heart sound. 1989.

123 Stapleton, J.F. (1985). Third and Fourth Heart Sounds. Signs and Symptoms in Cardiology, 214–226. Philadelphia, PA: Lippincott.

124 Kurfees, J.F. (1994). Heart sounds, murmurs, and valvular heart disease. In: Family Medicine,R.B.Taylor 617–625. Springer.

125 Bertrand, C.A., Milne, I.G., and Hornick, R. (1956). A study of heart sounds and murmurs by direct heart recordings. *Circulation* 13: 49–57.

126 Van Vollenhoven, E., Van Rotterdam, A., Dorenbos, T., and Schlesinger, F.G. (1969). Frequency analysis of heart murmurs. *Medical & Biological Engineering* 7: 227–232.

127 Evans, W. (1947). Heart murmurs part I. *British Heart Journal* 9: 1.

128 Smythe, J.F., Teixeira, O.H.P., Vlad, P., Demers, P.P., and Feldman, W. (1990). Initial evaluation of heart murmurs: Are laboratory tests necessary? *Pediatrics* 86: 497–500.

129 Cheitlin, M.D. and Byrd, R.C. (1981). The click-murmur syndrome: A clinical problem in diagnosis and treatment. *JAMA* 245: 1357–1361.

130 Gulotta Stephen, J., Gulco, L., Padmanabhan, V., and Miller, S. (1974). The syndrome of systolic click, murmur, and mitral valve prolapse – a cardiomyopathy? *Circulation* 49: 717–728. doi:10.1161/01.CIR.49.4.717.

131 Langley, P. and Murray, A. (2017). Heart sound classification from unsegmented phonocardiograms. *Physiological Measurement* 38: 1658–1670. doi:10.1088/1361-6579/aa724c.

132 Dwivedi, A.K., Imtiaz, S.A., and Rodriguez-Villegas, E. (2019). Algorithms for automatic analysis and classification of heart sounds – a systematic review. *IEEE Access* 7: 8316–8345. doi:10.1109/ACCESS.2018.2889437.

133 Lok, C.E., Morgan, C.D., and Ranganathan, N. (1998). The accuracy and interobserver agreement in detecting the 'gallop sounds' by cardiac auscultation. *Chest* 114: 1283–1288. https://doi.org/10.1378/chest.114.5.1283.

134 Martinez-Lopez, J.I. (1974). Sounds of the heart in diastole. *The American Journal of Cardiology* 34: 594–601. https://doi.org/10.1016/0002-9149(74)90133-7.

135 Sudhakar Reddy, P., Salerni, R., and Shaver, J.A. (1985). Normal and abnormal heart sounds in cardiac diagnosis: Part II. Diastolic sounds. *Current Problems in Cardiology* 10: 1–55. https://doi.org/10.1016/0146-2806(85)90027-1.

136 Luisada, A.A. and Maccanon, D.M. (1966). The physiologic basis of the heart sounds. *Diseases of the Chest* 49: 258–266.

137 Hanna, I.R. and Silverman, M.E. (2002). A history of cardiac auscultation and some of its contributors. *The American Journal of Cardiology* 90: 259–267.

138 Craige, E. and Smith, D. Heart sounds. Heart disease-a textbook of cardiovascular medicine. Philadelphia: WB Saunders 1980, 50.

139 Johnston, M., Collins, S.P., and Storrow, A.B. (2007). The third heart sound for diagnosis of acute heart failure. *Current Heart Failure Reports* 4: 164–169. doi:10.1007/s11897-007-0036-z.

140 Zhang, G., Liu, M., Guo, N., and Zhang, W. (2016). Design of the MEMS piezoresistive electronic heart sound sensor. *Sensors* 16. doi: 10.3390/s16111728.

141 Allataifeh, A. and Al Ahmad, M. (2020). Simultaneous piezoelectric noninvasive detection of multiple vital signs. *Scientific Reports* 10: 416. doi:10.1038/s41598-019-57326-6.

142 Goel, M. (2003). Electret sensors, filters and MEMS devices: New challenges in materials research. *Current Science* 85: 443–453.

143 Reed, T.R., Reed, N.E., and Fritzson, P. (2004). Heart sound analysis for symptom detection and computer-aided diagnosis. *Simulation Modelling Practice and Theory* 12: 129–146. https://doi.org/10.1016/j.simpat.2003.11.005.

144 Hu, Y. and Xu, Y. (2012). An ultra-sensitive wearable accelerometer for continuous heart and lung sound monitoring. *In Proceedings of 2012 Annual International Conference of the IEEE Engineering in Medicine and Biology Society* 28 Aug.–1 Sept.: 694–697. doi:10.1109/EMBC.2012.6346026.

145 Mubarak, Q.-U.-A., Akram, M.U., Shaukat, A., Hussain, F., Khawaja, S.G., and Butt, W.H. (2018). Analysis of PCG signals using quality assessment and homomorphic filters for localization and classification of heart sounds. *Computer Methods and Programs in Biomedicine* 164: 143–157. https://doi.org/10.1016/j.cmpb.2018.07.006.

146 Gupta, C., Gupta, S., Ayers, C., Thompson, B.S., Mammen, P.P., Markham, D.W., and Drazner, M.H. (2008). Reproducibility of acoustic cardiography in detecting a third heart sound. *Journal of Cardiac Failure* 14: S108. doi:10.1016/j.cardfail.2008.06.376.

147 Chen, T.E., Yang, S.I., Ho, L.T., Tsai, K.H., Chen, Y.H., Chang, Y.F., Lai, Y.H., Wang, S.S., Tsao, Y., and Wu, C.C. (2017). S1 and S2 heart sound recognition using deep neural networks. *IEEE Transactions on Biomedical Engineering* 64: 372–380. doi:10.1109/TBME.2016.2559800.

148 Siejko, K.Z., Thakur, P.H., Maile, K., Patangay, A., and Olivari, M.-T. (2013). Feasibility of heart sounds measurements from an accelerometer within an ICD pulse generator. *Pacing and Clinical Electrophysiology* 36: 334–346. https://doi.org/10.1111/pace.12059.

149 Lin, W.Y., Chou, W.C., Chang, P.C., Chou, C.C., Wen, M.S., Ho, M.Y., Lee, W.C., Hsieh, M.J., Lin, C.C., Tsai, T.H., et al. (2018). Identification of location specific feature points in a cardiac cycle using a novel seismocardiogram spectrum system. *IEEE Journal of Biomedical and Health Informatics* 22: 442–449. doi:10.1109/JBHI.2016.2620496.

150 Shafiq, G., Tatinati, S., Ang, W.T., and Veluvolu, K.C. (2016). Automatic identification of systolic time intervals in seismocardiogram. *Scientific Reports* 6: 37524. doi:10.1038/srep37524.

151 Giovangrandi, L., Inan, O.T., Wiard, R.M., Etemadi, M., and Kovacs, G.T.A. (2011). Ballistocardiography – A method worth revisiting. *In Proceedings of 2011 Annual International Conference of the IEEE Engineering in Medicine and Biology Society* 30 Aug.–3 Sept.: 4279–4282.

152 Gubner, R.S., Rodstein, M., and Ungerleider, H.E. (1953). Ballistocardiography; an appraisal of technic, physiologic principles, and clinical value. *Circulation* 7: 268–286. doi:10.1161/01.cir.7.2.268.

153 Alihanka, J., Vaahtoranta, K., and Saarikivi, I. (1981). A new method for long-term monitoring of the ballistocardiogram, heart rate, and respiration. *American Journal of Physiology-Regulatory, Integrative and Comparative Physiology* 240: R384–R392. doi:10.1152/ajpregu.1981.240.5.R384.

154 Bruser, C., Stadlthanner, K., Waele, S.D., and Leonhardt, S. (2011). Adaptive beat-to-beat heart rate estimation in ballistocardiograms. *IEEE Transactions on Information Technology in Biomedicine* 15: 778–786. doi:10.1109/TITB.2011.2128337.

155 Chung, G.S., Lee, J.S., Hwang, S.H., Lim, Y.K., Jeong, D., and Park, K.S. (2010). Wakefulness estimation only using ballistocardiogram: Nonintrusive method for sleep monitoring. *Proceedings of 2010 Annual International Conference of the IEEE Engineering in Medicine and Biology* 31 Aug. –4 Sept.: 2459–2462. doi:10.1109/IEMBS.2010.5626544.

156 Inan, O.T., Etemadi, M., Wiard, R.M., Kovacs, G.T.A., and Giovangrandi, L. (2009). Novel methods for estimating the ballistocardiogram signal using a simultaneously acquired electrocardiogram. *Proceedings of 2009 Annual International Conference of the IEEE Engineering in Medicine and Biology Society* 3-6 Sept: 5334–5347.

157 Wiard, R.M., Inan, O.T., Argyres, B., Etemadi, M., Kovacs, G.T.A., and Giovangrandi, L. (2011). Automatic detection of motion artifacts in the ballistocardiogram measured on a modified bathroom scale. *Medical & Biological Engineering & Computing* 49: 213–220. doi:10.1007/s11517-010-0722-y.

158 Conn, N.J., Schwarz, K.Q., and Borkholder, D.A. (2019). In-home cardiovascular monitoring system for heart failure: Comparative study. *JMIR Mhealth Uhealth* 7: e12419. doi:10.2196/12419.

159 Inan, O.T., Etemadi, M., Wiard, R.M., Giovangrandi, L., and Kovacs, G.T.A. (2009). Robust ballistocardiogram acquisition for home monitoring. *Physiological Measurement* 30: 169–185. doi:10.1088/0967-3334/30/2/005.

160 Elgendi, M. (2012). On the analysis of fingertip photoplethysmogram signals. *Current Cardiology Reviews* 8: 14–25. doi:10.2174/157340312801215782.

161 Jubran, A. (1999). Pulse oximetry. *Critical Care* 3: R11. doi:10.1186/cc341.

162 Azmal, G.M., Al-Jumaily, A., and Al-Jaafreh, M. (2006). Continuous measurement of oxygen saturation level using photoplethysmography signal. *Proceedings of 2006 International Conference on Biomedical and Pharmaceutical Engineering* 11–14 Dec.: 504–507.

163 Sviridova, N. and Sakai, K. (2015). Human photoplethysmogram: New insight into chaotic characteristics. *Chaos, Solitons, and Fractals* 77: 53–63. https://doi.org/10.1016/j.chaos.2015.05.005.

164 Masip, J., Gayà, M., Páez, J., Betbesé, A., Vecilla, F., Manresa, R., and Ruíz, P. (2012). Pulse oximetry in the diagnosis of acute heart failure. *Revista Española De Cardiologia (English Edition)* 65: 879–884. https://doi.org/10.1016/j.rec.2012.02.021.

165 Januzzi, J.L., Jr., Sakhuja, R., O'Donoghue, M., Baggish, A.L., Anwaruddin, S., Chae, C.U., Cameron, R., Krauser, D.G., Tung, R., Camargo, C.A., Jr., et al. (2006). Utility of amino-terminal pro–brain natriuretic peptide testing for prediction of 1-year mortality in patients with dyspnea treated in the emergency department. *Archives of Internal Medicine* 166: 315–320. doi:10.1001/archinte.166.3.315.

166 Anand Inder, S., Fisher Lloyd, D., Chiang, Y.-T., Latini, R., Masson, S., Maggioni Aldo, P., Glazer Robert, D., Tognoni, G., and Cohn Jay, N. (2003). Changes in brain natriuretic peptide and norepinephrine over time and mortality and morbidity in the Valsartan heart failure trial (Val-HeFT). *Circulation* 107: 1278–1283. doi:10.1161/01.CIR.0000054164.99881.00.

167 Chow Sheryl, L., Maisel Alan, S., Anand, I., Bozkurt, B., De Boer Rudolf, A., Felker, G.M., Fonarow Gregg, C., Greenberg, B., Januzzi James, L., Kiernan Michael, S., et al. (2017). Role of biomarkers for the prevention, assessment, and management of heart failure: A scientific statement from the American Heart Association. *Circulation* 135: e1054–e1091. doi:10.1161/CIR.0000000000000490.

168 Maisel, A.S., Krishnaswamy, P., Nowak, R.M., McCord, J., Hollander, J.E., Duc, P., Omland, T., Storrow, A.B., Abraham, W.T., Wu, A.H.B., et al. (2002). Rapid measurement of B-type natriuretic peptide in the emergency diagnosis of heart failure. *New England Journal of Medicine* 347: 161–167. doi:10.1056/NEJMoa020233.

169 Januzzi, J.L., Camargo, C.A., Anwaruddin, S., Baggish, A.L., Chen, A.A., Krauser, D.G., Tung, R., Cameron, R., Nagurney, J.T., Chae, C.U., et al. (2005). The N-terminal Pro-BNP investigation of dyspnea in the emergency department (PRIDE) study. *The American Journal of Cardiology* 95: 948–954. https://doi.org/10.1016/j.amjcard.2004.12.032.

170 McDonald, K., Troughton, R., Dahlström, U., Dargie, H., Krum, H., Van Der Meer, P., McDonagh, T., Atherton, J.J., Kupfer, K., San George, R.C., et al. (2018). Daily home BNP monitoring in heart failure for prediction of impending clinical deterioration: Results from the HOME HF study. *European Journal of Heart Failure* 20: 474–480. https://doi.org/10.1002/ejhf.1053.

171 Maisel, A., Barnard, D., Jaski, B., Frivold, G., Marais, J., Azer, M., Miyamoto Michael, I., Lombardo, D., Kelsay, D., Borden, K., et al. (2013). Primary results of the HABIT trial (Heart failure assessment with BNP in the home). *Journal of the American College of Cardiology* 61: 1726–1735. doi:10.1016/j.jacc.2013.01.052.

172 Klersy, C., De Silvestri, A., Gabutti, G., Regoli, F., and Auricchio, A. (2009). A meta-analysis of remote monitoring of heart failure patients. *Journal of the American College of Cardiology* 54: 1683–1694. doi:10.1016/j.jacc.2009.08.017.

173 Yun, J.E., Park, J.-E., Park, H.-Y., Lee, H.-Y., and Park, D.-A. (2018). Comparative effectiveness of telemonitoring versus usual care for heart failure: A systematic review and meta-analysis. *Journal of Cardiac Failure* 24: 19–28. https://doi.org/10.1016/j.cardfail.2017.09.006.

174 Conraads, V.M., Tavazzi, L., Santini, M., Oliva, F., Gerritse, B., Yu, C.-M., and Cowie, M.R. (2011). Sensitivity and positive predictive value of implantable intrathoracic impedance monitoring as a predictor of heart failure hospitalizations: The SENSE-HF trial. *European Heart Journal* 32: 2266–2273. doi:10.1093/eurheartj/ehr050.

175 Heist, E.K., Herre, J.M., Binkley, P.F., Van Bakel, A.B., Porterfield, J.G., Porterfield, L.M., Qu, F., Turkel, M., and Pavri, B.B. (2014). Analysis of different device-based intrathoracic impedance vectors for detection of heart failure events (from the Detect fluid early from intrathoracic impedance monitoring study). *The American Journal of Cardiology* 114: 1249–1256. https://doi.org/10.1016/j.amjcard.2014.07.048.

176 Hindricks, G., Taborsky, M., Glikson, M., Heinrich, U., Schumacher, B., Katz, A., Brachmann, J., Lewalter, T., Goette, A., Block, M., et al. (2014). Implant-based multiparameter telemonitoring of patients with heart failure (IN-TIME): A randomised controlled trial. *The Lancet* 384: 583–590. https://doi.org/10.1016/S0140-6736(14)61176-4.

177 Landolina, M., Perego Giovanni, B., Lunati, M., Curnis, A., Guenzati, G., Vicentini, A., Parati, G., Borghi, G., Zanaboni, P., Valsecchi, S., et al. (2012). Remote monitoring reduces healthcare use and improves quality of care in heart failure patients with implantable defibrillators. *Circulation* 125: 2985–2992. doi:10.1161/CIRCULATIONAHA.111.088971.

178 Anand, I.S., Tang, W.H.W., Greenberg, B.H., Chakravarthy, N., Libbus, I., and Katra, R.P. (2012). Design and performance of a multisensor heart failure monitoring algorithm: Results from the multisensor monitoring in congestive heart failure (MUSIC) study. *Journal of Cardiac Failure* 18: 289–295. https://doi.org/10.1016/j.cardfail.2012.01.009.

179 Cleland John, G.F., Louis Amala, A., Rigby Alan, S., Janssens, U., and Balk Aggie, H.M.M. (2005). Noninvasive home telemonitoring for patients with heart failure at high risk of recurrent admission and death. *Journal of the American College of Cardiology* 45 (1654–1664): doi:10.1016/j.jacc.2005.01.050.

180 Lyngå, P., Persson, H., Hägg-Martinell, A., Hägglund, E., Hagerman, I., Langius-Eklöf, A., and Rosenqvist, M. (2012). Weight monitoring in patients with severe heart failure (WISH). A randomized controlled trial. *European Journal of Heart Failure* 14: 438–444. https://doi.org/10.1093/eurjhf/hfs023.

181 Dovancescu, S., Saczynski, J.S., Darling, C.E., Riistama, J., Sert Kuniyoshi, F., Meyer, T., Goldberg, R., and McManus, D.D. (2015). Detecting heart failure decompensation by measuring transthoracic bioimpedance in the outpatient setting: Rationale and design of the SENTINEL-HF study. *JMIR Research Protocols* 4: e121. doi:10.2196/resprot.4899.

182 Kotb, A., Cameron, C., Hsieh, S., and Wells, G. (2015). Comparative effectiveness of different forms of telemedicine for individuals with heart failure (HF): A systematic review and network meta-analysis. *PLOS ONE* 10: e0118681. doi:10.1371/journal.pone.0118681.

183 Nouryan, C.N., Morahan, S., Pecinka, K., Akerman, M., Lesser, M., Chaikin, D., Castillo, S., Zhang, M., and Pekmezaris, R. (2018). Home telemonitoring of community-dwelling heart failure patients after home care discharge. *Telemedicine and e-Health* 25: 447–454. doi:10.1089/tmj.2018.0099.

184 Gingele, A.J., Ramaekers, B., Brunner-La Rocca, H.P., De Weerd, G., Kragten, J., Van Empel, V., Van Der Weg, K., Vrijhoef, H.J.M., Gorgels, A., Cleuren, G., et al. (2019). Effects of tailored telemonitoring on functional status and health-related quality of life in patients with heart failure. *Netherlands Heart Journal* 27: 565–574. doi:10.1007/s12471-019-01323-x.

185 Emani, S. (2017). Remote monitoring to reduce heart failure readmissions. *Current Heart Failure Reports* 14: 40–47. doi:10.1007/s11897-017-0315-2.

186 Khalil, S.F., Mohktar, M.S., and Ibrahim, F. (2014). The theory and fundamentals of bioimpedance analysis in clinical status monitoring and diagnosis of diseases. *Sensors* 14. doi: 10.3390/s140610895.

187 Maurizi, N., Faragli, A., Imberti, J., Briante, N., Targetti, M., Baldini, K., Sall, A., Cisse, A., Berzolari, F.G., Borrelli, P., et al. (2017). Cardiovascular screening in low-income settings using a novel 4-lead smartphone-based electrocardiograph (D-Heart®). *International Journal of Cardiology* 236: 249–252. doi:10.1016/j.ijcard.2017.02.027.

188 Raja, J.M., Elsakr, C., Roman, S., Cave, B., Pour-Ghaz, I., Nanda, A., Maturana, M., and Khouzam, R.N. (2019). Apple watch, wearables, and heart rhythm: Where do we stand? *Annals of Translational Medicine* 7: 417-417. doi:10.21037/atm.2019.06.79.

189 DeVore, A.D., Wosik, J., and Hernandez, A.F. (2019). The future of wearables in heart failure patients. *JACC. Heart Failure* 7: 922–932. https://doi.org/10.1016/j.jchf.2019.08.008.

190 Cleland, J.G.F. and Antony, R. (2011). It makes SENSE to take a safer road. *European Heart Journal* 32: 2225–2227. doi:10.1093/eurheartj/ehr120.

191 Inglis, S.C., Conway, A., Cleland, J.G.F., and Clark, R.A. (2014). Is age a factor in the success or failure of remote monitoring in heart failure? Telemonitoring and structured telephone support in elderly heart failure patients. *European Journal of Cardiovascular Nursing* 14: 248–255. doi:10.1177/1474515114530611.

192 Ware, P., Dorai, M., Ross, H.J., Cafazzo, J.A., Laporte, A., Boodoo, C., and Seto, E. (2019). Patient adherence to a mobile phone–based heart failure telemonitoring program: A longitudinal mixed-methods study. *JMIR Mhealth Uhealth* 7: e13259. doi:10.2196/13259.

193 Availabe online: https://www.cardiovascular.abbott/us/en/patients/treatments-therapies/pulmonary-artery-pressure-monitoring-for-heart-failure/managing-heart-failure.html (accessed on 15 April 2021).

6

Artificial Intelligence Techniques in Cardiology

An Overview

Ikram-Ul Haq and Bo Xu

6.1 Introduction

The unique marvel of human intelligence lies in its innate ability to reason, meta-reason, and seamlessly synthesize abstract concepts, distinct from the binary logic of computer science. Artificial intelligence (AI) is a rapidly evolving transdisciplinary field. It integrates computer science, statistics, psychology, neuroscience, material science, mechanical engineering, and computer hardware design to develop algorithms that aim to simulate human intuition, decision-making, and object recognition [1]. The concepts and methodologies underpinning AI have been well-established for some time, but recent technological advancements that support processing large volumes of data have driven a surge in interest in AI [2]. Machine learning (ML) refers to a collection of techniques which enable AI.

The overarching objectives of AI in medicine are threefold: to optimize patient care, to improve efficiency, and to improve clinical outcomes. More specifically, there are growing applications in the fields of basic science drug discovery, genetic-based treatments, radiology, and surgical specialties [1, 2]. In cardiology, there has been a growth in the potential sources of new patient data, as well as advances in investigations and therapies, which position the field well to uniquely benefit from AI: for clinicians, these benefits potentially translate into improving the accuracy of diagnosis, risk assessment, prognostication, and decision-making for treatments; for health systems, these benefits potentially translate into improved workflows and technical protocols, reducing medical errors and costs; for patients, these benefits potentially translate into promoting optimal prevention and treatment of cardiovascular disease.

This chapter aims to introduce the various AI techniques and their respective applications in cardiovascular medicine, to introduce the steps involved in building AI algorithms, as well as to discuss the current limitations and pitfalls.

Predicting Heart Failure: Invasive, Non-Invasive, Machine Learning, and Artificial Intelligence Based Methods, First Edition. Edited by Kishor Kumar Sadasivuni, Hassen M. Ouakad, Somaya Al-Maadeed, Huseyin C. Yalcin, and Issam Bait Bahadur.

6.2 Artificial Intelligence Techniques

6.2.1 Artificial Intelligence and Statistical Models

AI can be understood as an extension of statistical modeling, with the differences related less to methodologies and more to the respective objectives and the questions they aim to answer (Figure 6.1). Statistics is the mathematical study of data, and statistical models use data to infer relationships and extrapolate values [1]. However, statistical models emphasize understanding the relationships between data points rather than extrapolating values [2]. In comparison, the primary goal of AI is to predict future values using existing data, with less emphasis being placed on understanding the relationships between variables [3]. However, there are exceptions to this rule with some ML techniques, such as LASSO (least absolute shrinkage and selection operator) regression which allow relationships between data points to be analyzed.

At the most superficial level, AI can be divided into general and applied (or narrow) AI (Figure 6.2) [4]. General AI refers to the ability of an algorithmic system to process, learn, and solve previously unseen problems; this is yet to be achieved. Applied or narrow AI is more common and refers to algorithmic processes being developed for specific and specialized purposes [2].

6.2.2 Machine Learning

ML techniques vary in their objectives, applications, and architectures (Table 6.1). The type, structure, and depth of input data influence which algorithm is most appropriate in answering a research question. Some algorithms, such as supervised learning algorithms are better suited for analyzing structured data over languages, and others, including deep learning, are more suited to images with spatial resolution [5]. In brief, ML is an iterative process that involves approximating complex mathematical relationships between inputs and outputs by learning from a large data set to predict values from new, unseen data [6]. Supervised, unsupervised, semi-supervised, reinforcement, and deep learning are terms describing how ML algorithms learn from data.

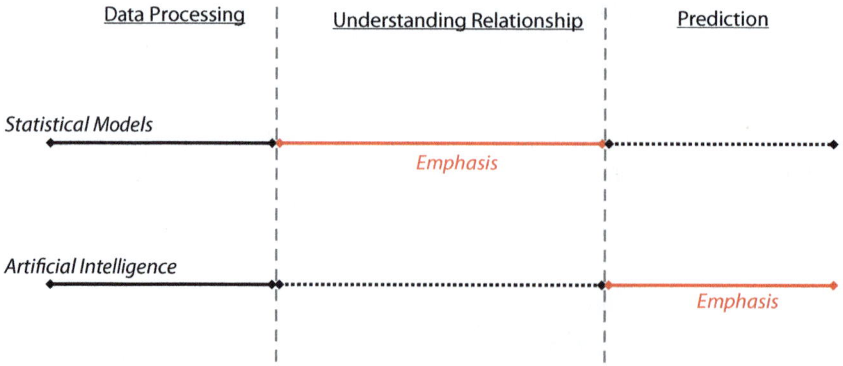

Figure 6.1 Relationship between statistical models and AI.

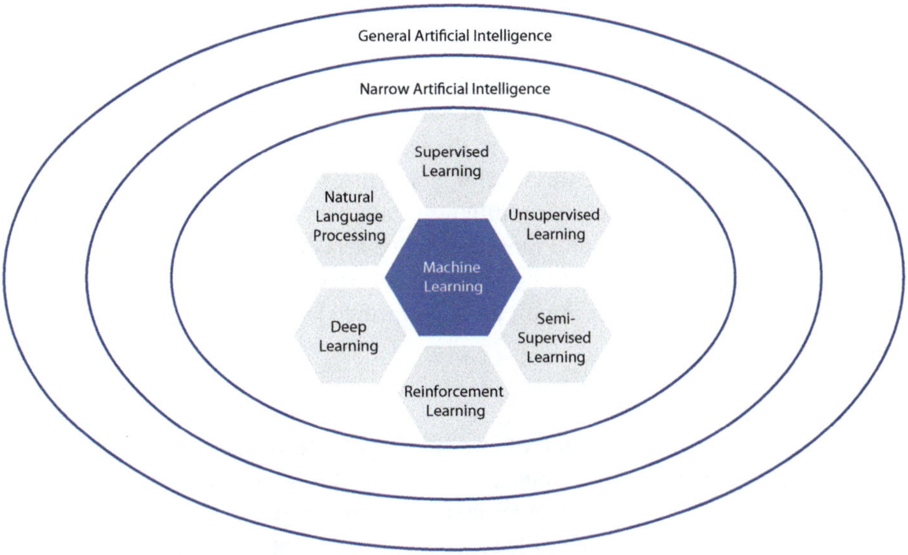

Figure 6.2 Relationship between AI and ML techniques.

Table 6.1 ML techniques.

Type of Learning	ML Algorithm	Outcomes
Supervised	Classification	Categorical
Labeled data with defined outputs	Regression	Continuous
Unsupervised	Clustering	Similarity of inputs
Unlabeled data with unknown outputs	Dimensionality reduction	Extract relevant features
	Association	Co-occurrence likelihood
	Anomaly reduction	Outliers
Semi-supervised	Generative	Combination of supervised and unsupervised outcomes
Reinforcement	Reward based	Sequential decision-making

6.2.2.1 Supervised Learning

Supervised learning refers to algorithms learning rules between a set of inputs and outputs using a labeled training data set (referred to as mapping) in order to predict outcomes for new inputs. The labeled training data set typically consists of predictor variables, features, and labeled outcomes (Table 6.1). Features refer to pieces of information that make up data and the quality, accuracy, and richness of features determine the overall effectiveness of supervised ML algorithms [7].

The aim in training a supervised ML algorithm is to optimize its generalizability such that the model defines the underlying relationship but not to the extent of introducing inadvertent bias from poorly curated data sets [1]. Hence, a variance-bias trade-off exists where variance refers to how well the model performs with new, subtly different data, and bias refers to how well the model fits to the training data [7]. Overfitting refers to a model with a high bias and a low variance: it is overfitted to the training data set such that it struggles to adapt to new, subtly different data. Obtaining large sets of reliably labeled data is often the hardest and most expensive aspect of creating supervised ML algorithms. It is important that training is monitored to ensure an optimal balance of bias and variance [7]. The most common tasks performed by supervised models include classification and regression.

6.2.2.1.1 Classification

Classification is used when the output of an ML algorithm is a categorical variable and involves classifying data points into one or more categories. Linear separability is a key concept underpinning this approach and refers to the notion of using a line or a plane to separate data (Figure 6.3). The line or plane separating data into classes is referred to as a decision boundary, and the area chosen to define a class is referred to as a decision surface (Figure 6.3). If a data point falls within a decision surface, it is assigned to that class.

Support vector machines (SVMs) are a commonly used technique in supervised classification ML algorithms and use hyperplanes to separate data points. An optimal hyperplane separates classes in a way that creates maximum separation between the different classes. SVMs are relatively straightforward but are less useful in analyzing more complex, multidimensional data. Instead, kernel methods are typically used for complex multidimensional data where samples cannot be linearly separated.

6.2.2.1.2 Regression

Regression is used when the output of a supervised ML model is a continuous variable; commonly used regression techniques include LASSO, rich regression, and elastic net

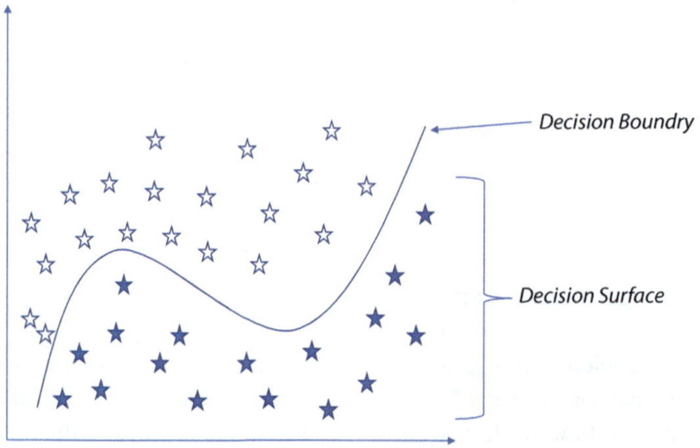

Figure 6.3 Linear and non-linear decision boundaries and surfaces.

regression. LASSO regression is an important regularization technique which uses shrinkage to avoid a regression model being overfitted [5, 6]. Shrinkage refers to data points being shrunk toward the mean. It remains an important type of regression for models which include multiple factors that are correlated or have a high level of multicollinearity [7].

6.2.2.1.3 Examples of Supervised Learning in Cardiology

There are a growing number of studies applying supervised ML algorithms to cardiology, including in personalized medicine, imaging, and disease prognostication. Personalized medicine involves tailoring investigations, treatments, and predictions to individual patients, thereby minimizing reductionism. Reductionism refers to treating all patients with the same disease states identically, irrespective of their genetics, lifestyle, background, and determinants of cardiovascular health [6]. One aspect of precision medicine involves creating a digital twin of the patient which integrates genomics, wearable devices, electronic health records, imaging data, and other data points to create a simulated model of the patient that is updated in real time through statistical and mechanistic modeling [2]. Traditional cardiovascular risk models extrapolate risk from a sample population, inevitably ignoring subtle clinical confounders. In contrast, AI algorithms can personalize risk calculations by including complex and subtle clinical factors.

One example is a study using supervised ML algorithms to predict 5-year all-cause mortality (ACM) in patients with suspected coronary artery disease (CAD) using cardiac computed tomographic angiography (CCTA) images [8]. Included in the development of this algorithm were 25 clinical and 44 CCTA parameters, and the algorithm was found to be superior to the Framingham risk score (FRS), segment stenosis score (SSS), segment involvement score (SIS), and the modified Duke index (MDI) in predicting 5-year ACM (ML: 0.79 vs. FRS: 0.61, SSS: 0.64, SIS: 0.64, DI: 0.62; $p < 0.001$) [8]. Another example is a study that combined CCTA stenosis and plaque measurements to develop a supervised ML algorithm to predict myocardial flow reserve (MFR) [9]. In the study, 153 arteries in 51 patients undergoing CCTA were analyzed to build this composite risk score and the algorithm was found to be superior to quantitative CCTA stenosis in predicting MFR by ^{13}N-ammonia PET scan (ML AUC = 0.83, CTA stenosis = 0.66; $p = 0.005$) [9]. A similar multicenter trial evaluated a boosted ensemble ML algorithm built from quantitative CCTA measurements to predict lesion-specific ischemia [10]. In the trial, 254 patients underwent CCTA and invasive coronary angiogram with fractional flow reserve (FFR) measurement in 484 vessels [10]. The ML algorithm had a superior area under the curve (AUC) of 0.84 compared with individual CCTA measurements (AUC: 0.76; $p < 0.006$) [10].

Supervised ML algorithms have also been applied to other cardiac imaging modalities. A recent study used a combination of supervised and deep learning to develop an ML algorithm using 91,232 single-lead ECGs from 53,549 patients to classify a single ambulatory electrocardiogram (ECG) monitoring lead into 12 rhythm classes with an AUC of 0.97, when tested in an independent data set with a consensus committee of board-certified cardiologists [11]. In echocardiography, supervised ML algorithms have been developed to identify and classify different echo views, including one study successfully classifying 15 standard views with an accuracy of 91.7% after training the supervised ML algorithm on 267 transthoracic echocardiogram (TTE) studies [12]. This was in comparison to an average accuracy of 79.4% for board-certified echocardiographers classifying a subset of the same test images ($p = 0.03$) [12]. Classification supervised ML algorithms have also been studied in echocardiography to differentiate hypertrophic cardiomyopathy from physiologic hypertrophy, and constrictive cardiomyopathy from restrictive cardiomyopathy [13–15]. In CCTA, supervised ML algorithms have also been applied to automatically quantify coronary artery calcification [16]. Algorithms have also been used to identify patients with hemodynamically significant CAD by analyzing the left ventricle (LV) [17]. For example, one study analyzed CCTA scans from 166 patients who underwent invasive FFR and used a series of ML algorithms to segment, classify, and identify ischemic changes in the LV myocardium [17]. After that, a SVM classifier was used to categorize patients according to the presence of functionally significant stenosis with an AUC of 0.74 when compared with invasive hemodynamic testing [17].

Another case of supervised ML algorithms is in disease prognostication. For example, algorithms have been successfully used to predict which patients with CAD will eventually undergo early revascularization [18]. A recent study evaluated 713 myocardial perfusion scans (MPSs) and associated invasive angiography to compare an ML algorithm with visual analysis by two experienced readers [18]. It found the specificity of the algorithm in predicting early both revascularization and 3-year major adverse cardiovascular events was superior ($74.7 \pm 4.2\%$) [18].

Other examples of regression-based supervised ML learning include a recent study illustrating that three-dimensional (3D) cardiac motion can predict survival in patients with newly diagnosed pulmonary hypertension [19]. In this study, 256 patients with newly diagnosed pulmonary hypertension underwent cardiac MRI, right heart catheterization and a 6-minute walk test [19]. A supervised ML algorithm was then applied to a 3D model of right ventricular motion and better predicted survival compared with conventional imaging, hemodynamic, functional, and clinical markers (AUC = 0.73 vs 0.60; $p < 0.001$) [19]. The study found impaired contractile motion in anatomically distinct but functionally synergistic areas of the right ventricle provided early signals as to the severity of pulmonary hypertension and hence mortality [19].

6.2.2.2 Unsupervised Learning

Unsupervised learning is a more advanced form of learning using unlabeled data to discover underlying relationships; it is often referred to as knowledge discovery [7]. Unsupervised learning holds great promise in clinical practice where coding large data sets can be prohibitively expensive and time-consuming. Common examples of unsupervised learning techniques include clustering, dimensionality reduction, association, and anomaly detection [2].

Clustering involves dividing objects into groups that share similar characteristics with the aim of finding subgroups within a larger data set. The most commonly used techniques include hierarchical clustering, K-means clustering, density-based spatial clustering of applications with noise, and model-based clustering [7]. Irrelevant features can compromise the efficacy, efficiency, and utility of ML algorithms and dimensionality reduction is a technique used to minimize irrelevant features by identifying the most important features in a data set [20]. Anomaly detection is a technique that identifies outliers in a data set and helps unsupervised ML algorithms remove anomalies and erroneous data entries [6].

6.2.2.2.1 Examples of Unsupervised Learning in Cardiology

Unsupervised learning is often combined with more advanced techniques, such as deep learning, when applied to large, complex data sets in cardiology. One example is a comprehensive unsupervised ML algorithm which was able to successfully differentiate heart failure with preserved ejection fraction (HFpEF) from healthy subjects by analyzing LV long axis myocardial velocity patterns on stress echocardiography [14]. This study built an unsupervised ML algorithm from 156 patients using 22 descriptors with 300 features collected from tissue Doppler-derived longitudinal myocardial velocity traces at rest and during exercise [14]. The algorithm found naturally occurring patterns and relationships within the details to identify a continuum of disease from normal cardiac function to patients with HFpEF [14]. The spectrum varied in age, body mass index, left ventricular mass index, and left ventricular filling pressures and symptom burden as measured by the 6-minute walk test [14].

Clustering-based algorithms are the more common examples of unsupervised learning in cardiology. One example is an unsupervised ML algorithm used to identify distinct hypertensive subgroups associated with the myocardial substrate for HFpEF [21]. The ML algorithm clustered 1273 patients into two mutually exclusive pheno-groups, based on 47 variables including clinical characteristics, cardiac structure, and function [21]. These subgroups may represent different genotypes that could benefit from targeted therapies to prevent HFpEF onset [21]. Another example is in type 2 diabetes mellitus where an unsupervised ML algorithm was applied to the echocardiographic images of 842 patients from two prospective cohorts to identify three clusters of patients from 12 echocardiographic variables [22]. Cluster 1 patients had the lowest LV mass index, the highest LV ejection fraction (LVEF), and were predominantly male; Cluster 2 patients were the oldest and had the highest strain and E/e' ratios; Cluster 3 patients had the highest LV mass index and the lowest LVEF [22]. A cluster analysis was then performed which found clusters 2 and 3 were associated with worse cardiovascular mortality and hospitalizations compared with cluster 1 (HR 2.37) [22]. Hierarchical clustering algorithms have also been studied to identify distinct clusters in diastolic heart failure. One study performed a cluster analysis and developed an ML model of LV diastolic dysfunction from 130 patients that was subsequently tested in a prospective cohort of 44 patients [23]. Speckle-tracking echocardiography (STE) was used to measure simultaneous changes in left atrial and ventricular volumes, longitudinal strains, and strain rates [23]. STE strongly correlated with conventional indices and clustered patients into three groups with differing severities of diastolic dysfunction and LV filling pressures [23]. Another example is a study that identified two distinct groups using an unsupervised, hierarchical cluster analysis of echocardiographic parameters of diastolic dysfunction in 866 patients [24]. Compared with conventional classification, the clustering algorithm improved prediction of all-cause and cardiac mortality [24]. Similarly, other studies have used unsupervised clustering-based ML algorithms to identify differences in clinical, structural, and invasive hemodynamics, which have been correlated with hospitalizations and with all-cause and cardiac mortality [3, 25].

6.2.2.3 Semi-Supervised Learning

Semi-supervised learning combines supervised and unsupervised learning techniques. One of the more costly and time-consuming aspects of supervised learning is accurately labeling large data sets [25]. Semi-supervised learning provides the ability to extrapolate and label a large data set from a smaller, manually labeled data set. This is performed by manually labeling a small portion of data and then employing unsupervised learning algorithms to extrapolate from this data. Generative adversarial networks (GAN) are a commonly used semi-supervised technique that employs two neural networks: a generator and discriminator [1, 2, 25]. Generators are trained to synthesize plausible data points as outputs, and the discriminator is a typical convolutional neural network that aims to distinguish between fake and real data [7].

6.2.2.3.1 Examples of Semi-Supervised Learning in Cardiology

Semi-supervised learning is a more novel technique that requires knowledge of various learning techniques. Several studies have employed this in cardiology that have focused on using semi-supervised ML algorithms to quantify chamber dimensions on echocardiography. An example are algorithms developed to automatically quantify left atrium (LA), LV volumes, and LVEF from 3D TTE images [26, 27]. One study applied this algorithm to 159 patients and found automated LVEF measurements using a semi-supervised algorithm had a strong correlation both with manual 3D volumetric measurements from three readers ($r = 0.87–0.96$) and with cardiac magnetic resonance (CMR) ($r = 0.84–0.95$) [26]. Another example is a study which included apical four- and two-chamber views from 255 patients across four centers and applied a semi-supervised ML algorithm to assess EF and LV longitudinal strain. The fully automated algorithm was compared with manual estimation, and the study found the algorithm to be feasible in 98% of studies with an average analysis time of 8 seconds per patient [27].

6.2.2.4 Reinforcement Learning

Reinforcement learning is a technique in which an algorithm is trained to learn an action that gains maximum reward. The algorithm is given input data and a specific outcome to optimize, learning through trial and error. This technique is seldom used in cardiology, but is more commonly used in computer gaming programs; a notable example is AlphaGo (a computer program that uses reinforcement learning to play Go) [1]. However, one example of reinforcement learning in cardiology is a study which aimed to use this technique to detect eight anatomical landmarks, including bony structures, organs, and vessel bifurcations, from 1487 3D-CT scans from 532 patients [28].

6.2.3 Deep Learning

Deep learning is another subfield of ML of which artificial neural networks (ANNs), recurrent neural networks (RNNs), and convolutional neural networks (CNNs) are the most commonly used techniques [25]. In comparison with traditional ML algorithms, deep learning requires minimal data arbitration or feature engineering (Figure 6.4). Feature engineering is a key step in building an ML model and consists of extracting all the required features for a problem statement (feature extraction) and selecting the most important features that will improve the ML model (feature selection). Deep learning automates the process of feature engineering and interrogates the input data directly.

ANNs are modeled on the neural structures of the brain and consist of interconnected perceptrons with varying weights, indicating the strength of each connection (Figure

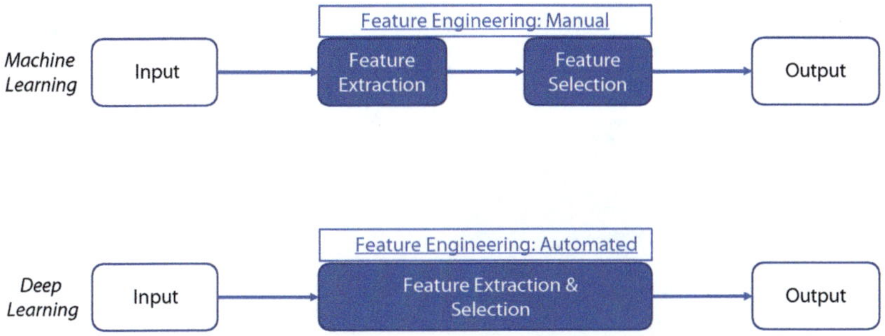

Figure 6.4 Comparing ML and deep learning.

6.5). By providing an ANN with a large training data set, these weights are fine-tuned, and the ANN is optimized to better establish the relationship between input and output [7]. ANNs typically consist of three layers – input, hidden, and output layer – and process inputs in a forward direction to solve problems related to tabular, image, or textual data [25]. ANNs can use many hidden layers to produce increasingly abstracted and non-linear representations of underlying data [1].

When a looping constraint is applied to a hidden layer of an ANN, it becomes an RNN [7]. RNNs are particularly well suited to processing sequential data, such as speech and language.

CNNs are fully connected neural networks that have learnable weights and biases. They employ kernels for automatic feature extraction which are a series of convolutional operations which progressively extract relevant features. CNNs are particularly useful in processing large and complex data sets such as imaging data [25]. Traditional ML algorithms struggle with imaging data as they are highly dimensional, and it is extremely difficult to assign individual weights for each feature.

For example, an image with a pixel size of 750 × 750 and three channels has nearly 2 million features (750 × 750 × 3). Additionally, a single-pixel does not carry enough useful information, but rather a patch of pixels will need to be analyzed [1]. Convolutional layers in a CNN attempt to overcome these difficulties. Each convolutional layer uses a set of filters that forms a small grid of weights and performs a weighted sum nonlinear transformation. The same filter is applied to all possible locations in the whole input. In this way, the number of weights to train is significantly reduced [7].

6.2.3.1 Examples of Deep Learning in Cardiology

Deep learning has been widely studied and applied to various aspects of cardiovascular medicine. One example is its application to ECGs. ECGs are routinely used in the evaluation of patients, and are relatively low-cost and widely available. Deep learning algorithms have been developed to detect structural heart disease, arrhythmias, phenotypic patterns and electrolyte disturbances [11, 29–34]. For example, CNN-derived ML algorithms applied to ECGs have been validated to detect LV systolic dysfunction [30, 34]. One study trained a CNN algorithm to detect LV dysfunction using paired 12-lead ECG and echocardiogram data from 44,959 patients [30]. The algorithm was then tested on an independent sample of 52,870 patients, and was found to have a sensitivity, specificity, and accuracy of 93%, 86.3%, and 85.7%, respectively [30]. Another example is a

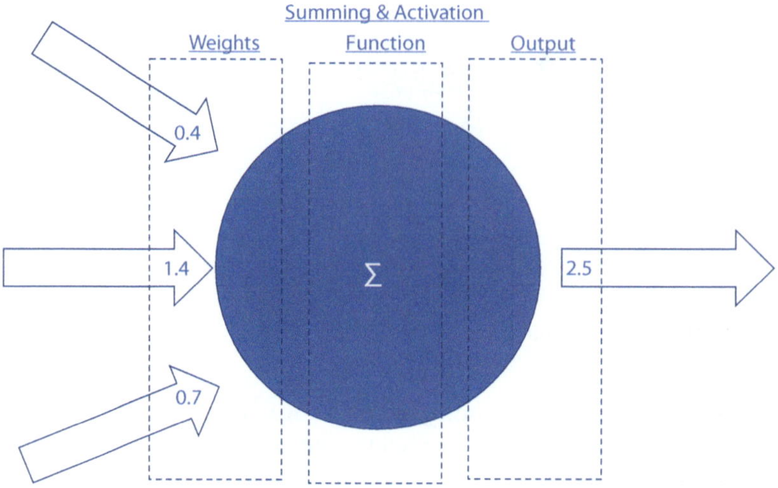

Figure 6.5 A perceptron and a simple ANN with interconnected perceptrons.

retrospective study which used a CNN algorithm to detect LV hypertrophy in 21,286 patients in two hospitals who underwent 12-lead ECG and echocardiography 4 weeks apart [35]. The AUCs of the AI ECG algorithm were 0.880 (95% CI: 0.877–0.883) and 0.868 (95% CI: 0.865–0.871) in the internal and external validation cohorts respectively, when compared with echocardiography [35]. Unsupervised learning CNN-based ML algorithms have been validated to detect and predict arrhythmias. A recent study developed a CNN-based ML algorithm from 180,922 patients to predict the probability of developing atrial fibrillation from normal sinus rhythm by studying temporal ECGs from these patients [31]. The study split the patients into a training data set (126,526 patients with 454,789 ECGs), internal validation data set (18,116 patients with 64,340 ECGs), and testing data set (36,280 patients with 130,802 ECGs). The algorithm had an AUC of 0.87 (95 % CI: 0.86–0.88), a sensitivity of 79%, and a specificity of 79.5% [31, 36].

CNN has also been validated in detecting obstructive CAD from myocardial perfusion imaging (MPI), compared with total perfusion deficit (TPD). The study included 1638 patients undergoing stress 99mTc-sestamibi or tetrofosmin MPI in nine sites who also underwent invasive coronary angiogram within 6 months [37]. The CNN algorithm was trained using raw and quantified polar maps to evaluate and predict obstructive CAD using stratified 10-fold cross-validation [37]. The AUC for disease prediction by the CNN was higher than for TPD (per patient: 0.80 vs 0.78; per vessel: 0.76 vs 0.73; $p < 0.01$) [37]. Moreover, the time needed for the evaluation of a new patient with the pre-trained model was < 1 second, even without the dedicated graphics board used during the training of the system [37]

6.2.4 Natural Language Processing

Most information in electronic health records is unstructured and in free text. Recent technological advances have allowed narrative text to be extracted using a technique called natural language processing (NLP), which converts unstructured text into a structured form [38]. NLP is a multistep process with the first and most important step being lexical analysis. There are various techniques which can be employed in lexical analysis, and these include part of speech (POS) tagging, hidden Markov model (HMM), names entity recognition (NER) and parsing or syntactic analysis (PSA) [38]. In POS tagging, each word is tagged to a corresponding category of words that share grammatical properties. HMM remembers the sequence of words in a sentence and tagged as nouns, verbs, and determiners. In NER, words are tagged by the type of entity the word represents. These entities can be persons, companies, times, or locations. PSA analyzes the grammar of the text and the way the words are arranged. It uses predefined grammatical rules to test whether a sentence string conforms to these set rules [38]. Examples of its current applications in cardiology include extracting information from clinical notes, radiology reports, and pathology reports.

6.3 Steps in Building an AI Algorithm

Building a clinically meaningful and effective ML algorithm is a multifaceted, complex process, and requires the input of a multidisciplinary team with diverse skills and talents. Most notably, clinicians are at the forefront of delivering healthcare and are most in tune with the problems arising in clinical care. However, clinicians often lack the technical capabilities to develop and test ML algorithms and thus require data scientists. The process can be broken down into six steps (Figure 6.6) [1]. The first is identifying the problem and often requires multidisciplinary input from clinicians, data scientists, data engineers, patients, and other stakeholders [2]. The second is collecting the appropriate data with features and labels of interest; this is often the most time-consuming and expensive aspect. The third is preparing the data through a combination of feature selection and feature engineering [4]. This step is closely linked with the next step, as the type of ML algorithms that can be used is often dictated by the type, quality, and preparation of the data. The fifth step involves developing and building the ML algorithm using a training data set. The final step is validating the ML algorithm through a process of internal and external validation using independent and separate data sets [7].

6.4 Limitations, Challenges, and Opportunities

It is important to appreciate the challenges associated with AI, and these can be broadly divided into limitations relating to existing research, limitations inherent with AI technology, and challenges in clinical translation.

6.4.1 Limitations of Existing Studies

Most studies thus far employ narrow AI and apply ML algorithms to predefined and preselected variables with parameter adjustments in testing cohorts to obtain a good

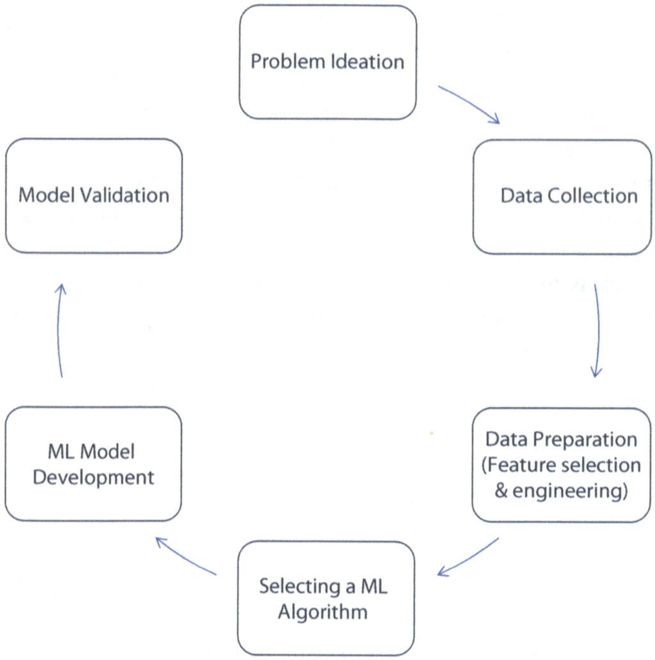

Figure 6.6 Steps in building AI algorithms in cardiology.

performance. Hence, the bulk of ML algorithms have been studied on retrospectively collected and curated data. The major limitation with this approach is the obvious risk of developing models that are overfitted to the target data that do not generalize well to previously unseen external data. There are also the inherent biases which are inadvertently introduced into algorithms that are built and validated solely on retrospective, single-center data. ML algorithms require large data sets, and therefore subtle biases are introduced, such as a lack of diversity leading to unintended downstream consequences of the algorithms being inherently skewed to identify the dominant types of patients contributing to the model development. Another related limitation is the lack of existing frameworks and guidelines in conducting AI research. This lack of data set, methodological, and reporting standardization leads to an inability to comprehensively evaluate for methodological bias in analyses, and often masks biases. Moreover, this makes institutional cross-collaboration more difficult.

The natural next step is to study these ML algorithms on external data sets, not involved in model development, in a multicenter prospective study design. These future prospective studies will need to evaluate patient outcomes and treatment pathways.

6.4.2 Pitfalls with the Technology

As with all technologies, AI remains susceptible to privacy, security, and data breach concerns. Patient data used for algorithm development need to remain de-identified and handled with care. Another unique limitation is the black-box phenomenon, which a lot of ML algorithms suffer from. This refers to the notion that certain ML algorithms, such as deep learning, are inherently opaque where there is a lack of clarity as to how the algorithm processes input data to generate outcomes. This adds to the complexity and difficulty in being able to rigorously critique the methodological validity of ML algorithms. Without this insight, it becomes increasingly difficult to sense-check an algorithm to see if it is in line with real-world observations. An example of this is in risk prediction ML algorithms, where it is important to understand why the algorithm has classified a patient as high risk to help tailor interventions appropriately.

6.4.3 Challenges in Clinical Translation

The novelty of AI algorithms and the lack of prospective, multicenter randomized trials mean that large gaps in evidence exist currently. Most notably, the clinical translational ability of ML algorithms remains relatively unknown, with the practical difficulties of deploying such technologies in real-world clinical practice still not fully investigated. Important considerations include the cost-benefit analysis, the risks of false-positives, and the longer-term clinical outcomes of AI technologies compared with current clinical standards of care. At present, in accordance with the Food and Drug Administration, diagnostic software tools are classified as Class 2 (medium risk devices). If ML algorithms are to be used to guide treatment in addition to diagnosis, they would require a further level of evidence and validation, potentially enabling them to be classified as Class 3 medical devices.

6.5 Conclusions

- Clinical decision-making is reliant on synthesizing high-quality data to help solve patient problems. As the amount of available patient data increases, it is likely clinical decision-making will be augmented by AI techniques in the future.
- AI offers the potential to summarize and synthesize this growth of patient data to potentially guide individualized therapy.
- There is a large variety of ML approaches that can be employed as detailed in this chapter. The most appropriate algorithm choice will be guided by the research question and the type of data available.

References

1 Lopez-Jimenez, F., Attia, Z., Arruda-Olson, A.M., et al. (2020). Artificial Intelligence in Cardiology: Present and Future. *Mayo Clinic Proceedings. Mayo Clinic* 95: 1015–1039.

2 Corral-Acero, J., Margara, F., Marciniak, M., et al. (2020). The "Digital Twin" to enable the vision of precision cardiology. *European Heart Journal* 41: 4556–4564.

3 Dey, D., Slomka, P.J., Leeson, P., et al. (2019). Artificial intelligence in cardiovascular imaging: JACC State-of-the-Art Review. *Journal of the American College of Cardiology* 73: 1317–1335.

4 Johnson, K.W., Torres Soto, J., Glicksberg, B.S., et al. (2018). Artificial intelligence in cardiology. *Journal of the American College of Cardiology* 71: 2668–2679.

5 Xu, B., Kocyigit, D., Grimm, R., Griffin, B.P., and Cheng, F. (2020). Applications of artificial intelligence in multimodality cardiovascular imaging: A state-of-the-art review. *Progress in Cardiovascular Diseases* 63: 367–376.

6 Leopold, J.A. and Loscalzo, J. (2018). Emerging role of precision medicine in cardiovascular disease. *Circulation Research* 122: 1302–1315.

7 Deng, C., Ji, X., Rainey, C., Zhang, J., and Lu, W. (2020). Integrating machine learning with human knowledge. *iScience* 23: 101656.

8 Motwani, M., Dey, D., Berman, D.S., et al. (2017). Machine learning for prediction of all-cause mortality in patients with suspected coronary artery disease: A 5-year multicentre prospective registry analysis. *European Heart Journal* 38: 500–507.

9 Dey, D., Diaz Zamudio, M., Schuhbaeck, A., et al. (2015). Relationship between quantitative adverse plaque features from coronary computed tomography angiography and downstream impaired myocardial flow reserve by 13N-Ammonia positron emission tomography: A pilot study. *Circulation. Cardiovascular Imaging* 8: e003255.

10 Dey, D., Gaur, S., Ovrehus, K.A., et al. (2018). Integrated prediction of lesion-specific ischaemia from quantitative coronary CT angiography using machine learning: A multicentre study. *European Radiology* 28: 2655–2664.

11 Hannun, A.Y., Rajpurkar, P., Haghpanahi, M., et al. (2019). Cardiologist-level arrhythmia detection and classification in ambulatory electrocardiograms using a deep neural network. *Nature Medicine* 25: 65–69.

12 Madani, A., Arnaout, R., Mofrad, M., and Arnaout, R. (2018). Fast and accurate view classification of echocardiograms using deep learning. *NPJ Digital Medicine* 1.

13 Narula, S., Shameer, K., Salem Omar, A.M., Dudley, J.T., and Sengupta, P.P. (2016). Machine-learning algorithms to automate morphological and functional assessments in 2D echocardiography. *Journal of the American College of Cardiology* 68: 2287–2295.

14 Sanchez-Martinez, S., Duchateau, N., Erdei, T., et al. (2018). Machine learning analysis of left ventricular function to characterize heart failure with preserved ejection fraction. *Circulation. Cardiovascular Imaging* 11: e007138.

15 Sengupta, P.P., Huang, Y.M., Bansal, M., et al. (2016). Cognitive machine-learning algorithm for cardiac imaging: A pilot study for differentiating constrictive pericarditis from restrictive cardiomyopathy. *Circulation. Cardiovascular Imaging* 9.

16 Wolterink, J.M., Leiner, T., de Vos, B.D., van Hamersvelt, R.W., Viergever, M.A., and Isgum, I. (2016). Automatic coronary artery calcium scoring in cardiac CT angiography using paired convolutional neural networks. *Medical Image Analysis* 34: 123–136.

17 Zreik, M., Lessmann, N., van Hamersvelt, R.W., et al. (2018). Deep learning analysis of the myocardium in coronary CT angiography for identification of patients with functionally significant coronary artery stenosis. *Medical Image Analysis* 44: 72–85.

18 Arsanjani, R., Dey, D., Khachatryan, T., et al. (2015). Prediction of revascularization after myocardial perfusion SPECT by machine learning in a large population. *Journal of Nuclear Cardiology: Official Publication of the American Society of Nuclear Cardiology* 22: 877–884.

19 Dawes, T.J.W., de Marvao, A., Shi, W., et al. (2017). Machine learning of three-dimensional right ventricular motion enables outcome prediction in pulmonary hypertension: A cardiac MR imaging study. *Radiology* 283: 381–390.

20 Leiner, T., Rueckert, D., Suinesiaputra, A., et al. (2019). Machine learning in cardiovascular magnetic resonance: Basic concepts and applications. *Journal of Cardiovascular Magnetic Resonance* 21: 61.

21 Katz, D.H., Deo, R.C., Aguilar, F.G., et al. (2017). Phenomapping for the identification of hypertensive patients with the myocardial substrate for heart failure with preserved ejection fraction. *Journal of Cardiovascular Translational Research* 10: 275–284.

22 Ernande, L., Audureau, E., Jellis, C.L., et al. (2017). Clinical implications of echocardiographic phenotypes of patients with diabetes mellitus. *Journal of the American College of Cardiology* 70: 1704–1716.

23 Omar, A.M.S., Narula, S., Abdel Rahman, M.A., et al. (2017). Precision phenotyping in heart failure and pattern clustering of ultrasound data for the assessment of diastolic dysfunction. *JACC. Cardiovascular Imaging* 10: 1291–1303.

24 Lancaster, M.C., Salem Omar, A.M., Narula, S., Kulkarni, H., Narula, J., and Sengupta, P.P. (2019). Phenotypic clustering of left ventricular diastolic function parameters: Patterns and prognostic relevance. *JACC. Cardiovascular Imaging* 12: 1149–1161.

25 Kagiyama, N., Shrestha, S., Farjo, P.D., and Sengupta, P.P. (2019). Artificial intelligence: Practical primer for clinical research in cardiovascular disease. *Journal of the American Heart Association* 8: e012788.

26 Tsang, W., Salgo, I.S., Medvedofsky, D., et al. (2016). Transthoracic 3D echocardiographic left heart chamber quantification using an automated adaptive analytics algorithm. *JACC. Cardiovascular Imaging* 9: 769–782.

27 Knackstedt, C., Bekkers, S.C., Schummers, G., et al. (2015). Fully automated versus standard tracking of left ventricular ejection fraction and longitudinal strain: The FAST-EFs multicenter study. *Journal of the American College of Cardiology* 66: 1456–1466.

28 Ghesu, F.C., Georgescu, B., Zheng, Y., et al. (2019). Multi-Scale Deep Reinforcement Learning for Real-Time 3D-Landmark Detection in CT Scans. *IEEE Transactions on Pattern Analysis and Machine Intelligence* 41: 176–189.

29 Attia, Z.I., Friedman, P.A., Noseworthy, P.A., et al. (2019). Age and sex estimation using artificial intelligence from standard 12-lead ECGs. *Circulation. Arrhythmia and Electrophysiology* 12: e007284.

30 Attia, Z.I., Kapa, S., Lopez-Jimenez, F., et al. (2019). Screening for cardiac contractile dysfunction using an artificial intelligence-enabled electrocardiogram. *Nature Medicine* 25: 70–74.

31 Attia, Z.I., Noseworthy, P.A., Lopez-Jimenez, F., et al. (2019). An artificial intelligence-enabled ECG algorithm for the identification of patients with atrial fibrillation during sinus rhythm: A retrospective analysis of outcome prediction. *Lancet* 394: 861–867.

32 Strodthoff, N. and Strodthoff, C. (2019). Detecting and interpreting myocardial infarction using fully convolutional neural networks. *Physiological Measurement* 40: 015001.

33 Galloway, C.D., Valys, A.V., Shreibati, J.B., et al. (2019). Development and validation of a deep-learning model to screen for hyperkalemia from the electrocardiogram. *JAMA Cardiology* 4: 428–436.

34 Jentzer, J.C., Kashou, A.H., Attia, Z.I., et al. (2021). Left ventricular systolic dysfunction identification using artificial intelligence-augmented electrocardiogram in cardiac intensive care unit patients. *International Journal of Cardiology* 326: 114–123.

35 Kwon, J.M., Jeon, K.H., Kim, H.M., et al. (2020). Comparing the performance of artificial intelligence and conventional diagnosis criteria for detecting left ventricular hypertrophy using electrocardiography. *Europace: European Pacing, Arrhythmias, and Cardiac Electrophysiology: Journal of the Working Groups on Cardiac Pacing, Arrhythmias, and Cardiac Cellular Electrophysiology of the European Society of Cardiology* 22: 412–419.

36 Kashou, A.H., Rabinstein, A.A., Attia, I.Z., et al. (2020). Recurrent cryptogenic stroke: A potential role for an artificial intelligence-enabled electrocardiogram? *HeartRhythm Case Reports* 6: 202–205.

37 Betancur, J., Commandeur, F., Motlagh, M., et al. (2018). deep learning for prediction of obstructive disease from fast myocardial perfusion SPECT: A multicenter study. *JACC. Cardiovascular Imaging* 11: 1654–1663.

38 Koleck, T.A., Dreisbach, C., Bourne, P.E., and Bakken, S. (2019). Natural language processing of symptoms documented in free-text narratives of electronic health records: A systematic review. *Journal of the American Medical Informatics Association : JAMIA* 26: 364–379.

7

Utilizing Data Mining Classification Algorithms for Early Diagnosis of Heart Diseases

Ahmad Mousa Altamimi and Mohammad Azzeh

7.1 Introduction

Great attention has been paid to medical research to identify heart disease. Heart disease diagnosis is based on the patient's signs and symptoms and is affected by several factors such as cholesterol level, blood pressure, obesity, smoking habit, and other factors [1]. This creates a challenge to provide quality services with low costs. Quality service involves diagnosing patients properly to get effective treatments. According to the World Heart Federation and the World Health Organization, heart diseases are top of the list of various life-threatening diseases, taking around 17.9 million lives each year [2]. However, 90% of those deaths were estimated to have been preventable if patients had been correctly diagnosed early and had improved their habits [3].

In traditional healthcare environments, diagnosing heart diseases is done in the conventional way, whereby physicians review the symptoms and order some tests, such as blood tests, electrocardiogram, and echocardiogram. However, this conventional way leads to uncertainty of diagnosis, which in turn produces complicated therapy and more medical costs. The misdiagnosis results from many physicians not following the known guidelines for evaluating and managing heart failure [4]. Therefore, the high rates of inaccuracy reported in different studies are not surprising [5].

The core element for treatment success is a reliable and precise diagnosis. Expert systems [6] could be applied to emulate the ability of experts to answer not only simple questions like "What is the average age of patients who have heart disease?" or "Identify the patients who have been treated for heart diseases and complaining from other diseases?" but also complex ones like "Given patient records, predict the probability of patients who will be diagnosed with a heart disease?"or "Find the most significant risk factor that results in a heart disease?" Using such systems could decrease medical examination errors, reduce practice variation, and enhance diagnosis outcomes.

The main use of machine learning algorithms is to discover huge volumes of data by detecting patterns and summarizing data into a format that can be understood. Three main data mining techniques can classify previously unorganized data into predefined

Predicting Heart Failure: Invasive, Non-Invasive, Machine Learning, and Artificial Intelligence Based Methods, First Edition. Edited by Kishor Kumar Sadasivuni, Hassen M. Ouakad, Somaya Al-Maadeed, Huseyin C. Yalcin, and Issam Bait Bahadur.

classes or categorize new data into pre-existing categories: examining previously classified data, learning the classification rules, and applying these rules to new data. The same process is also used to identify relationships between them and to develop a pattern of these relationships. These patterns can be then used as a reference for predicting future behavior. Surveys such as those by Abdelrazek et al. [7] and Ranjan et al. [8] investigated the impact and power of machine learning algorithms in predicting systems.

In this chapter, we focus on data mining classification techniques for predicting heart diseases. Five classifiers (Naive Bayes (NB), support vector machine (SVM), random forest (RF), decision tree (DT), and linear discriminant analysis (LDA)) have been used to analyze a medical data set recorded to diagnose cardiovascular diseases. The data set used in this study has 14 clinical attributes with a different full-size training set. Multiple evaluation measures have been used to compare each classifier's performance: the accuracy, the sensitivity, area under the curve (AUC), and specificity. For this, several experiments have been conducted. Results reported that SVM and NB outperform other classifiers with an accuracy rate above 80% and a large AUC, providing a more effective and comprehensive forecasting mechanism. We believe that these models can be integrated with medical information systems to assist in diagnosing heart diseases in the earlier stages.

The rest of the chapter is structured as follows. Previous studies are discussed in Section 7.2. Section 7.3 presents various classification algorithms. Section 7.4 discusses the research methodology, and the results and discussions are given in Section 7.5. Finally, the conclusions and future works are introduced in Section 7.6.

7.2 Previous Studies

Many data mining investigations have been carried out for diagnosing heart diseases [9–11]. In this context, researchers have applied different machine learning algorithms, such as the association rules technique, clustering, and classification algorithms, to extract significant patterns for predicting heart diseases with good levels of accuracy. The association rules mining technique, for example, has been utilized in many works to find frequent items among large patient data sets to diagnose the presence of heart diseases. Panda and Dash [12] and Ordonez [13] used association rules to build a model for determining relations amongst patients' attributes values in order to discover interesting relations between variables in the data set. Others have followed the same principle with little modification in their models. Ahmed and Hannan [14], for instance, optimized the association rules in the case of a huge generated set to save prediction time and avoid unwanted rules, while Jabbar et al. [15] proposed a new approach based upon sequence number and clustering a small amount of data at a time to produce scalable and efficient prediction of heart diseases. Soni et al. used an integrated approach of association and classification to discover and then use rules in the database, to construct an efficient classifier [16]. However, in Moreno et al.'s study, while association algorithms were successfully applied for prediction in the health area of interest, they also discovered a large number of rules (some of them of no interest); in addition, the performance of association algorithms was generally low [17].

On the other hand, in Karegowda et al.'s study [18], clustering was employed to partition patients data into a set of meaningful clusters, each of which discovers the overall distribution pattern and correlations among the data attributes, thus helping practitioners to understand the natural grouping of patients' data in order to diagnose the presence of heart diseases correctly. However, clustering is very expensive for processing large data sets, so it is better used as a preprocessing step enabling other classification algorithms to get insights into the data distribution. That being said, clustering techniques have been applied to discover hidden patterns with reference to heart patients. Some studies have used K-means to group and extract data relevant to heart disease [19, 20]. The maximal frequent itemset algorithm (MAFIA) has also been applied to discover heart attack predictions rules [20]. It is important to mention that many clustering algorithms in the literature were implemented with a tool called Weka [21], a set of algorithms and tools used for preprocessing data, classification, clustering, and visualization. However, the main drawbacks of such methods are that they do not work well with dense data, it is difficult to predict the number of clusters, and, in the case where different initial partitions are chosen, different final clusters will be produced [22, 23].

The genetic algorithm was also used by Masilamani et al. [24] to get the optimal subset amongst patients' attribute values adequate for heart disease prediction. The genetic algorithm's global optimization benefit was also used by Amin et al. [25] to implement a hybrid system for initializing neural network weights based on a set of risk elements such as hypertension, high cholesterol, obesity, and others. In another system [26], a layered neuro-fuzzy approach produced a very low error rate in predicting heart diseases.

Classification methods have been extensively applied in developing prediction models for heart diseases. Popular classification algorithms such as SVM, DT, NB, and neural networks (NNs) have been used in this context. Mixed results were presented in Xing et al. [27] and Peter and Somasundaram [28] when these algorithms were employed to develop prediction models. For instance, Xing et al. [27] used SVMs, NNs, and DTs with 502 cases. Their experiments showed that SVM was the best prediction model, followed by NN. In contrast, other studies proved that the NB produced more accurate predictions than other popular algorithms such as DT and NN [28]. Furthermore, another study reported that NN was recognized as the best prediction model with 15 prominent features as risk factors in the literature [29]. The hybrid intelligent technique binds to NNs in Chitra and Seenivasagam [30] to produce a prediction model to improve prediction accuracy. The results show that the hybrid intelligent technique offer improvement in terms of accuracy.

Recently, Toughui et al.'s study [31] compared multiple machine learning algorithms implemented in the following tools: RapidMiner, Orange, MATLAB, Knime, Weka, and Scikit-Learn. The results showed that MATLAB was the best tool.

After reviewing the classification related literature, we were motivated to use the classification algorithms to develop a heart disease prediction model based on a clinical data set. Our work is different from the works presented above in two ways: firstly, five classifiers were applied to analyze medical data sets with different sizes; secondly, extensive analysis has been conducted using the MATLAB tool. The simulated implementation produced a very low error rate when calculating the prediction's accuracy.

7.3 Choice of Machine Learning Algorithms

The healthcare environment generally includes rich data about patients and their treatment stored in health management systems. Such data is valuable, especially if we transfer the existing information into good practices. Machine learning algorithms are widely used to extract valuable knowledge from hidden relationships and trends among the data. In fact, machine learning algorithms have been extensively used in healthcare research as a stage of the knowledge discovery process [32], which presents favorable ways to discover the hidden relationship in the health data [33]. They have been applied to a diversity of healthcare domains to improve and accelerate decision-making [32]. Classification methods are the most widely used algorithms in the healthcare sector as they help predict patient status by classifying patient records to find the class that matches the new patient record [3]. Classification is a supervised learning technique, which requires the data to be initially labeled [33]. These data are the entered into a classification algorithm to be learned, as shown in Figure 7.1, to discover the relationship between input variables and the target variable. In this phase, the classification algorithms build the classifier from the training data. Each observation that forms the training set is referred to as a class label. When a new case is received, the constructed classification algorithm is used to classify it into one of the predefined labels, as shown in Figure 7.2.

In the literature, many classification algorithms are used for healthcare data sets. Among them, we have chosen five common machine learning algorithms that are widely

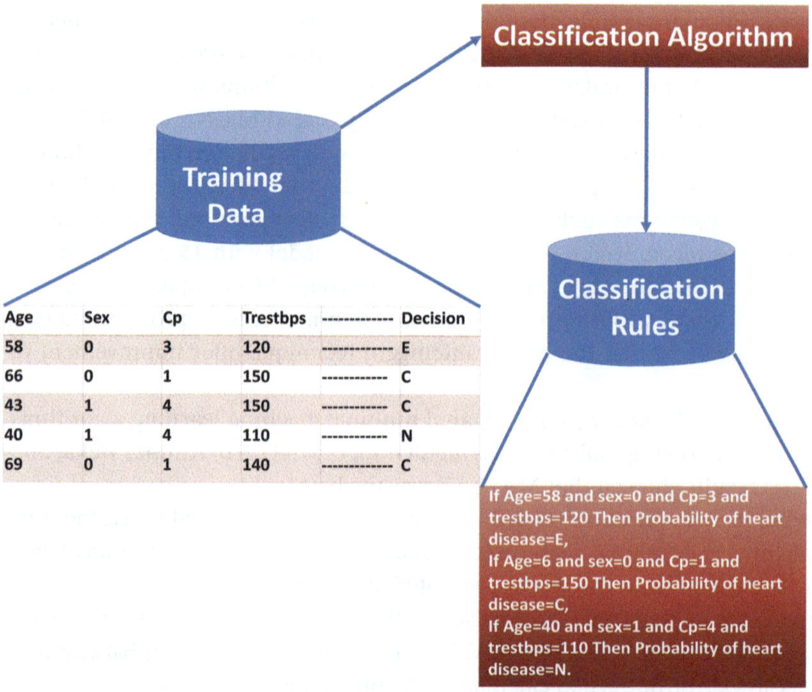

Figure 7.1 Building the classifier phase.

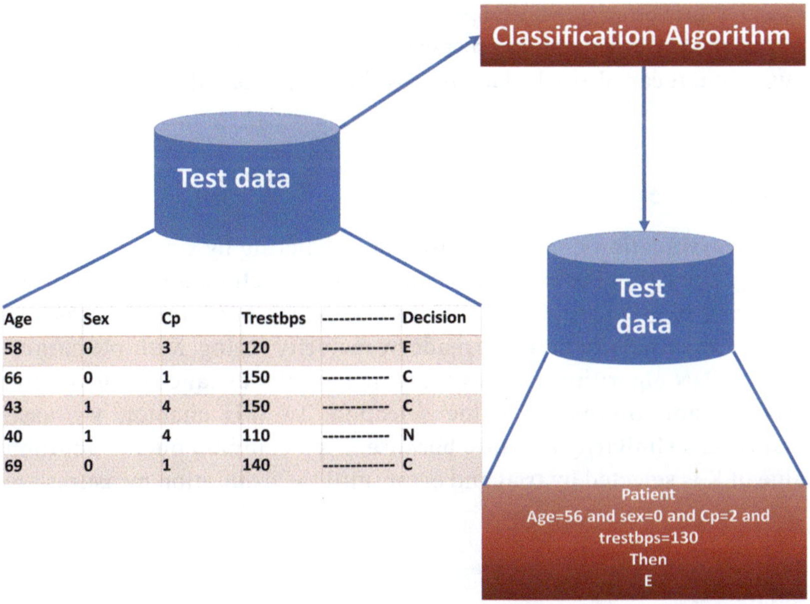

Figure 7.2 Using the classifier for prediction.

used in healthcare studies: (i) K-nearest neighbor (k-NN), (ii) DT), (iii) RF, (iv) NB, and (v) SVM. We now give an overview of each of these employed classification algorithms. As we stated in the introduction, the study investigates the classification algorithms' stability and performance for predicting patient status from previous known patient data, using heart disease related data.

7.3.1 Decision Tree

The DT is used for classification and regression tasks that accept different input feature types [34]. The principle behind constructing a DT is quite simple. The DT model is constructed using the binary recursive partitioning technique, which iteratively divides the data into groups and then divides it up on each branch. The least-squares error is used as a loss function to determine when the process of fitting must terminate. A powerful DT algorithm known as the classification and regression trees (CART) algorithm was used in this study. The CART algorithm consists of three main stages:

1. Building a tree that contains coherent data in each branch.
2. Pruning the DT to reduce overfitting.
3. Using a smoothing technique to prevent sharp discontinuities between adjacent linear models at the pruned tree leaves.

7.3.2 Naive Bayes

The NB classifier is a probabilistic algorithm based on Bayes' theorem, with independence assumptions [34]. It considers that the presence/absence of a particular attribute of a class is unrelated to any other attribute's presence/absence when the class variable is given. It helps to make the computation process very easy, and it has better speed and accuracy for huge data. It can also calculate the possible output based on the input and add new raw data at run time [35].

7.3.3 K-Nearest Neighbor

K-NN is a simple classification algorithm based on predicting by similarity [36]. It is considered a lazy algorithm because it consumes time searching for similar cases. This algorithm's basic idea is to find within historical data a set of similar K cases to the new case, where the final prediction is made by majority voting. Multiple parameters calibrate the k-NN algorithm's accuracy, which are the distance measure, the feature importance, and optimal K value selection. In this chapter, we used Euclidean distance as a similarity measure because it is a common one. In addition to that, the value of K is selected by trial and error until the evaluation measures are improved.

7.3.4 Random Forest

RF is an ensemble learning algorithm based on constructing a forest of DT classifiers. Each DT in the forest is constructed from different training data sets. The final prediction is usually measured by voting. The RF has several advantages, notably computation efficacy and better accuracy than a DT without significantly increasing computational cost. It can also predict up to thousands of explanatory variables [34].

7.3.5 Support Vector Machine

The main idea of SVM is to build an optimal hyperplane with a maximum margin that can separate class labels efficiently. Maximizing the margin and producing the largest possible distance between the hyperplane and the instances on each side have been proven to reduce an upper bound on the expected generalization error. Since healthcare data are often nonlinear, the SVM uses kernel functions to map data from low dimensionality to higher dimensionality, facilitating optimal hyperplane [37].

7.4 Research Methodology

The current research aims to improve the diagnosis of heart diseases by examining the patient's symptoms using data mining classification methods. A literature review was carried out to review the data mining works related to diagnosing heart diseases to achieve this goal. After that, five classifiers (NB, DT, LDA, RF, and SVM) were selected to build various classifiers. Each technique has a different way of building classifiers, ensuring that they behave differently and produce different results, underscoring the practical viability of our approach. In all conducted experiments, the leave-one-out cross-validation (holdout) model was adopted to evaluate algorithms' performance where original data sets are partitioned into different training and testing sets. One observation is held out in each validation cycle, whereas the remaining observations act as a training set and build the classifier model. This step is repeated until all observations act as test observations. Accordingly, each iteration's performance errors are calculated, and the average performance is calculated at the end of validation.

7.4.1 Data Sets Description

Two data sets were used in this study. The first one was obtained from the Cleveland Clinic Foundation [38] and contained 303 records; 297 are complete and 6 have missing/ unknown values. The second one was the Statlog data set available at the UCI Machine Learning Repository [39] and contains 270 completed records. Originally, the two data sets shared the same 76 features, but they were preprocessed to produce 14 attributes in an effort to reduce the number of variables. Consequently, we used these specific attributes for the two data sets described in Table 7.1 to facilitate comparison and replication studies. The statistical properties of numerical features for the Cleveland and Statlog data sets are presented in Tables 7.2 and 7.3, respectively.

Figure 7.3 shows the target variable's bar plot, demonstrating that both labels of yes and no have a relatively close number of records. This means that we do not need to use class imbalance techniques to distribute the data well. The number of heart disease patients is slightly larger than normal patients in the Cleveland data set, but the opposite can be found for the Statlog data set. This variety enables us to understand better the data set structure and its impact on classification accuracy.

Figure 7.4 shows the number of records distributed based on target and sex. It is clear from the figure that the number of females is less than the number of males in both target labels in both data sets. Interestingly the number of male patients with heart disease is smaller than normal patients for Cleveland data set, but the opposite can be found for Statlog.

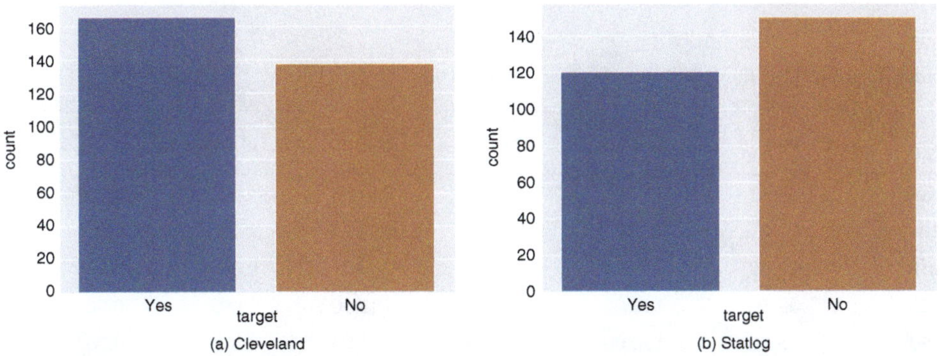

Figure 7.3 Bar plot of target variable.

Table 7.1 Heart failure data set with 14 attributes.

Attribute	Description
age	Age of the patient in years_
sex	Represented as a binary number. 1 =male, 0 = female.
cp	Chest pain type. Values range from 1 to 4. { 1: typical angina, 2: atypical angina, 3: non-anginal pain, 4: asymptomatic}.
trestbps	Resting blood pressure measured in mmHg on admission to the hospital.
chol	Serum cholesterol of the patient measured in mg/d1_
fbs	Fasting blood sugar of the patient. If greater than 120 mg/di the attribute value is 1 (true), else the attribute value is 0 (false). {1: true, 0_ false}.
restecg	Resting electrocardiographic results for the patient_ This attribute can take 3 integer values 0, 1, CT 2_ {0: normal, 1: having ST-T wave abnormality, 2: showing probable or definite left ventricular hypertrophy by Estes criteria}
thalach	Maximum heart rate achieved of the patient.
exang	Exercise induced angina. Values can be {0: No CT 1: true}.
oldpeak	ST depression induced by exercise relative to rest.
slope	Measure of slope for peak exercise. Values can be 1, 2, or 3. {1: up sloping, 2: flat, 3: down sloping}.
ca	Number of majorvessels (0-3) colored by fluoroscopy. Attributevalues can be 0 to 3.
thal	Represents heart rate of the patient. It can take values 3, 6, or 7_ {3: normal, 6: fixed defect, 7: reversable defect}.
num	Contains a numeric value between 0 and 4. Each value represents a heart disease CT absence of all of them. { 0 <50% diameter narrowing_ (Absence of heart disease). 1 to 4: >50% diameter narrowing_ (Presence of different heart diseases)

Table 7.2 Statistical description of Cleveland data set.

	age	trestbps	chol	thalach	oldpeak	ca
mean	54.37	131.62	246.26	149.65	1.04	0.73
std	9.08	17.54	51.83	22.91	1.16	1.02
min	29.00	94.00	126.00	71.00	0.00	0.00
0.25	47.50	120.00	211.00	133.50	0.00	0.00
0.50	55.00	130.00	240.00	153.00	0.80	0.00
0.75	61.00	140.00	274.50	166.00	1.60	1.00
max	77.00	200.00	564.00	202.00	6.20	4.00

Table 7.3 Statistical description of Statlog data set.

	age	trestbps	chol	thalach	oldpeak	ca
mean	54.44	131.34	249.66	149.68	1.05	0.67
std	9.10	17.86	51.69	23.17	1.15	0.94
min	30.00	94.00	126.00	71.00	0.00	0.00
0.25	48.00	120.00	213.00	133.00	0.00	0.00
0.50	55.00	130.00	245.00	153.50	0.80	0.00
0.75	61.00	140.00	280.00	166.00	1.60	1.00
max	77.00	200.00	564.00	202.00	6.20	3.00

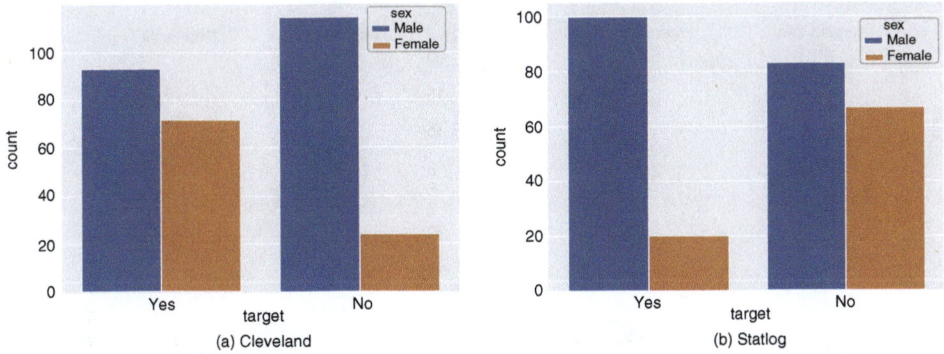

Figure 7.4 Bar plot for the relationship between target and sex.

Figure 7.5 shows the average age for males and females distributed based on the target label. We can notice that the average age for male patients is slightly smaller than females for both target labels in both data sets, which means that men are likely to have heart disease earlier than females during their lives. This finding is also confirmed in Figure 7.6, which shows that males' age distribution is much more normal than the distribution of females' age in both data sets. Most females are likely to have heart problems in the late stage of their lives.

Figure 7.7 demonstrates the distribution of resting blood pressure for heart and normal patients, classified based on sex variables. We can notice that both data sets have relatively the same distribution. The main observation is that there is no significant difference between heart patients and normal patients for males, but there is a significant difference between the two distributions for females.

7.4.2 Data Preprocessing

The data sets were preprocessed to handle noise, inconsistency, and missing values. The noises and inconsistencies were corrected manually. However, the missing values had to be treated before being used as they could have led to failure in classification or

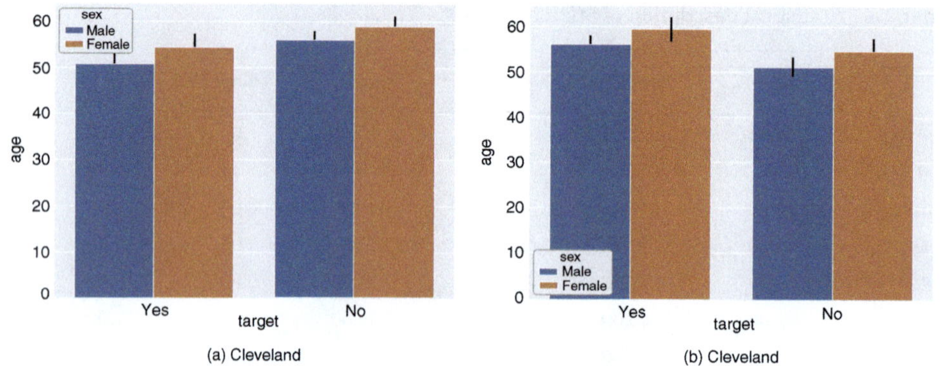

Figure 7.5 Bar plot for the relationship between target, sex, and age.

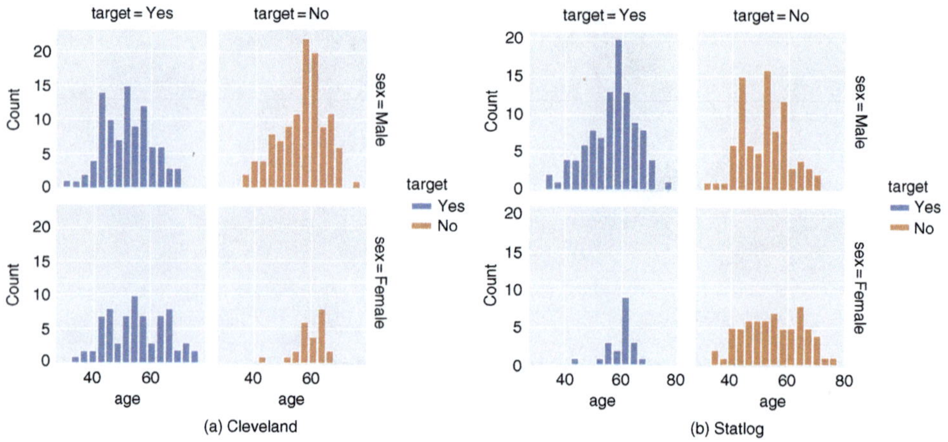

Figure 7.6 Histogram of age variables classified based on sex and target.

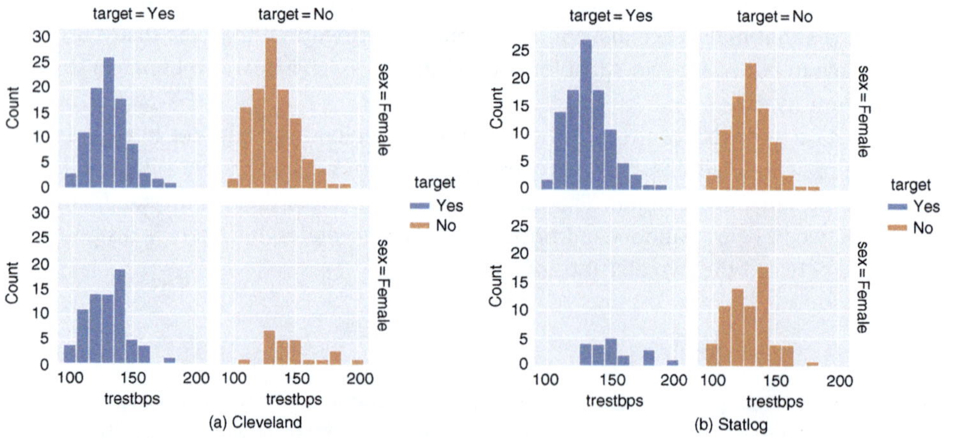

Figure 7.7 Histogram of resting blood pressure classified based on sex and target.

incorrect disease prediction [40]. Two common techniques could be applied for handling the data sets: deletion and imputation. Removing missing instances is the most used way for treating missing values, whereby cases that cannot be processed are removed. Despite the simple implementation of this method, it can remove useful information. On the other hand, the imputation method is used where missing values are replaced with estimated values. In our research, the second approach was used. Specifically, we used the nearest neighbor algorithm with k = 5 to impute missing values where a case is imputed using values from the majority of the complete five nearest cases.

7.4.3 Performance Measures

Five common evaluation measures were used to assess the efficiency of the prediction models. These evaluation measures were selected as they are widely used to evaluate the efficiency of prediction models. The first measure is Recall, as shown in Equation 7.1, which measures how well a binary classification predicts positive labels. The second measure is precision, as shown in Equation 7.2, which measures the probability that a positive prediction is correct. The third measure is accuracy, as shown in Equation 7.3, which measures the performance of classification. The fourth measure is specificity, as shown in Equation 7.4, which measures how well a binary classification test correctly identifies the negative cases. The last measure is the F-measure, as shown in Equation 7.5, which measures the probability that a positive prediction is correct [32].

$$Recall = \frac{t_p}{t_p + f_n} \tag{7.1}$$

$$Precision = \frac{t_p}{t_p + f_p} \tag{7.2}$$

$$Accuracy = \frac{t_p + t_n}{t_p + t_n + f_p + f_n} \tag{7.3}$$

$$sepcificity = \frac{t_n}{t_n + f_p} \tag{7.4}$$

$$F - measure = \frac{2 \times precision \times recall}{precision + recall} \tag{7.5}$$

Where:

- t_p is true positive.
- t_n is true negative.
- f_p is false positive.
- f_n is false negative.

7.5 Results

In traditional healthcare systems, doctors rely on the signs or symptoms of patients to diagnose heart diseases. However, many signs and symptoms are non-specific, leading to unwanted errors and affecting the quality of the provided health services. To overcome this issue, expert systems were developed to emulate health decision-making with improved accuracy. This involves correlating various pieces of patients' information, followed by obtaining specific patterns. In this research, we applied five classification algorithms for predicting heart diseases based on pre-selected attributes.

For each data set, we ran the five classification algorithms using 10-fold cross-validation. The obtained results are shown in Tables 7.4 and 7.5. The results in Table 7.4 for the Cleveland data set show that all models can produce good predictions and good performance. We notice that all performance measures, except recall, suggest that NB is the most predictive for the Cleveland data set. Figure 7.8 demonstrates the receiver operating characteristic (ROC) for all models over the Cleveland data set. It is clear that that SVM and NB are the most superior ones for the Cleveland data set.

The results obtained for the Statlog data set, shown in Table 7.5, are similar to those obtained for the Cleveland data set. Accuracy, Precision, and Specificity performance measures indicate that SVM is the most accurate algorithm while AUC, Recall, and F1 measures recommend NB is the most accurate one, as shown in Table 7.5. Another important issue that should be emphasized in this study is the ranking stability of the classification algorithm over both data sets and across multiple performance measures. Ranking algorithm stability means that this algorithm should always produce accurate results and rank high overall data sets across all evaluation

Table 7.4 Performance measures using the Cleveland data set.

	AUC	Accuracy	Recall	Precision	F1	Specificity
k-NN	0.61	0.61	0.66	0.64	0.65	0.56
SVM	0.90	0.82	0.86	0.82	0.84	0.77
NB	0.91	0.84	0.85	0.85	0.85	0.83
DT	0.76	0.76	0.75	0.80	0.77	0.78
RF	0.88	0.82	0.85	0.82	0.84	0.78

Table 7.5 Performance measures using the Statlog data set.

	AUC	Accuracy	Recall	Precision	F1	Specificity
k-NN	0.72	0.67	0.58	0.65	0.61	0.75
SVM	0.90	0.83	0.77	0.83	0.80	0.87
NB	0.91	0.83	0.81	0.82	0.81	0.85
DT	0.69	0.68	0.61	0.65	0.63	0.73
RF	0.89	0.81	0.75	0.81	0.78	0.86

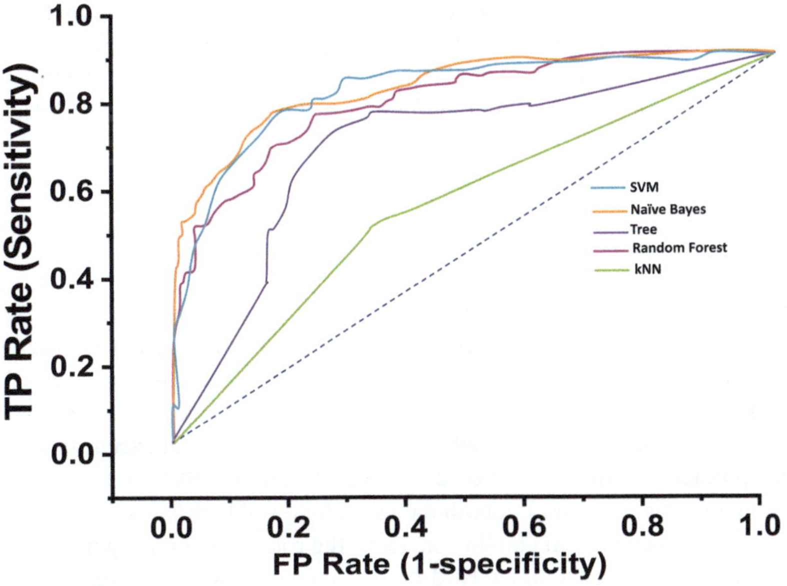

Figure 7.8 ROC for all models over the Cleveland data set.

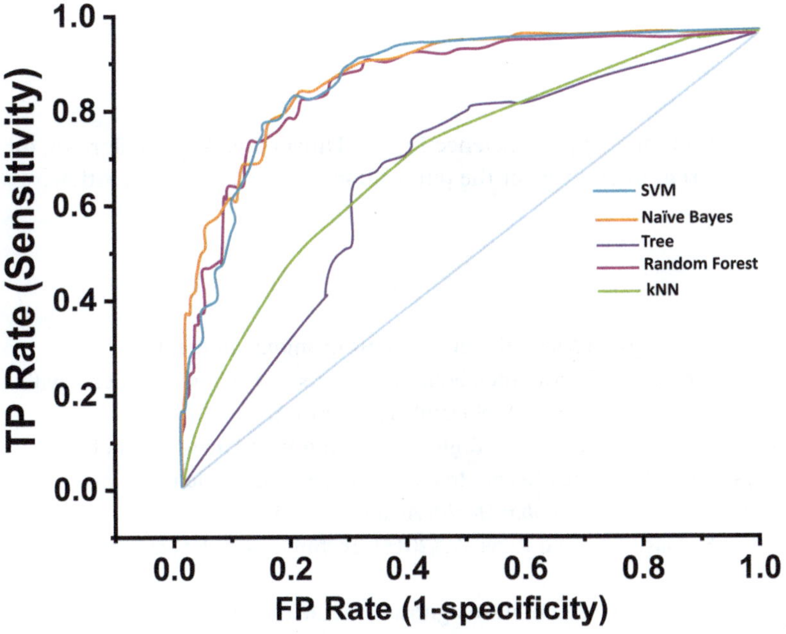

Figure 7.9 ROC for all models over the Statlog data set.

measures. Our results show that the NB has ranked first across all evaluation measures and, in the Cleveland data set, is followed by SVM in the second position. At the same time, SVM and NB obtained the best rank in the Statlog data set. Although ensemble learning like RF has been proved to produce superior results, in our case, the NB and SVM have outperformed this ensemble version. Finally, we can conclude from the above results that k-NN obtained the worst results in both data sets.

Figure 7.9 demonstrates the ROC for all models over the Statlog data set. It is clear that SVM, NB, and RF are superior, confirming the findings in Table 7.5. The DT and k-NN are the worst models over the Statlog data set.

7.6 Conclusion and Future Work

In this study, different machine learning algorithms were studied to enhance the early detection of heart diseases. Specifically, five classifiers were utilized to improve the accuracy of heart disease predictions. Moreover, an extensive experiment was performed using two data sets. For each data set, the classifiers were applied using leave-one-out cross-validation. Results demonstrated that all classification algorithms are accurate and can produce good predictions. However, it confirms that the NB and SVM were ranked first across all evaluation measures and in both data sets, followed by RF in second position. This can lead us to an important conclusion about the role of uncertainty in classifying data. SVM and NB have completely different mechanisms for building the relationship between inputs and output. In future work, we will study the impact of feature selection and weighting on the overall performance of classifiers.

Acknowledgment

The authors are grateful to the Applied Science Private University, Amman-Jordan, for the full financial support granted to cover the publication fee of this research article.

References

1 Lampignano, L., et al. (2020). Cross-sectional relationship among different anthropometric parameters and cardiometabolic risk factors in a cohort of patients with overweight or obesity. *PLoS One* 15 (11) (November): e0241841.

2 Gyawali, B., Khanal, P., Mishra, S.R., Van Teijlingen, E., and Wolf Meyrowitsch, D. (2020). Building strong primary health care to tackle the growing burden of non-communicable diseases in Nepal. *Global Health Action* 13 (1): Dec.

3 Ahmad, P., Qamar, S., Qasim, S., and Rizvi, A. (2015). Techniques of data mining in healthcare: A review.

4 Salmasi, M.Y., et al. (2020). The risk of misdiagnosis in acute thoracic aortic dissection: A review of current guidelines. *Heart*.106 (12): 885-889

5 Kapłon-Cieślicka, A., et al. (2020). Is heart failure misdiagnosed in hospitalized patients with preserved ejection fraction? From the European Society of Cardiology – Heart Failure Association EURObservational research programme heart failure long-term registry. *ESC Heart Failure* 7 (5) (Oct): 2098–2112.

6 Ali, F., et al. (2020). A smart healthcare monitoring system for heart disease prediction based on ensemble deep learning and feature fusion. *Information Fusion* 63: 208–222.

7 Abdelrazek, S., El-Henawy, I.M., Ismail, A., Abdlerazek, S., and El-Henawy, I.M. (2020). Big data analytics in heart diseases prediction. *Artic. Journal of Theoretical and Applied Information Technology* 15 (11).

8 Ranjan, R., Yadav, R.K., and Rao, T.S. (2020). A comparative study for predicting heart diseases using data mining techniques. *International Journal of Research and Analytical Reviews*. 7 (1); 168–172.

9 Kumar, A., Kumar, P., Srivastava, A., Ambeth Kumar, V.D., Vengatesan, K., and Singhal, A. (2020). Comparative analysis of data mining techniques to predict heart disease for diabetic patients. *Communications in Computer and Information Science* 1244 (CCIS): 507–518.

10 Nalluri, S., Vijaya Saraswathi, R., Ramasubbareddy, S., Govinda, K., and Swetha, E. (2020). Chronic heart disease prediction using data mining techniques. *Advances in Intelligent Systems and Computing* 1079: 903–912.

11 Panda, D. and Dash, S.R. (2020). Predictive system: Comparison of classification techniques for effective prediction of heart disease. *Smart Innovation, Systems and Technologies* 159: 203–213.

12 Ordonez, C. (2006). Association rule discovery with the train and test approach for heart disease prediction. IEEE Xplore. *ieeexplore.ieee.org*.

13 Jabbar, M.A., Chandra, P., and Deekshatulu, B.L. (2012). Prediction of risk score for heart disease using associative classification and hybrid feature subset selection. *International Conference on Intelligent Systems Design and Applications, ISDA* 628–634.

14 Ahmed, A. and Hannan, S.A. (2012). Data mining techniques to find out heart diseases: An overview. *(Sem Qualis) International Journal of Innovative Technology and Exploring Engineering (IJITEE)* 1 (4): 18–23.

15 Jabbar, M., Chandra, P., Dr., and Deekshatulu, B.L. (2011). Cluster based association rule mining for heart attack prediction. *Journal of Theoretical and Applied Information Technology* 32 (2): 196–201.

16 Soni, J., Ansari, U., Sharma, D., and Soni, S. (2011). Predictive data mining for medical diagnosis: An overview of heart disease prediction. *International Journal of Computer Applications* 17 (8): 43–48.

17 Moreno, M.N., Segrera, S., and López, V.F. (2005). Association rules: Problems, solutions and new applications. *Knowl. Creat. Diffus. Util.* 317–323.

18 Karegowda, A.G., Jayaram, M.A., and Manjunath, A.S. (2012). Cascading K-means clustering and K-nearest neighbor classifier for categorization of diabetic patients. *International Journal of Engineering and Advanced Technology (IJEAT)* 1 (3): 147–151.

19 Dbritto, R., Srinivasaraghavan, A., and Joseph, V. (2016). Comparative analysis of accuracy on heart disease prediction using classification methods. *International Journal of Applied Information Systems* 11 (2): 22–25.

20 Patil, S.B. and Kumaraswamy, Y.S. (2009). Extraction of significant patterns from heart disease warehouses for heart attack prediction. *International Journal of Computer Science and Network Security* 9 (2): 228–235.

21 Weka 3 – Data mining with open source machine learning software in Java.

22 Fahad, A., et al. (2014). A survey of clustering algorithms for big data: Taxonomy and empirical analysis. *IEEE Transactions on Emerging Topics in Computing* 2 (3): 267–279.

23 Peizhuang, W. (2013). Pattern Recognition with Fuzzy Objective Function Algorithms.

24 Masilamani, A., Anbarasi, M., and Anupriya, E. (2010). Enhanced prediction of heart disease with feature subset selection using genetic algorithm.

25 Amin, S.U., Agarwal, K., and Beg, R. (2013). Genetic neural network based data mining in prediction of heart disease using risk factors. *2013 IEEE Conference on Information and Communication Technologies, ICT 2013* 1227–1231.

26 Sen, A.K., Patel, S.B., and Shukla, D.P. (2013). A data mining technique for prediction of coronary heart disease using neuro-fuzzy integrated approach two level. *International Journal of Engineering and Computer Science* 2 (9): 1663–1671.

27 Xing, Y., Wang, J., Zhao, Z., and Gao, Y. (2007). Combination data mining methods with new medical data to predicting outcome of coronary heart disease. *2007 International Conference on Convergence Information Technology, ICCIT 2007* 868–872.

28 Peter, T.J. and Somasundaram, K. (2012). An empirical study on prediction of heart disease using classification data mining techniques. *IEEE-International Conference on Advances in Engineering, Science and Management, ICAESM-2012* 514–518.

29 Srinivas, K., Raghavendra Rao, G., and Govardhan, A. (2010). Analysis of coronary heart disease and prediction of heart attack in coal mining regions using data mining techniques. *ICCSE 2010-5th International Conference on Computer Science and Education, Final Program and Book of Abstracts* 1344–1349.

30 Chitra, R. and Seenivasagam, S. (2013). Review of heart disease prediction system using data mining and hybrid intelligent techniques. *ICTACT Journal on Soft Computing (IJSC)* 03 (04): 605–609.

31 Tougui, I., Jilbab, A., and El Mhamdi, J. (2020). Heart disease classification using data mining tools and machine learning techniques. *Health and Technology* 10 (5): 1137–1144.

32 Gupta, S., Kumar, D., and Sharma, A. (2011). Performance analysis of various data mining classification techniques on healthcare data. *International Journal of Computer Science and Information Technology (IJCSIT)* 3 (4).

33 Han, J., Kamber, M., and Pei, J. (2012). *Data Mining: Concepts and Techniques.*

34 Li, L., Wu, Y., and Ye, M. (2015). Experimental comparisons of multi-class classifiers. *Inform* 39 (1): 71–85.

35 Nalini Jagtap, N., Shevatekar, P.P., and Mustary, N. A comparative study of classification techniques in data mining algorithms. *International Journal of Modern Trends in Engineering and Research* 4 (7): 58–63. 2017.

36 Sharma, S., Sharma, V., and Sharma, A. (2016). Performance based evaluation of various machine learning classification techniques for chronic kidney disease diagnosis. Jun.

37 Vaghela, C., Bhatt, N., and Mistry, D. (2015). A survey on various classification techniques for clinical decision support system. *International Journal of Computer Applications* 116 (23): 14–17.

38 UCI. (2019). UCI Machine Learning Repository: Heart Disease Data Set. UCI.

39 UCI Machine Learning Repository. Statlog (Heart) data set. *UCI Machine Learning Repository*. https://archive.ics.uci.edu/ml/datasets/statlog+(heart).

40 UshaRani, Y. and Sammulal, P. (2016). A novel approach for imputation of missing attribute values for efficient mining of medical datasets – class based cluster approach. *Revista Tecnica de la Facultad de Ingenieria Universidad del Zulia* 39 (May): 184–195.

8

Applications of Machine Learning for Predicting Heart Failure

Sabri Boughorbel, Yassine Himeur, Huseyin Enes Salman, Faycal Bensaali, Faisal Farooq, and Huseyin C. Yalcin

8.1 Introduction

Heart failure (HF) is a chronic disease in which the cardiac system fails to pump the normal blood level in the body, leading to a reduced oxygen level in organs and tissues. It is a global health burden that creates a major challenge for the healthcare systems worldwide. The global prevalence of HF is 64.34 million cases, corresponding to 8.52 cases per 1000 inhabitants. This translates to 9.9 million years lost due to disability. In terms of costs, the HF burden accounts for US$346.17 billion [1]. In the Arab Gulf Region, the prevalence of HF is about 1–2% of the population [2] accounting for more than 4 million patients. The average affected population is 10 years younger than in developed countries [2, 3]. Some of the main risk factors of HF are sex, obesity, hypertension, diabetes, smoking, and previous heart conditions. While, the prevalence of HF as a function of age peaks for older people over 70, a recent study showed that HF risk in the younger population is higher for obesity, hypertension, diabetes, and smoking. These results emphasize the importance of preventive measures across adult life [4, 5].

Due to the progressive and chronic nature of HF, high hospitalization rates and emergency visits are reported for HF patients. About one-fourth of HF patients are readmitted for medical care within a month, and at least half of these readmissions are related to HF symptoms [6]. High hospitalization rates increase the work burden of medical professionals and also increase healthcare expenditure. The healthcare costs of HF management are estimated to be about 1–2% of all healthcare expenditure [7, 8].

The early prediction of HF risk is important in enabling preventive action and limiting the consequences of HF. The traditional method for developing risk factor models for HF is typically using logistic regression models with general health data. Such an approach suffers from a limited predictive power when a large population is used to fit the models. Since logistic regression is a linear model, it cannot capture non-linearity in complex and noisy data. Machine learning (ML) approaches provide good alternatives to traditional HF risk scoring and prediction. High model capacity allows for a better predictive performance limiting the underfitting problem observed with logistic regression models. Several ML approaches incorporate interpretability elements to help the user

Predicting Heart Failure: Invasive, Non-Invasive, Machine Learning, and Artificial Intelligence Based Methods, First Edition. Edited by Kishor Kumar Sadasivuni, Hassen M. Ouakad, Somaya Al-Maadeed, Huseyin C. Yalcin, and Issam Bait Bahadur.

understanding which variables are the most predictive. In the section 8.2, we provide the reader with a brief introduction to the field of ML. In the following sections we give an introduction to the use of ML for the diagnosis of HF.

8.2 Brief Explanation of ML Techniques for Medicine

ML is the field responsible for developing methods and tools that can learn and make decisions based on data. It can be viewed as the intersection of several fields such as computer science and statistics. Software development has recently contributed significantly to the rapid progress of the field. Before the emergence of ML, intelligent programs were hard-coding rules derived from domain experts. These expert systems quickly became very complex and incapable of coping with real-world applications. ML automatically derives these rules from the data. Hidden patterns can be discovered in the data and be used to detect disease, anomalies, and other events. In ML, there is no need to explicitly write these rules as ML inherently captures them during model training.

Because of the digitalization of healthcare, capturing, sharing, and delivering massive amounts of data has become a high priority. ML plays an essential role by addressing the challenges posed by the huge quantity of data. It tends to demonstrate that collecting and processing various data types from different sources, such as electronic health record data, raw patient data, diagnosis results, resource/patients provision, healthcare personnel information, along with a variety of "big data" pertaining to human-to-human interactions (from cellular operators, traffic, airlines, social media, etc.) can efficiently improve healthcare services [9]. In this context, ML helps healthcare organizations meet the growing demand for medical care, improving operations, and lowering costs. At the same time, ML innovation helps healthcare experts in (i) effectively predicting, detecting, and treating diseases, (ii) speeding up decision-making while guaranteeing more accurate, precise, and personalized cares, and (iii) optimizing the use and allocation of scarce healthcare resources [10, 11]. ML techniques are capable of automating tedious and repetitive tasks such as speech-to-text translation, structuring clinical notes, finding landmarks in radiology and pathology images, generating alerts and reminders, etc. Recently, chatbots have been successfully used to initiate remote consultations and tackle the growing demand for medical care during the pandemic. ML can offload many tasks from clinicians, allowing them to free up time to improve patient care.

The first step in building ML models for HF diagnosis is to prepare a training data set. We consider the example of HF diagnosis using electrocardiogram (ECG) data. The training dataset is retrospectively collected and here the subject outcomes are known. This means that for each recorded ECG in the data set, it is already known whether it corresponds to a patient with HF or it corresponds to a subject who did not have HF. The information attached to each ECG sample (HF or no HF) is typically called the labels. This scenario, where labels are available, is known as supervised learning. When labels are not available, an unsupervised learning problem is addressed. Once the data is annotated and ready, an ML model can be trained to classify whether the ECG corresponds to HF or not. There is extensive literature and also prior work on the different types of ML models. Each model has a set of parameters to be estimated based on the training data. Once trained, the model can be applied to new data and predict the label (HF event or no HF event).

8.3 Detection and Diagnosis of HF

The growing number of HF patients and increasing healthcare costs indicate the importance of the early diagnosis of HF for efficient treatment planning. For the diagnosis of HF, several clinical tests including blood tests, chest radiography, echocardiography, and ECG are performed in addition to physical examination and disease history investigation of the patient [12, 13]. A research study has shown that the deep learning model trained with ECG alone has high sensitivity and specificity in detecting HF [14]. Several criteria, such as Framingham, Boston, European Society of Cardiology (ESC), and the Gothenburg criteria, are employed by evaluating the clinical test data to decide on the presence of HF [15]. According to the ESC guidelines, the patient's clinical history, observed symptoms, physical activity, and resting ECG are examined at the first step [10]. The symptoms of HF can be summarized as ankle swelling, dyspnea, fatigue due to elevated jugular venous pressure, pulmonary crackles, and peripheral edema [16–18]. If all examinations mentioned are normal, the presence of HF is not expected. If any of the initial stage evaluations are abnormal, plasma natriuretic peptides are recommended to be measured and, after this measurement, the clinicians decide on whether there is a further need for echocardiography [14]. Brain natriuretic peptide (BNP) is a protein secreted by the ventricular musculature in response to volume or pressure overload. The natriuretic peptide family is important for volume and blood pressure regulation. The presence of BNP in blood plasma is being used as a biomarker for diagnosing HF. Studies have shown that the use of BPN can improve HF diagnosis compared with the use of echocardiography [19]. An effective technique for HF diagnosis is to measure the intracardiac filling pressures using implantable pressure sensors by means of cardiac catheterization [20] but the invasive nature of catherization limits the routine usage of this method [21].

8.4 Prediction of HF

After the diagnosis of HF, the severity of the condition is clinically predicted and classified using either the New York Heart Association (NYHA) or the American College of Cardiology/American Heart Association (ACC/AHA) guidelines [22]. These guidelines are constituted to accurately predict the state of the disease and to plan the most appropriate treatment methods. NYHA guidelines basically use the physical activity capabilities and observed symptoms of the patient for the classification of HF [13]. On the other hand, in the ACC/AHA guidelines, the structural changes and symptoms are described for HF stages [19]. In other words, NYHA guidelines define the exercise capacity and symptomatic status of the patient [14], and ACC/AHA guidelines focus on the developmental stage and progression of HF [10]. These two methods are complementary and provide important information for deciding the presence and severity of HF. NYHA guidelines can be considered to be more subjective compared to ACC/AHA guidelines due to the observer variability during the evaluation [23]. An objective evaluation of HF severity can be performed using the combination of 2D ECG and Doppler flow imaging [17].

With the advances in sensor technologies, it is also possible to predict the HF worsening state remotely before the hospitalization and clinical tests. For this purpose, noninvasive or minimally invasive sensor measurements are performed via remote patient monitoring (RPM) systems [15]. These RPM methods continuously measure the blood pressure [24], body weight [25], physical activity [19], bioimpedance [26–28], and ventricular filling pressures [29–31] of HF patients remotely, and predict the impending HF decompensation before there are serious symptoms. It is reported that RPM trials have reduced the all-cause and HF-related mortality of HF patients [32, 33], prevented unnecessary HF-related hospitalizations [34], and increased the life quality of HF patients [35].

8.5 ML Techniques for Detection and Diagnosis of HF

In recent years, ML has gained a growing importance in cardiovascular medicine, especially for the detection and diagnosis of HF. This is mainly due to the huge amounts of data recorded using different medical devices, such as electronic health records (EHRs), multimodality images, and mobile health sensors, which requires powerful and smart algorithms to extract pertinent information, predict HF, and detect and classify HF [36, 37]. Based on the nature of the ML algorithms used for detection and diagnosis of HF, four classes can be identified:

1. **Supervised learning models**: Annotated datasets are used to train this kind of model, in which for each item of input data there is a label referring to the nature of HF. After training the ML model, a test data set is used for its validation which includes labels. Accordingly, different ML metrics are then used to estimate the accuracy, precision, recall, specificity, etc. Classification and regression are notable supervised learning models [38].
2. **Unsupervised learning models**: Data sets employed for training this kind of model do not include labels. Their main role is to discriminate between the different HF types by using algorithms relying on clustering, one-class classification, dimensionality reduction, etc. [39].
3. **Semi-supervised learning models**: These combine supervised learning and unsupervised learning through the use of both unlabeled data and labeled data during the training process. Explicitly, this is usually achieved by using a lesser amount of annotated data with a hefty amount of unlabeled data [9].
4. **Reinforcement learning models**: The main advantage of these models is that they do not require an annotated data set for their training. In addition, the results are not directly associated with the input data, hence these models can learn from experience. Specifically, these models can detect the HF by (i) improving their presentation using their association with the environment, and (ii) figuring out the manner for discussing their faults and getting the adequate outcome by assessing and testing different prospects [39].

Table 8.1 summarizes the different ML paradigms and how they can support care givers in the identification and treatment of HF.

In this context, ML and big data analytics play an essential role in modern medicine. ML provides efficient solutions to alleviate the difficulties usually encountered by physicians when they are struggling to compute and analyze big data recorded using medical devices [40]. For instance, using ML in the field of cardiology means that detection, diagnosis, and prediction of HF can be effectively conducted. In doing so, different steps should be carefully followed:

1. **Data collection**: Different kinds of data can be collected to help in predicting HF. Usually, they are classified into three categories: *personal data*, such as gender, age, weight, smoking/no-smoking, etc.; *clinical data*, which are gleaned using wearables, imaging techniques, echocardiography (ECG), and EHRs; and *omics data*, which are gathered by analyzing cardiac tissue or blood and include genomics, translatomics, transcriptomics, metabolomics, proteomics, and lipidomics [41].
2. **Data preprocessing**: This step is important as it is responsible for cleaning data. Therefore, it removes noise, filters data by removing uncomplete samples, irrelevant and redundant features, and/or replaces incomplete data with the mean or median of their neighbors. This step helps later in simplifying the data analysis process and ensuring data quality and consistency [42].
3. **Feature extraction and selection**: This is of significant importance in most classification and regression applications as it aims to extract the most relevant features that enable an accurate and robust HF analysis. Based on the objective of the ML-based solution and collected data, various kinds of data can be extracted in time domain, frequency domain, entropy domain, multimodal domain, etc. in order to rank the features corresponding to the most important HF risk factors [42].
4. **Classification**: This aims to categorize and classify extracted features into different classes with reference to the nature of the ML model deployed (supervised, unsupervised, semi-supervised, or reinforcement learning), and hence identify the HF (left-sided, right-sided, diastolic, or systolic). Conventional ML models have been widely used in the previous two decades, such as support vector machine (SVM), decision tree (DT), K-nearest neighbor (k-NN), random forest (RF), Naive Bayes, and ensemble classifiers. However, nowadays, increasing attention is devoted to using deep learning models such as convolutional neural networks (CNNs), recurrent neural networks (RNNs), denoising autoencoder (DAE), deep belief networks (DBNs), and long short-term memory (LSTM). Moreover, deep reinforcement learning has more recently begun to receive much attention for developing data-driven clinical decision support tools [43].

Table 8.1 ML paradigms and how they can help tackle HF.

Approach	Contribution to the Care of HF
Unsupervised learning	Patient clustering, triage, and HF subtype identification
Semi-supervised learning	HF prediction, HF phenotyping
Supervised learning	HF prediction, HF phenotyping
Reinforcement learning	Treatment planning and new treatment discovery

Each of the steps listed above is important in obtaining a high performance ML system. While data preprocessing and feature extraction can be standardized and reduced effort can be required to build them, data collection and classification could be considered as the most critical components of the system. The collected data should be representative of real-world scenarios in terms of variability across subjects, noise in the data, and the distribution shift of time. Modern classification techniques based on deep learning have shown superiority over traditional ML when coupled with large data sets. The accuracy of classifier based deep learning has reached human-level accuracy in various applications, such as in computer vision or natural language processing. The ability of deep learning to model complex data while being computationally efficient has overtaken classical ML classifiers.

Figure 8.1 illustrates the overall architecture of an HF detection and diagnosis system based on ML.

8.6 HF Diagnosis Using Biopsy Images

The diagnosis of HF usually relies on physical examination, lab tests, and clinical history. However, in some patients, these diagnosis methods fail to identify signs of HF. Alternatively, endomyocardial biopsy (EMB) is the gold standard for identifying and grading HF. Nirschl et al. proposed an automated deep learning model for the recognition of HF from whole slide images of hematoxylin and eosin (H&E) tissue [44]. The introduced neural network architecture is an adaptation of the work of Janowczyk and Madabhushi [45]. The network is formed by alternating convolutional, batch normalization, and rectified linear unit (ReLU) activation layers. The model has more than 13,000 tunable weights trained based on a data set of 1144 regions of interests (ROI) from 209 whole slide images from 94 patients with HF and 115 subjects without HF. Several CNN architectures were used such as AlexNet, GoogLeNet, ResNet50, and ResNet50. These models were compared with the traditional feature engineered approach using WND-CHARM [46]. The latter extracts 4059 features and an RF classifier is trained based on these features. The held-out test set was blindly and independently evaluated by two expert pathologists to compare with the ML models. The clinicians were given unlimited time to complete the task. Cohen's kappa inter-rater agreement between the two pathologists was 0.40 with an individual accuracy of 75% at patient level. The performance metrics used are accuracy, sensitivity, specificity, positive predictive value, and AUC (area under ROC curve). The performance of the deep learning model in terms of AUC was 0.97 compared to 0.95 for RF and 0.75 for the pathologists. The CNN model shows 99% sensitivity and 94% specificity. These results are obtained at ROI level. The analysis at patient level also showed an advantage of the deep learning approach.

8.7 HF Case Identification from EHR Data

The use of EHR is an important research direction for predicting HF. The availability of large EHR data sets allows the training of accurate deep learning models as well classical ML models. Structured data in EHR such as International Classification of Diseases

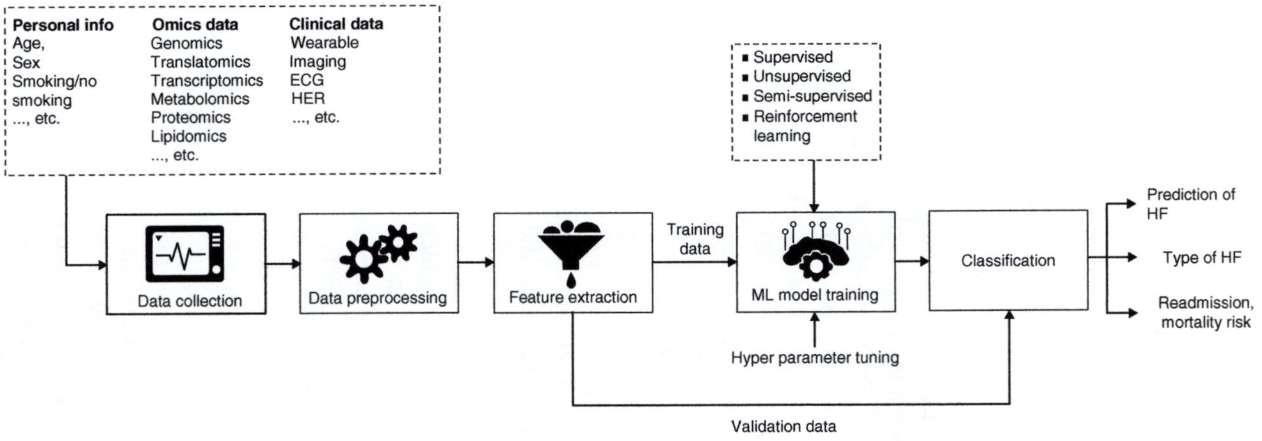

Figure 8.1 Overall architecture of HF diagnosis/prediction using ML models.

(ICD), medication, lab orders, etc. can be represented as a sequence of categorical variables over time, when each patient visit is an element of this sequence. Hence, there is similarity between EHR data representation and natural language representation where the text is represented as a sequence of words or sentences. Therefore, ML models developed in the area of language understanding can readily be applied to EHR data.

In Rasmy et al. [47], a large EHR data set is used for the predictive modeling of HF onset risk. The data set included more than 150,000 HF patients and over 1,000,000 controls from about 400 hospitals. Patients are defined based on the two criteria: (i) at least three encounters with related HF had to occur within 12 months; (ii) the first HF diagnosis occurred when they were over 50 years old. For each case, 10 matched controls are identified based on the primary care hospital, sex, and age. Furthermore, the time span of the control and case data were matched by ensuring that the first visit of the controls were within one year of the first visit of the matched case and there was at least one visit a month before or any time after the diagnosis date of the matched case. Each visit is represented by the medical codes related to diagnoses, medication, and surgical procedure data. For diagnoses and surgical procedures, ICD-9 and ICD-10 were used. For medication information, the National Drug Codes (NDC) were used.

A known deep learning model called RETAIN (reverse time attention model) has been previously used for HF prediction [48] based on a relatively small data set compared with the one used in Rasmy et al. [47]. The model was designed to predict the diagnosis of HF at the next visit. Hence at each visit, the model gives a probability score for the patient having an HF. RETAIN is a two-branch neural attention model on top of an embedding layer. It takes as input the sequence of recorded events in the patient's EHR. First, an embedding layer is responsible for reducing the dimensionality of the input representation and converting the multi-hot vector input to a real-valued smaller size vector representation. Then two gated recurrent unit (GRU) RNNs are derived in parallel. The first RNN (RNNα) is responsible for deriving attention weights of the visits, which is a vector α where length is the number of visits. Therefore, it is possible to infer which visits are most important for predicting HF. The second RNN (RNNβ) is used to derive the clinical code level attention. Hence, it is possible to know which event (diagnosis, medication, surgical procedure) is most relevant for the prediction of HF. These two RNNs can be applied to new patients not seen during model training. They provide good interpretability properties of the model.

In order to compare the RETAIN model with classical ML approaches, a baseline logistic regression model using an aggregated feature vector on the temporal dimension was adapted. Each dimension represents the count of each code event in the subject's history. L1 and L2 regularization terms were evaluated in the experimental analysis. Also, the embedding from RETAIN was used as input to train the logistic regression. EHRs from multiple hospitals were gathered for the Cerner Health Facts database. For each hospital the cohort was divided into training, validation, and test sets with a ratio of 7:1:2. A regularized logistic regression model was used as a baseline model. The feature vector for the baseline was the codes' occurrence of the aggregated data on the temporal dimension. The RETAIN model achieved an AUC of 82% compared with 79% for logistic regression. The generalizability of the model across hospitals was performed by training

RETAIN using a single hospital data and evaluating the model on other hospital data. This led to a 3.6% reduction in AUC. The combination of deep learning and EHR is a promising future direction for building accurate predictive models for clinical decision support tools for HF.

8.8 ML Techniques for Predicting HF

Predicting of HF risks using ML is becoming one of the top priorities for medical doctors and physicians. Specifically, when ML is applied to different kinds of medical records, it helps in predicting survival in patients who have HF symptoms, and detecting the main clinical features leading to HF. However, much work is still needed to improve the accuracy of HF predictors as most of them have failed to reach high performance levels [49, 50]. In addition to the traditional ML models, deep learning algorithms are gaining much popularity because of their supremacy in terms of performance compared with conventional models, especially if they are trained with huge amounts of data, and their ability to improve on human specialists' performance.

To predict HF risks, data sets including medical records of HF patients are usually used for training the ML algorithms. The process is similar to the diagnosis and detection of HF already explained in Figure 8.1, but with some differences regarding the types of input data that need to be fed into the ML models and the output to be produced. Therefore, the objectives are also different, as they are more oriented to predicting HF mortality and severity risks, HF destabilizations, HF relapses, and/or HF readmission [37, 51]. In this context, in addition to the EHR data (e.g. demographics, admission characteristics, medical history, visits to emergency departments, history of medication use, and healthcare services out of hospital), telemonitoring data can be utilized for identifying and predicting different HF risks (e.g. readmission risks) [52]. Moreover, by combining EHR data with tele-HF data and wearable sensor data the accuracy of predicting HF risks can be improved as discussed in Mortazavi et al. [53].

8.8.1 Prediction of In-Hospital Mortality

J. Kwon et al. have developed an ML model to predict in-hospital mortality for a patient with heart conditions based on echocardiography [54]. The cohort was based on a multicenter retrospective data set. The data from hospital A was used to train a deep learning model while data from hospital B was used for validation. The study size was 25,776 patients, with 1026 registered in-hospital mortalities. Predictor variables were extracted from the echocardiography first raw text reports. First extracted were 11 continuous variables, such as age, weight, height, left or right ventricular systolic dysfunction (LVSD/ RVSD), left atrial dimension (LAD), etc. First, these continuous variables were zero-mean and standard-deviation-one normalized. Then 54 categorical variables were parsed from the report. These variables are counts on the occurrence of specific keywords in the raw text. For example, mitral valve description gathers 10 variables for keywords such as stenosis [5 possible values: absent/trace/mild/moderate/severe], calcification [2 possible values: Y/N], prosthesis [2 possible values: Y/N], etc. The input feature vector formed by the concatenation of the continuous and categorical variables were passed to the deep learning model for training. The model consists of three dense layers with batch normalization and dropout. Comparison with logistic regression and random forests models were conducted, and additional validation of results for coronary heart disease and HF subgroups were conducted in the experimental analysis. The test set included 3840 patients from hospital A and 1560 patients from hospital B. The used performance metrics are the area under ROC curve (AUROC) and the area under precision recall curve (AUPRC). Based on the hospital A held-out set, the deep learning model (AUROC: 0.912, AUPRC: 0.143) outperformed RFs (AUROC: 0.893, AUPRC: 0.134) and logistic regression (AUROC:0.841, AUPRC: 0.205) in the prediction of in-hospital mortality. For the hospital B test set, the deep learning model (AUROC: 0.898, AUPRC: 0.280) outperformed RFs (AUROC: 0.848, AUPRC: 0.186) and logistic regression (AUROC: 0.841, AUPRC: 0.20) in the prediction of in-hospital mortality. The previous results were based on the general cohort of the heart disease cohort. For the subgroup of HF patients, the chosen baselines were the Meta-Analysis Global Group in Chronic Heart Failure deep learning model (MAGGIC) and the Get With The Guidelines-Heart Failure (GWTG-HF) program [55, 56]. The deep learning model (AUROC: 0.913, AUPRC: 0.351) significantly outperformed both MAGGIC (AUROC: 0.806, AUPRC: 0.154) and GWTG-HF (AUROC: 0.783, AUPRC: 0.285).

8.8.2 Prediction of 30-Day HF Readmission

HF readmission is a major healthcare problem. Patient deterioration is correlated with 30-day readmission and significant costs are attached to it. The early prediction of readmission risk can contribute to the reduction of this problem. Scheduling early follow-up based on this predictive model can play an important role in preventing patient readmission and health complications. J. Frizzel et al. proposed a comparison of MLapproaches for this task [57, 58]. The following models were compared: tree-augmented Naive Bayesian network (TAN), an RF algorithm, a gradient-boosted model (GBM), and logistic regression models (LR and LASSO). The baseline models are statistical models built using EHR data (EHR model) [59] and administrative claims model (CMS) [60]. The cohort included 56,477 patients from the GWTG-HF data set. The study population's overall 30-day readmission rate was 21.2%. The variables included in the analysis were extracted from patient EHRs and cover demographics, socioeconomic status, medical history, characterization of HF, lab results, etc. In total, about 250 variables were used as features in the analysis. The data set was randomly divided into training (70%) and validation (30%). The models' performance was assessed based on the validation set. The C statistic was used as a performance measure to distinguish between a readmission or not. The performance of the ML models and the statistical models are respectively TAN(0.62), LR(0.62), LASSO(0.62), RF(0.61), GBM(0.61), EHR model (0.59), and CMS (0.6). The experimental results revealed that there is no significant difference between ML models and statistical models in this context. One limitation of this study is the use of only C statistics as performance metrics. It is possible that additional metrics might better reveal a difference between the studied models.

8.9 Future Direction

HF is a serious cardiovascular disorder affecting a wide range of the population worldwide. The prevalence of HF increases with age, with the prevalence of HF in people over 75 and over 85 years of age being more than 8% and 10%, respectively. The cost burden for the management of HF is significantly high – about 2% of all healthcare expenditure is estimated to be for HF-related cases. This high expenditure is due to the high prevalence and rehospitalization rates of HF patients because of its chronic nature. It is expected that the number of HF patients in the future will increase as the average life expectancy has increased in developed countries. In order to tackle the excessive cost of HF healthcare and the increased work burden on healthcare professionals, advanced modalities are required, particularly to assist clinicians in the diagnosis and decision-making stages of HF, as is the ability to predict the outcomes of the treatments administered. Early diagnosis of HF and prediction of impending HF decompensation are critically important in preventing high mortality and rehospitalization rates and in increasing the quality of life of HF patients. For example, the use of wearable devices can support the continuous remote monitoring of someone with elevated risk, at reduced cost. It is also an excellent example of implementing an early prediction system that can be easily scaled to a large population of vulnerable subjects. The use of ECG on smartwatches has been shown to be capable of identifying several types of heart attacks with an accuracy of 93–95% [61]. Wearable devices are an important future direction that could leverage ML and artificial intelligence tools to provide time-critical prediction to caregivers.

8.10 Conclusion

In modern medicine, the quantity and complexity of huge medical data lead to challenges in solving complex clinical problems. It is here that artificial intelligence and ML applications have important benefits that can help clinicians in the diagnosis, therapeutic decisions, and prediction of the outcomes of HF. Such ML applications guide clinicians to diagnose HF early and prevent the condition from worsening. ML applications have the potential to reduce HF rates and save lives, because these algorithms enable the prediction of HF disease onset months before the clinical diagnosis.

ML applications involve analysis and classification of medical data. Data mining techniques are applied to classify the controls and HF patients, to differentiate HF subtypes with reduced ejection fraction, and to predict the HF severity. In this study, we reviewed the existing ML techniques and their advantages for the diagnosis and prediction of HF, as well as for the prediction of outcomes such as in-hospital mortality and 30-day HF readmission. The results of ML applications demonstrate the high potential of these methods in the diagnosis and prediction of HF. With the development of non-invasive sensor technologies, RPM systems are being introduced to continuously monitor HF patients, and ML algorithms are necessary to discern the markers of HF before observing the symptoms. All these facts point to a revolution in the clinical application of artificial intelligence and ML in cardiovascular medicine that might be seen in the near future. In this chapter we reviewed the following points:

- We gave a brief explanation of ML techniques for medicine, introducing ML principles and the building blocks of an ML system.
- We discussed traditional methods used by clinicians for the diagnosis and prediction of HF.

After we discussed the common clinical practice for both the diagnosis and prediction of HF, we similarly presented ways in which ML and artificial intelligence can contribute to improving the diagnosis and prediction of HF:

- We discussed ML approaches for the detection and diagnosis of HF; we covered ML models trained on biopsy images and how HF can be identified using model trained with large collection of EHRs.
- We considered ML and artificial intelligence methods for the prediction of HF; we focused on approaches for in-hospital mortality prediction, and also examined models for the prediction of 30-day HF readmission.

Acknowledgments

This study was made possible by National Priorities Research Program (NPRP) grant No. NPRP13S-0108-200024 from the Qatar National Research Fund (a member of Qatar Foundation). The statements made herein are solely the responsibility of the authors.It was also supported with a Qatar University International Research Collaboration Co-Fund (IRCC) program (IRCC-2020-002).

References

1 Gouveia, M., Ascenção, R., Fiorentino, F., Costa, J., Caldeira, D., Broeiro-Gonçalves, P., Fonseca, C., and Borges, M. (2019). The current and future burden of heart failure in Portugal. *ESC Heart Failure* 6: 254–261. https://doi.org/10.1002/ehf2.12399.

2 Coke, R. (2019). Heart of Middle East. Routledge. doi: 10.4324/9781315828152.

3 Elasfar, A.A., Alhabeeb, W., and Elasfar, S. (2020). Heart failure in the Middle East Arab countries: Current and future perspectives. *Journal of the Saudi Heart Association (JSHA)* 32: 236–241. doi: 10.37616/2212-5043.1040.

4 Tromp, J., Paniagua, S.M., Lau, E.S., Allen, N.B., Blaha, M.J., Gansevoort, R.T., Hillege, H.L., Lee, D.E., Levy, D., Ramachandran, V.S., and Van Der Harst, P. (2021). Age dependent associations of risk factors with heart failure: Pooled population based cohort study. *The BMJ* 372 (Mar. 23).

5 Bragazzi, N.L., Zhong, W., Shu, J., Abu Much, A., Lotan, D., Grupper, A., Younis, A., and Dai, H. (2021). Burden of heart failure and underlying causes in 195 countries and territories from 1990 to 2017. *European Journal of Preventive Cardiology*. doi: 10.1093/eurjpc/zwaa147.

6 Inan Omer, T., Baran Pouyan, M., Javaid Abdul, Q., Dowling, S., Etemadi, M., Dorier, A., Heller, J.A., Bicen, A.O., Roy, S., De Marco, T., et al. (2018). Novel wearable seismocardiography and machine learning algorithms can assess clinical status of heart failure patients. *Circulation. Heart Failure* 11: e004313. doi: 10.1161/CIRCHEARTFAILURE.117.004313.

7 Ponikowski, P., Voors, A.A., Anker, S.D., Bueno, H., Cleland, J.G.F., Coats, A.J.S., Falk, V., González-Juanatey, J.R., Harjola, V.-P., Jankowska, E.A., et al. (2016). 2016 ESC Guidelines for the diagnosis and treatment of acute and chronic heart failure: The Task Force for the diagnosis and treatment of acute and chronic heart failure of the European Society of Cardiology (ESC) developed with the special contribution of the Heart Failure Association (HFA) of the ESC. *European Heart Journal* 37: 2129–2200. doi: 10.1093/eurheartj/ehw128.

8 Farré, N., Vela, E., Clèries, M., Bustins, M., Cainzos-Achirica, M., Enjuanes, C., Moliner, P., Ruiz, S., Verdú-Rotellar, J.M., and Comín-Colet, J. (2016). Medical resource use and expenditure in patients with chronic heart failure: A population-based analysis of 88 195 patients. *European Journal of Heart Failure* 18: 1132–1140. https://doi.org/10.1002/ejhf.549.

9 Ray, A. and Chaudhuri, A.K. (2021). Smart healthcare disease diagnosis and patient management: Innovation, improvement and skill development. *Machine Learning with Applications* 3 (Mar. 15): 100011.

10 Uddin, S., Khan, A., Hossain, M.E., and Moni, M.A. (2019). Comparing different supervised machine learning algorithms for disease prediction. *BMC Medical Informatics and Decision Making* 19 (1) (Dec.): 1–6.

11 Krittanawong, C., Virk, H.U., Bangalore, S., Wang, Z., Johnson, K.W., Pinotti, R., Zhang, H., Kaplin, S., Narasimhan, B., Kitai, T., and Baber, U. (2020). Machine learning prediction in cardiovascular diseases: A meta-analysis. *Scientific Reports* 10 (1) (Sep. 29): 1-1.

12 Hunt Sharon, A., Abraham William, T., Chin Marshall, H., Feldman Arthur, M., Francis Gary, S., Ganiats Theodore, G., Jessup, M., Konstam Marvin, A., Mancini Donna, M., Michl, K., et al. (2009). 2009 focused update incorporated into the ACC/AHA 2005 guidelines for the diagnosis and management of heart failure in adults. *Journal of the American College of Cardiology* 53: e1–e90. doi: 10.1016/j.jacc.2008.11.013.

13 Tripoliti, E.E., Papadopoulos, T.G., Karanasiou, G.S., Naka, K.K., and Fotiadis, D.I. (2017). Heart failure: Diagnosis, severity estimation and prediction of adverse events through machine learning techniques. *Computational and Structural Biotechnology Journal* 15: 26–47. https://doi.org/10.1016/j.csbj.2016.11.001.

14 Kim, K. and Kwon, J. (2019). Deep learning for diagnosing heart failure from ECG signals. *The Journal of Heart and Lung Transplantation* 38 (4): S375.

15 Roger, V.L. (2010). The heart failure epidemic. *International Journal of Environmental Research and Public Health* 7. doi: 10.3390/ijerph7041807.

16 Ponikowski, P., Voors, A.A., Anker, S.D., Bueno, H., Cleland, J.G.F., Coats, A.J.S., Falk, V., González-Juanatey, J.R., Harjola, V.P., Jankowska, E.A., et al. (2016). 2016 ESC guidelines for the diagnosis and treatment of acute and chronic heart failure: The Task Force for the diagnosis and treatment of acute and chronic heart failure of the European Society of

Cardiology (ESC) developed with the special contribution of the Heart Failure Association (HFA) of the ESC. *European Heart Journal* 37: 2129–2200. doi: 10.1093/eurheartj/ehw128.

17 Yancy Clyde, W., Jessup, M., Bozkurt, B., Butler, J., Casey Donald, E., Colvin Monica, M., Drazner Mark, H., Filippatos Gerasimos, S., Fonarow Gregg, C., Givertz Michael, M., et al. (2017). 2017 ACC/AHA/HFSA focused update of the 2013 ACCF/AHA guideline for the management of heart failure. *Journal of the American College of Cardiology* 70: 776–803. doi: 10.1016/j.jacc.2017.04.025.

18 Faragli, A., Abawi, D., Quinn, C., Cvetkovic, M., Schlabs, T., Tahirovic, E., Düngen, H.D., Pieske, B., Kelle, S., Edelmann, F., et al. (2020). The role of non-invasive devices for the telemonitoring of heart failure patients. *Heart Failure Reviews*. doi: 10.1007/s10741-020-09963-7.

19 Gackowski, A., Isnard, R., Golmard, J.L., Pousset, F., Carayon, A., Montalescot, G., Hulot, J.S., Thomas, D., Piwowarska, W., and Komajda, M. (2004). Comparison of echocardiography and plasma B-type natriuretic peptide for monitoring the response to treatment in acute heart failure. *European Heart Journal* 25 (20) (1): 1788–1796.

20 Le Jemtel, T.H. and Alt, E.U. (2006). Are hemodynamic goals viable in tailoring heart failure therapy? Hemodynamic goals are outdated. *Circulation* 113: 1027–1032. discussion 1033.

21 Smeets, C.J.P., Lee, S., Groenendaal, W., Squillace, G., Vranken, J., De Cannière, H., Van Hoof, C., Grieten, L., Mullens, W., Nijst, P., et al. (2020). The added value of in-hospital tracking of the efficacy of decongestion therapy and prognostic value of a wearable thoracic impedance sensor in acutely decompensated heart failure with volume overload: Prospective cohort study. *JMIR Cardiology* 4: e12141.

22 Dickstein, K., Cohen-Solal, A., Filippatos, G., McMurray, J.J., Ponikowski, P., Poole-Wilson, P.A., Strömberg, A., Van Veldhuisen, D.J., Atar, D., Hoes, A.W., et al. (2008). ESC guidelines for the diagnosis and treatment of acute and chronic heart failure 2008: The Task Force for the diagnosis and treatment of acute and chronic heart failure 2008 of the European Society of Cardiology developed in collaboration with the Heart Failure Association of the ESC (HFA) and endorsed by the European Society of Intensive Care Medicine (ESICM). *European Journal of Heart Failure* 10: 933–989. doi: 10.1016/j.ejheart.2008.08.005.

23 Fleg Jerome, L., Piña Ileana, L., Balady Gary, J., Chaitman Bernard, R., Fletcher, B., Lavie, C., Limacher Marian, C., Stein Richard, A., Williams, M., and Bazzarre, T. (2000). Assessment of functional capacity in clinical and research applications. *Circulation* 102: 1591–1597. doi: 10.1161/01.CIR.102.13.1591.

24 Koehler, F., Koehler, K., Deckwart, O., Prescher, S., Wegscheider, K., Winkler, S., Vettorazzi, E., Polze, A., Stangl, K., Hartmann, O., et al. (2018). Telemedical interventional management in Heart Failure II (TIM-HF2), a randomised, controlled trial investigating the impact of telemedicine on unplanned cardiovascular hospitalisations and mortality in heart failure patients: Study design and description of the intervention. *European Journal of Heart Failure* 20: 1485–1493. https://doi.org/10.1002/ejhf.1300.

25 Inglis, S.C., Clark, R.A., Dierckx, R., Prieto-Merino, D., and Cleland, J.G.F. (2015). Structured telephone support or non-invasive telemonitoring for patients with heart failure. *Cochrane Database of Systematic Reviews*. doi: 10.1002/14651858.CD007228.pub3.

26 Amir, O., Ben-Gal, T., Weinstein, J.M., Schliamser, J., Burkhoff, D., Abbo, A., and Abraham, W.T. (2017). Evaluation of remote dielectric sensing (ReDS) technology-guided therapy for decreasing heart failure re-hospitalizations. *International Journal of Cardiology* 240: 279–284. https://doi.org/10.1016/j.ijcard.2017.02.120.

27 Murphy, N., Shanks, M., and Alderman, P. (2019). Management of heart failure with outpatient technology. *The Journal for Nurse Practitioners* 15: 12–18. https://doi.org/10.1016/j.nurpra.2018.07.004.

28 Chouvarda, I., Philip, N.Y., Natsiavas, P., Kilintzis, V., Sobnath, D., Kayyali, R., Henriques, J., Paiva, R.P., Raptopoulos, A., Chételat, O., et al. (2014). WELCOME — Innovative integrated care platform using wearable sensing and smart cloud computing for COPD patients with comorbidities. *Proceedings of 2014 36th Annual International Conference of the IEEE Engineering in Medicine and Biology Society* 26-30, Aug: 3180–3183. doi: 10.1109/EMBC.2014.6944298.

29 Abraham, W.T., Adamson, P.B., Bourge, R.C., Aaron, M.F., Costanzo, M.R., Stevenson, L.W., Strickland, W., Neelagaru, S., Raval, N., Krueger, S., et al. (2011). Wireless pulmonary artery haemodynamic monitoring in chronic heart failure: A randomised controlled trial. *The Lancet* 377: 658–666. https://doi.org/10.1016/S0140-6736(11)60101-3.

30 Shavelle, D.M., Desai, A.S., Abraham, W.T., Bourge, R.C., Raval, N., Rathman, L.D., Heywood, J.T., Jermyn, R.A., Pelzel, J., Jonsson, O.T., et al. (2020). Lower rates of heart failure and all-cause hospitalizations during pulmonary artery pressure-guided therapy for ambulatory heart failure: One-year outcomes from the CardioMEMS post-approval study. *Circulation. Heart Failure* 13: e006863. doi: 10.1161/circheartfailure.119.006863.

31 Abraham, J., McCann, P.J., Guglin, M.E., Bhimaraj, A., Benjamin, T.-A.S., Robinson, M.R., Jonsson, O.T., Feitell, S.C., Bhatt, K.A., Bennett, M.K., et al. (2020). Management of the patient with heart failure and an implantable pulmonary artery hemodynamic sensor. *Current Cardiovascular Risk Reports* 14: 12. doi: 10.1007/s12170-020-00646-4.

32 Klersy, C., De Silvestri, A., Gabutti, G., Regoli, F., and Auricchio, A. (2009). A meta-analysis of remote monitoring of heart failure patients. *Journal of the American College of Cardiology* 54: 1683–1694. doi: 10.1016/j.jacc.2009.08.017.

33 Zhu, Y., Gu, X., and Xu, C. (2020). Effectiveness of telemedicine systems for adults with heart failure: A meta-analysis of randomized controlled trials. *Heart Failure Reviews* 25: 231–243. doi: 10.1007/s10741-019-09801-5.

34 Nouryan, C.N., Morahan, S., Pecinka, K., Akerman, M., Lesser, M., Chaikin, D., Castillo, S., Zhang, M., and Pekmezaris, R. (2018). Home telemonitoring of community-dwelling heart failure patients after home care discharge. *Telemedicine and e-Health* 25: 447–454. doi: 10.1089/tmj.2018.0099.

35 Ware, P., Ross, H.J., Cafazzo, J.A., Laporte, A., Gordon, K., and Seto, E. (2018). Evaluating the implementation of a mobile phone–based telemonitoring program: Longitudinal study guided by the consolidated framework for implementation research. *JMIR Mhealth Uhealth* 6: e10768. doi: 10.2196/10768.

36 Muhammad, Y., Tahir, M., Hayat, M., and Chong, K.T. (2020). Early and accurate detection and diagnosis of heart disease using intelligent computational model. *Scientific Reports* 10 (1) (Nov. 12): 1–7.

37 Tripoliti, E.E., Papadopoulos, T.G., Karanasiou, G.S., Naka, K.K., and Fotiadis, D.I. (2017). Heart failure: Diagnosis, severity estimation and prediction of adverse events through machine learning techniques. *Computational and Structural Biotechnology Journal* 15 (Jan. 1): 26–47.

38 Alonso-Betanzos, A. and Bolón-Canedo, V. (2018). Big-data analysis, cluster analysis, and machine-learning approaches. *Sex-Specific Analysis of Cardiovascular Function* 1065: 607–626.

39 Ren, H., Yu, S., Li, X., Qiu, W., Zhong, A., Guo, N., and Li, Q. (2019). Personalized treatment for heart failure with preserved ejection fraction using deep reinforcement learning. *Circulation* 140 (Suppl. 1) (Nov. 19): A15036.

40 Hussain, L., Awan, I.A., Aziz, W., Saeed, S., Ali, A., Zeeshan, F., and Kwak, K.S. (2020). Detecting congestive heart failure by extracting multimodal features and employing machine learning techniques. *BioMed Research International* 2020: (Feb. 18).

41 Lanzer, J.D., Leuschner, F., Kramann, R., Levinson, R.T., and Saez-Rodriguez, J. (2020). Big data approaches in heart failure research. *Current Heart Failure Reports* https://doi.org/10.1007/s11897-020-00469-9.

42 Katarya, R. and Meena, S.K. (2021). Machine learning techniques for heart disease prediction: A comparative study and analysis. *Health and Technology* 11 (1) (Jan): 87–97.

43 Olsen, C.R., Mentz, R.J., Anstrom, K.J., Page, D., and Patel, P.A. (2020). Clinical applications of machine learning in the diagnosis, classification, and prediction of heart failure. *American Heart Journal* 229: (Jul. 16). doi: 10.1016/j.ahj.2020.07.009. PMID: 32905873.

44 Nirschl, J.J., Janowczyk, A., Peyster, E.G., Frank, R., Margulies, K.B., Feldman, M.D., and Madabhushi, A. (2018). A deep-learning classifier identifies patients with clinical heart failure using whole-slide images of H&E tissue. *PLOS ONE* 13: e0192726. doi: 10.1371/journal.pone.0192726.

45 Janowczyk, A. and Madabhushi, A. (2016). Deep learning for digital pathology image analysis: A comprehensive tutorial with selected use cases. *Journal of Pathology Informatics* 7: 29. doi: 10.4103/2153-3539.186902.

46 Orlov, N., Shamir, L., Macura, T., Johnston, J., Eckley, D.M., and Goldberg, I.G. (2008). WND-CHARM: Multi-purpose image classification using compound image transforms. *Pattern Recognition Letters* 29: 1684–1693. https://doi.org/10.1016/j.patrec.2008.04.013.

47 Rasmy, L., Wu, Y., Wang, N., Geng, X., Zheng, W.J., Wang, F., Wu, H., Xu, H., and Zhi, D. (2018). A study of generalizability of recurrent neural network-based predictive models for heart failure onset risk using a large and heterogeneous EHR data set. *Journal of Biomedical Informatics* 84: 11–16. https://doi.org/10.1016/j.jbi.2018.06.011

48 Choi, E., Bahadori, M.T., Kulas, J.A., Schuetz, A., Stewart, W.F., and Sun, J. (2016). RETAIN: An interpretable predictive model for healthcare using reverse time attention mechanism. *arXiv Preprint arXiv:1608.05745.*

49 Al'Aref, S.J., Anchouche, K., Singh, G., Slomka, P.J., Kolli, K.K., Kumar, A., Pandey, M., Maliakal, G., Van Rosendael, A.R., Beecy, A.N., Berman, D.S., Leipsic, J., Nieman, K., Andreini, D., Pontone, G., Schoepf, U.J., Shaw, L.J., Chang, H.-J., Narula, J., Bax, J.J., Guan, Y., and Min, J.K. (2018). Clinical applications of machine learning in cardiovascular disease and its relevance to cardiac imaging. *European Heart Journal* 40 (24): 1975–1986.

50 Al'Aref, S.J., Singh, G., Van Rosendael, A.R., Kolli, K.K., Ma, X., Maliakal, G., Pandey, M., Lee, B.C., Wang, J., Xu, Z., Zhang, Y., Min, J.K., Wong, S.C., and Minutello, R.M. (2019). Determinants of in-hospital mortality after percutaneous coronary intervention: A machine learning approach. *Journal of the American Heart Association* 8 (5): 011160.

51 Guo, A., Pasque, M., Loh, F., Mann, D.L., and Payne, P.R. (2020). Heart failure diagnosis, readmission, and mortality prediction using machine learning and artificial intelligence models. *Current Epidemiology Reports* (Oct. 31): 1–8.

52 Awan, S.E., Bennamoun, M., Sohel, F., Sanfilippo, F.M., and Dwivedi, G. (2019). Machine learning-based prediction of heart failure readmission or death: Implications of choosing the right model and the right metrics. *ESC Heart Failure* 6 (2) (Apr.): 428–435.

53 Mortazavi, B.J., Downing, N.S., Bucholz, E.M., Dharmarajan, K., Manhapra, A., Li, S.X., Negahban, S.N., and Krumholz, H.M. (2016). Analysis of machine learning techniques for heart failure readmissions. *Circulation. Cardiovascular Quality and Outcomes* 9 (6) (Nov.): 629–640.

54 Kwon, J.-M., Kim, K.-H., Jeon, K.-H., and Park, J. (2019). Deep learning for predicting in-hospital mortality among heart disease patients based on echocardiography. *Echocardiography* 36: 213–218. https://doi.org/10.1111/echo.14220.

55 Wong, C.M., Hawkins, N.M., Petrie, M.C., Jhund, P.S., Gardner, R.S., Ariti, C.A., Poppe, K.K., Earle, N., Whalley, G.A., Squire, I.B., et al. (2014). Heart failure in younger patients: The Meta-analysis Global Group in Chronic Heart Failure (MAGGIC). *European Heart Journal* 35: 2714–2721. doi: 10.1093/eurheartj/ehu216.

56 Bergethon Kristin, E., Ju, C., DeVore Adam, D., Hardy, N.C., Fonarow Gregg, C., Yancy Clyde, W., Heidenreich Paul, A., Bhatt Deepak, L., Peterson Eric, D., and Hernandez Adrian, F. (2016). Trends in 30-day readmission rates for patients hospitalized with heart failure. *Circulation. Heart Failure* 9: e002594. doi: 10.1161/CIRCHEARTFAILURE.115.002594.

57 Frizzell, J.D., Liang, L., Schulte, P.J., Yancy, C.W., Heidenreich, P.A., Hernandez, A.F., Bhatt, D.L., Fonarow, G.C., and Laskey, W.K. (2017). Prediction of 30-day all-cause readmissions in patients hospitalized for heart failure: Comparison of machine learning and other statistical approaches. *JAMA Cardiology* 2: 204–209. doi: 10.1001/jamacardio.2016.3956.

58 Golas, S.B., Shibahara, T., Agboola, S., Otaki, H., Sato, J., Nakae, T., Hisamitsu, T., Kojima, G., Felsted, J., Kakarmath, S., et al. (2018). A machine learning model to predict the risk of

30-day readmissions in patients with heart failure: A retrospective analysis of electronic medical records data. *BMC Medical Informatics and Decision Making* 18: 44. doi: 10.1186/s12911-018-0620-z.

59 Eapen Zubin, J., Liang, L., Fonarow Gregg, C., Heidenreich Paul, A., Curtis Lesley, H., Peterson Eric, D., and Hernandez Adrian, F. (2013). Validated, electronic health record deployable prediction models for assessing patient risk of 30-day rehospitalization and mortality in older heart failure patients. *JACC. Heart Failure* 1: 245–251.

60 Keenan Patricia, S., Normand Sharon-Lise, T., Lin, Z., Drye Elizabeth, E., Bhat Kanchana, R., Ross Joseph, S., Schuur Jeremiah, D., Stauffer Brett, D., Bernheim Susannah, M., Epstein Andrew, J., et al. (2008). An administrative claims measure suitable for profiling hospital performance on the basis of 30-day all-cause readmission rates among patients with heart failure. *Circulation. Cardiovascular Quality and Outcomes* 1: 29–37. doi: 10.1161/CIRCOUTCOMES.108.802686.

61 Spaccarotella, C.S., Polimeni, A.P., Principe, E.P., Curcio, A.C., Migliarino, S.M., Mongiardo, A.M., De Rosa, S.D., and Indolfi, C. (2020). Multichannel electrocardiograms obtained by a smartwatch for the diagnosis of acute coronary syndromes: The SMARTAMI TRIAL. *European Heart Journal* 41 (Suppl. 2): ehaa946–3441.

9

Machine Learning Techniques for Predicting and Managing Heart Failure

Dafni K. Plati, Evanthia E. Tripoliti, Georgia S. Karanasiou, Aidonis Rammos, Aris Bechlioulis, Chris J. Watson, Ken McDonald, Mark Ledwidge, Yorgos Goletsis, Katerina K. Naka, and Dimitrios I. Fotiadis

9.1 State of the Art of Machine Learning Applications in HF

In the first part of this chapter a brief definition of heart failure (HF) is presented along with the various classifications, evaluation, and diagnosis of HF. Moreover, an extended review of the state of the art of applications of machine learning (ML) in HF diagnosis, severity estimation, and the prediction of adverse events (mortality or rehospitalization) is demonstrated.

9.1.1 Introduction

9.1.1.1 Background

According to the American College of Cardiology and the American Heart Association, HF "is a complex clinical syndrome that results from any structural or functional impairment of ventricular filling or ejection of blood" [1]. In simple words, HF is a chronic clinical syndrome, where the heart is unable to pump enough blood to deal with the systemic needs of the body [2]. It usually occurs because the heart has become either too weak or stiff.

Most patients with HF have symptoms due to impaired left ventricular myocardial function [2]. Patients with HF deal with various symptoms that affect their quality of life: dyspnea, fatigue, exercise intolerance, fluid retention, pulmonary hypertension, or other heart conditions, such as an irregular heartbeat and heart valve disease [1].

Although HF is the result of a number of problems affecting the heart, the predominant causes are the presence of myocardial ischemia (reduced coronary blood flow leading to reduced oxygen preventing the heart from functioning properly [3]) and high blood pressure (the risk for HF doubles in patients with blood pressure > 160/100 mmHg [4]). Moreover, patients may have more than one causative factor for HF. Conditions that can lead to HF include [5, 6]:

- Ischemic heart disease due to coronary artery disease
- Toxic damage due to recreational substance use (alcohol, narcotics, steroids, heavy metals, medications,) and chemotherapy

Predicting Heart Failure: Invasive, Non-Invasive, Machine Learning, and Artificial Intelligence Based Methods, First Edition. Edited by Kishor Kumar Sadasivuni, Hassen M. Ouakad, Somaya Al-Maadeed, Huseyin C. Yalcin, and Issam Bait Bahadur.

- Immune and inflammatory diseases
- Infiltrative diseases such as amyloidosis or sarcoidosis
- Metabolic causes (thyroid dysfunction, nutritional deficiencies)
- Genetic abnormalities
- Arrhythmias
- Valvular and structural abnormalities
- Hypertension [5]
- Life style habits such as the lack of exercise, smoking, and obesity, can exacerbate an existing problem [6].

HF is one of the most common causes of admission to hospital and is the cause of more than $30 billion spent in the US annually [7]. A total increase of 46% is estimated to be associated with more than 8 million adults with HF and can be compared to a global epidemic [8]. HF represents the primary cause of hospitalization in patients aged 65 years or older in the western world, and is accountable for more than 1 million hospitalizations per year in the US [8]. As presented in Figure 9.1 the HF prevalence is a worldwide phenomenon [9, 10].

HF imposes a significant burden on both patients and healthcare systems, with costly hospitalizations and high mortality rates [11, 12]. Hospitalizations due to HF represent 1–2% of all hospital admissions [13]. More than 20% of patients are rehospitalized within 30 days and up to 50% within 6 months [14], and 40% of patients die within a year of their first hospitalization [15]. Occurring more frequently in people over 65 [16], HF prevalence in the general population is estimated to be 4.2% [17]. Although HF is perceived as a disease of the elderly, studies have indicated that HF incidents are increasing in young people [18, 19].

Therefore, there is a great interest in reducing hospital readmissions due to HF; attempts to achieve this take different forms, from the introduction of penalties on hospitals that exceed the expected readmission rates [20] to specialized decision models [21].

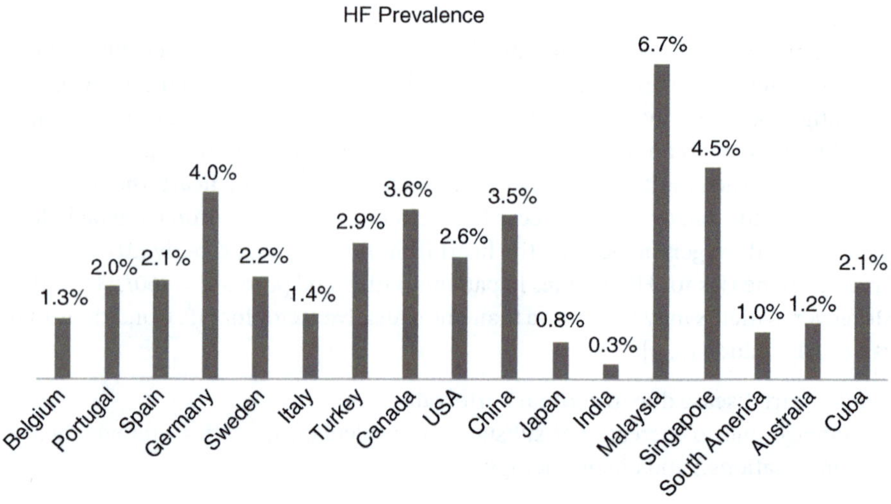

Figure 9.1 Prevalence of HF worldwide (data from Lund and Savarese [9] and Groenewegen et al. [10]).

9.1.1.2 HF Classifications

The American College of Cardiology/American Heart Association guidelines (2013) have classified HF into two categories according to the measurement of the left ventricle ejection fraction (EF): HF with preserved (≥50%) ejection fraction (HFpEF) – the heart pumps blood normally but is too stiff to fill properly that leads to impaired filling of the chambers of the heart; and HF with reduced (≤40%) ejection fraction (HFrEF) – the heart is too weak to efficiently pump blood out of the left ventricle [1, 22]. Ejection fraction reflects the pump function of the heart; it represents the amount of blood being pumped from the left ventricle (the heart's main pumping chamber) with each contraction and is expressed as a percentage. HF with mid-range or mildly reduced EF (HFmrEF) is an intermediate stage with an EF of 40–49%, that generally progresses either to HFpEF at 25% of cases or HFrEF at 33% of cases [23].

The most common classification for HF severity is the New York Heart Association (NYHA) classification. The NYHA classification has been widely used for almost a century and was updated in 1994 [24]. It is a fundamental tool for stratifying the risk of HF and also determines if a patient is eligible for a clinical trial or if the type of medication and devices are appropriate [25]. It classifies HF into the categories shown in (Figure 9.2 [26].

Depending on the time of onset, HF can be classified as acute or chronic. Acute HF can be defined as "the rapid onset or change of symptoms and signs of HF that requires urgent medical care" [5]. Furthermore, acute HF is a condition with an unfavorable prognosis and is characterized by high mortality and rehospitalization rates [27]. Patients who have stable HF for some time, without change in clinical status, are often said to have chronic HF [5].

9.1.1.3 Evaluation and Diagnosis

Due to the increased incidence and the large financial costs required to diagnose HF, the diagnosis and treatment of the disease are extremely critical issues. The diagnosis of HF can be difficult, especially in the early stages and there is not a single diagnostic test for HF. Furthermore, it might be particularly difficult to recognized and associate symptoms and signs in obese patients, in elderly people, and in patients who suffer from chronic lung disease and need to be assessed at each visit meticulously [16].

Initially, clinical symptoms and signs are estimated by clinicians by performing a physical examination of the patient. Also, standard biochemical and hematological tests have to be requested. These tests include complete blood analysis, urinalysis, and a

Class I – HF does not cause limitations to physical activity. Ordinary activities do not cause fatigue or shortness of breath.

Class II – HF causes slight limitation to physical activity with symptoms such as fatigue and shortness of breath. Patients with NYHA class II show no symptoms at rest.

Class III – HF causes marked limitations of physical activity. Patients with NYHA class III show no symptoms at rest, but less than ordinary activity causes symptoms of HF.

Class IV – HF patients are unable to carry on any physical activity without HF symptoms and even have symptoms when at rest.

Figure 9.2 NYHA classification. Based on The Criteria Committee of the New York Heart Association [24].

complete metabolic profile for levels of serum electrolytes (including sodium, potassium, calcium, and magnesium), serum urea nitrogen, serum creatinine, glucose, fasting lipid profile, and thyroid-stimulating hormone. Moreover the kidney and liver function have to be tested [28]. Apart from a detailed medical history, the electrocardiogram (ECG) is fundamental to reveal arrhythmias, conduction delays, or ischemia, while the echocardiogram is also a standard test to confirm systolic or diastolic dysfunction [29]. Also, the initial evaluation may include a chest X-ray, a coronary angiography (or a computed tomography coronary angiography (CTCA)) when coronary artery disease is suspected. In addition, cardiac magnetic resonance (CMR) imaging has become a very useful tool for investigating HF due to its a high spatial resolution and the use of late gadolinium enhancement (LGE) [30, 31]. Static images using T1 and T2 weighted black blood algorithms are valuable for tissue characterization. With CMR, clinicians are informed about anatomic structures, perfusion, and ventricular function while LGE can specify the exact causes of HF, depending on the pattern of scar formation such as amyloidosis, sarcoidosis, eosinophilic myocarditis, etc. and provide important prognostic information beyond other biomarkers [32, 33].

The measurement of serial natriuretic peptide (B-type natriuretic peptide (BNP) or N-terminal pro–B-type natriuretic peptide (NTproBNP)) is also included in the HF-specific laboratory tests (specifically in patients with suspected HF) in order to address the management of HF. According to the European Society of Cardiology (ESC) [5], systolic HF can be effectively ruled out with the levels of BNP or NTproBNP. As BNP levels increase, the specificity increases and the diagnosis of HF becomes easier [34]. Standard management of the HF patient involves a follow-up 2–12 times a year and patients are advised to self-monitor their weight and symptoms.

9.1.2 Applications of ML in HF

9.1.2.1 ML in Medicine

Medicine has always been characterized by (big) data that is suitable for the application of ML. ML is appropriate to clinical research since it is more flexible than traditional statistical methods. ML provides great potential for healthcare experts to exploit massive amounts of data from numerous sources, integrate them in a single system, curate them, and provide assessment and recommendations.

ML models have the potential to improve healthcare efficiency in numerous ways. Prognostic models could empower healthcare experts to select better treatment options for their patients. Additionally, diagnostic models could be used in screening, risk stratification, and recommending appropriate tests. This would decrease the burden on clinicians, save resources, and reduce costs.

According to Obermeyer and Emanuel [35], increasing the ability to transform data into knowledge will affect at least three areas of medicine: (i) it will dramatically improve prognosis, (ii) it will improve diagnostic accuracy and (iii) it will reduce much of the work of radiologists and anatomical pathologists, since these clinicians mainly focus on analyzing digitized images that can easily be processed by algorithms instead.

ML techniques can be grouped into two subcategories: supervised learning and unsupervised learning [36, 37]. In supervised learning, the model is trained by having as input a data set comprised of instances; every instance has a known outcome. The data set may consist of various features (discrete or continuous). The goal of the model is to predict a certain output that can also be discrete or continuous. In the case of a discrete output, we are referring to a classification problem and in the case where the output has a continuous value (range), we have a regression problem. By contrast, in unsupervised learning there is not a single output to predict; the data are unlabeled. The algorithms try to find patterns in the data. Clustering, the most common application, uses algorithms that try to group data in clusters based on similarities they might have.

Early diagnosis of HF, outcome prediction, hospital readmission, and mortality prediction in HF patients are the areas that benefit from the application of supervised ML techniques in the medical field with a discrete outcome.

9.1.2.2 ML Applications in HF Diagnosis/Prediction

Models based on ML techniques can be useful in helping physicians in HF diagnosis. Several studies have been conducted to build a model that can diagnose and detect HF at an early stage based on various ML algorithms (Table 9.1).

In 2010, Yang et al. [38] proposed a model based on support vector machines (SVM) to diagnose HF at an early stage using 289 patient cases. Samples were classified into three groups: the control group (70 subjects), the HF-prone group (59 subjects), and the HF group (160 subjects). The accuracy of the model was 87.50% and 65.85% in identifying subjects in HF-prone group and HF group, respectively. In 2012, Son et al. [39] tested an approach that combined rough set (RS)-based model with decision trees on 88 control subjects and 71 subjects with congestive HF. In their study, they utilized data with no missing values and features consisting of demographics information and clinical laboratory findings. The experimental results showed that their method performed with an accuracy of 97.50%, sensitivity 97.20%, and specificity 97.70%. In 2017, Choi et al. [40] applied deep learning (DL) methods and more specifically implemented a recurrent neural network (RNN) for the early detection of HF in 3884 HF subjects and 28,903 controls using electronic health record (EHR) data. The EHR data set included demographics, habits, clinical and laboratory findings, medications, and International Classification of Diseases (ICD)-9 codes. Their model achieved 77.70% area under the ROC curve (AUC), with a 12-month observation window, higher than regularized logistic regression (LR), neural network (NN), SVM and K-nearest neighbor (k-NN) classifier approaches. More recently, in 2020, Le et al. [41] implemented a multilayer perceptron (MLP) NN achieving an accuracy of 88.00%. The data set (299 subjects) they utilized comprised demographics, laboratory findings, lifestyle habits, and ejection fraction. Also in 2020, Potter et al. 2020 [42] applied the RF classifier to build a model able to predict Stage B HF based on energy waveform ECG. They utilized 254 subjects as the training set (135 with HF, 119 controls) and 65 subjects as the test set (27 with HF, 38 controls). Their model achieved AUC 76.00%, sensitivity 93.00%, and specificity 61.00%. Pecchia et al. [43] conducted a study utilizing the short-term heart rate variability (HRV) measures. They analyzed 1914.40 hours of ECG signals from 83 patients, of which 54 were used as controls and 29 were subjects suffering from chronic HF with NYHA classification I, II, and III. They designed a classifier based on the classification and regression trees (CART) method with 94.80% accuracy, 89.70% sensitivity, and 100% specificity on identifying normal subjects vs. subjects with NYHA classification I, II and III.

Table 9.1 State of the art of ML for HF diagnosis.

HF Diagnosis					
Study	**Target**	**Method**	**Features**	**Data Set**	**Evaluation Measures**
Yang et al. 2010	HF diagnosis Healthy vs. HF-prone vs. HF	SVM	Blood test, HRV measurements, echocardio-graphic and ECG features, chest radiography test, 6-minutes walk distance test and physical test.	289 subjects 70 controls 59 HF-prone 160 with HF	Accuracy 78.79% for the control group Accuracy 87.50% for the HF-prone group Accuracy 65.85% for the HF group
Pecchia et al. 2011	HF diagnosis Healthy vs. HF	CART method	HRV measures	83 subjects 29 with chronic HF 54 as controls	Accuracy 94.80%, Sensitivity 89.70% Specificity 100%
Son et al. 2012	HF diagnosis Healthy vs. HF	Combination of rough set based model with decision trees	Demographics, clinical laboratory findings	159 subjects 88 controls 71 with congestive HF	Accuracy 97.50% Sensitivity 97.20% Specificity 97.70
Austin et al. 2013	Healthy vs. HFpEF vs. HFrEF	RF	Demographics, vital signs, symptoms, laboratory results and medical history	EFFECT study data set 3697 subjects for training 4515 subjects for testing	69.60% positive predictive value
Zheng et al. 2015	Chronic HF diagnosis Healthy vs. chronic HF	Least squares-SVM model	Cardiac reserve and heart sound characteristics	152 subjects 88 controls 64 with chronic HF	Accuracy 95.39% Sensitivity 96.59% Specificity 93.75%
Masetic et al. 2016	HF diagnosis Healthy vs. HF	C4.5, k-NN, SVM, artificial NNs, RF	ECG signals	31 subjects 18 with congestive HF 13 controls	RF classifier gives 100.00% accuracy

(Continued)

Table 9.1 (Continued)

HF Diagnosis					
Study	**Target**	**Method**	**Features**	**Data Set**	**Evaluation Measures**
Chen et al. 2017	HF diagnosis Healthy vs. congestive HF	Sparse auto-encoder-based deep learning	HRV measures	116 subjects 44 with congestive HF 72 controls	Accuracy 72.41% Sensitivity 49.09% Specificity 85.62%
Choi et al. 2017	HF diagnosis Healthy vs. HF	RNN models	Demographics, habits, clinical and laboratory values, ICD-9 codes, medications	3884 with HF 28,903 controls	RNN model AUC 77.70%
Samuel et al. 2017	HF diagnosis Healthy vs. HF	Hybrid decision support method based on artificial NNs and fuzzy analytic hierarchy process technique	Demographics, symptoms, clinical and laboratory values, ECG results	Cleveland heart disease database 297 subjects 137 with HF 160 controls	Accuracy 91.10%
Reddy et al. 2018	HFpEF diagnosis Healthy vs. HFpEF	LR	Demographics, medications, echocardio graphic features, physical examination features	414 subjects 267 with HFpEF 147 controls	AUC 88.60%
Mohan et al. 2019	HF diagnosis Healthy vs. HF	Hybrid RF with a linear model	Demographics, symptoms, clinical and laboratory values	Cleveland heart disease database 297 subjects 137 with HF 160 controls	Accuracy 88.40% Sensitivity 92.80% Specificity 82.60%
Ali et al. 2019	HF diagnosis Healthy vs. HF	Stacked SVM	Demographics, symptoms, clinical and laboratory values	Cleveland heart disease database 297 subjects 137 with HF 160 controls	Accuracy 92.22% Sensitivity 100.00% Specificity 82.92%

(Continued)

Table 9.1 (Continued)

HF Diagnosis					
Study	**Target**	**Method**	**Features**	**Data Set**	**Evaluation Measures**
Javeed et al. 2019	HF diagnosis Healthy vs. HF	Random search algorithm for features selection and RF for HF diagnosis.	Demographics, symptoms, clinical and laboratory values	Cleveland heart disease database 297 subjects 137 with HF 160 controls	Accuracy 93.33% Sensitivity 95.12% Specificity 89.79%
Kim et al. 2019	HF diagnosis Healthy vs. HF	DL-based analysis	ECG features	2209 subjects with chronic HF 18,196 controls	ROC + 4 to + 6 with specificity 98.00% positive predictive value 95.00%
Kwon et al. 2019	HF diagnosis Healthy vs. HF	DNN	ECG features, demographics, heart rate, the presence of AF or AFL, QT interval, and QRS duration	22,765 subjects 1391 with HFrEF 21,374 controls	AUC 84.30%
Wang et al 2019	HF diagnosis Healthy vs. congestive HF	DL via short-term RR interval. Combined the LSTM network and convolution net architecture	HRV measures based on the RR interval	156 subjects 44 with congestive HF 112 controls	Accuracy 99.22%
Acharya et al. 2019	HF diagnosis Healthy vs. HF	CNN	ECG signals	73 subjects 15 with congestive HF 58 controls	Accuracy 98.97% Specificity 99.01% Sensitivity 98.87%
Liu et al. 2019	HFpEF diagnosis Healthy vs. HFpEF	ELM	Heart sound signals	842 subjects 441 with HFpEF 401 controls	Accuracy 96.32% Sensitivity 95.48% Specificity 97.10%
Le et al. 2020	HF diagnosis Healthy vs. HF	Multilayer perceptron NN	Demographics, laboratory findings, lifestyle habits, ejection fracture	299 patients	Accuracy 88.00%

(Continued)

Table 9.1 (Continued)

HF Diagnosis					
Study	**Target**	**Method**	**Features**	**Data Set**	**Evaluation Measures**
Potter et al. 2020	HF diagnosis Healthy vs. HF	RF	Demographics, symptoms, echocardiogram features, physical examination features, medications	Training set 254 subjects 135 with HF Test set 65 subjects 27 with HF	AUC 76.00% Sensitivity 93.00% Specificity 61.00%
Pires et al. 2020	Diagnosis of HF	NN, C4.5, k-NN, SVM, SGD	Heart rate features	270 subjects	Accuracy 87.69%
Gjoreski et al. 2020	Chronic HF diagnosis Healthy vs. chronic HF	ML and end-to-end DL	Heart sound characteristics	947 subjects	Accuracy 92.90% Sensitivity 82.30% Specificity 96.20%
Lal et al. 2020	HF diagnosis Healthy vs. HF	SVM, k-NN, decision trees, ensemble classifiers	HRV measures	116 subjects 44 with congestive HF 72 controls	SVM gives accuracy 93.10%
Ning et al. 2020	HF diagnosis Healthy vs. HF	DL method that is composed of a CNN and an RNN.	ECG signals	15 chronic HF patients 18 controls	Accuracy 99.93% Sensitivity 99.85% Specificity 100.00%
Choi et al. 2020	Healthy vs. HFrEF vs. HFmrEF vs. HFpEF	Hybrid approach (expert-driven and machine-learning driven)	Demographics, symptoms, clinical history, physical examination, ECG and echocardio-graphic features, NT-proBNP	1198 subjects	Accuracy 98.30%

Furthermore, many studies focused on detecting HF based on heart sound characteristics. A healthy heart has two sounds: the first heart sound (S1) and the second heart sound (S2). Extra heart sounds can be found in both normal and abnormal situations. The third heart sound, or protodiastolic gallop, (S3) that correlates with dysfunction or volume overload of the ventricles and the fourth heart sound (S4) that reflects left ventricular stiffness are both associated with HF [44]. In 2015, Zheng et al. [45] suggested a system for chronic HF prediction based on the analysis of cardiac reserve and heart sound characteristics. They applied the LS-SVM (least-squares SVM) classifier in 88 control subjects and 64 with chronic HF with an accuracy of 95.39%, sensitivity 96.59%, and specificity 93.75% of the proposed system for the detection of chronic HF. In 2020, Gjoreski et al. [46] combined classic ML and end-to-end DL to detect chronic HF. The classic ML learned from a large set of features and the DL learned both from the time-domain representation of the signal and the spectral representation of the signal. Their model achieved an accuracy of 92.90%, sensitivity 82.30%, and specificity 96.20%.

A large number of studies focus on predicting HF utilizing HRV measures. Lal et al. [47], Wang et al. [48], and Chen et al. [49] utilized HRV measures to predict congestive HF. Lal et al. implemented an SVM model with 93.10% accuracy on 116 subjects (44 with congestive HF and 72 controls), while Wang et al. applied the long short-term memory (LSTM) network on 156 subjects (44 with congestive HF and 112 controls) achieving 99.22% accuracy. Chen et al. applied the sparse auto-encoder-based deep learning (SAE-based DL) algorithm on 116 subjects (44 with congestive HF and 72 controls), and the results showed that the model achieved 72.41% accuracy. In 2020, Pires et al. [50] analyzed various features of heart rate from 270 subjects by applying NN, a C4.5 decision tree, k-NN, SVM, and stochastic gradient descent (SGD). The highest accuracy (87.69%) was achieved with the implementation of fivefold cross-validation with SGD, the same as was achieved with 20-fold cross-validation and 10-fold cross-validation implementing C4.5 and SVM.

In addition, other researchers have focused on analyzing ECG signals. Masetic et al. in 2016 [51] implemented C4.5, k-NN, SVM, artificial NN, and random forest (RF), classifying ECG signals from 18 patients with congestive HF and 13 controls. RF outperformed the others with 100.00% accuracy. In 2019, Acharya et al. [52] implemented a convolutional neural network (CNN) on ECG signals from 73 patients (15 with congestive HF and 58 controls) with accuracy 98.97%, specificity 99.01%, and sensitivity 98.87%. Also in 2019, Kim et al. [53] analyzed ECG features data from 2209 subjects with chronic HFrEF (1006 subjects) and HFmrEF (1103 subjects) and 18,196 controls. They applied a DL-based analysis with 98.00% specificity and 95.00% positive predictive value. In the same year, Kwon et al. [54] developed an algorithm using a deep neural network (DNN). They analysed ECG features and demographic information (age, sex, weight, height), heart rate, the presence of atrial fibrillation (AF) or atrial flutter (AFL), QT interval, and QRS duration in 22,765 patients, of whom 1391 had HFrEF. The AUC for identification of HFrEF was 84.30%. In a 2020 study, Ning et al. [55] analyzed ECG signals from 15 chronic HF patients and 18 controls, applying a DL technique which consisted of a CNN and an RNN with an accuracy of 99.93%, sensitivity 99.85%, and specificity 100.00%.

Many studies applied various ML techniques on the Cleveland heart disease database that consists of demographic characteristics, symptoms, clinical and laboratory values, and electrocardiographic results used as input features, from 297 subjects (137 with HF and 160 controls). In 2017, Samuel et al. [56] applied a hybrid decision support method based on an artificial NN and the fuzzy analytic hierarchy process (fuzzy AHP) technique to detect the presence of HF with 91.10% accuracy. Two years later, Mohan et al. [57] applied a hybrid RF on the Cleveland heart disease database. Their model achieved an accuracy of 88.40%, sensitivity 92.80%, and specificity 82.60%. Moreover, in 2019, Ali et al. [58] applied stacked SVM with an accuracy of 92.22%, sensitivity 100.00%, and specificity 82.92%, while Javeed et al. [59] applied a random search algorithm (RSA) for features selection and RF for HF prediction with an accuracy of 93.33%, sensitivity 95.12%, and specificity 89.79%.

Furthermore, a number of studies have focused on identifying the three subtypes of HF (HFrEF, HFmrEF, HFpEF). Reddy et al. [60] and Liu et al. [61] built diagnostic tools to detect the presence of HFpEF. Reddy et al. [60] performed LR on 414 patients with unexplained dyspnea (267 with HFpEF and 147 controls) achieving AUC 88.60% in the independent test cohort. Obesity, AF, age, medications, and echocardiographic features were retained for diagnosing patients with HFpEF. Liu et al. [61] applied an extreme learning machine (ELM) on heart sound signals from 842 subjects (401 healthy subjects used as control group, and 441 HFpEF patients). The results showed an accuracy of 96.32%, sensitivity 95.48%, and specificity 97.10%. Choi et al. [62] developed a hybrid approach (expert-driven and machine-learning driven) to classify subjects in four classes – HFrEF, HFmrEF, HFpEF, and healthy subjects – and achieved 98.30% accuracy. Demographics, symptoms, clinical history, physical examination, ECG and echocardiogram features, and NT-proBNP were used as input features from 1198 subjects. In 2013, Austin et al. [63] focused on classifying subjects according to disease subtype: HFpEF or HFrEF. To evaluate their model they utilized the Enhanced Feedback for Effective Cardiac Treatment (EFFECT) study data set. The data set consisted of subjects with acute HF that could be further classified as HFpEF or HFrEF. For the HF subtype classification, they selected 34 features, such as demographics, symptoms, physical examination features, laboratory findings, and medical history. The results indicated that the RF classifier could classify cases into one of the two subtypes with a 69.60% positive predictive value.

9.1.2.3 ML Applications in Severity Estimation

Due to the fact that HF is one of the main causes of hospitalization in western society and its increased mortality rate, it is becoming imperative to be able to assess the severity of HF at its early stages. HF might be asymptomatic in the early stages and can usually be expressed only by dyspnea or fatigue. Several studies propose a model that estimates the severity of patients suffering from HF (Table 9.2). In 2011, Pecchia et al. [64] designed a platform to enhance the effectiveness and efficiency of home monitoring, using ML for the early detection of patient deterioration. Their study, proposed a remote health monitoring platform that supported HF severity assessment, based on the CART method. The data set they used was based on HRV measures and ECG signals from 29 subjects with HF (12 with mild HF and 17 with severe HF) and 54 subjects used as controls. Their model achieved an accuracy of 79.30%, sensitivity 82.30% and specificity 75.00%.

In 2012, Guidi et al. [65] built an artificial intelligence-based computer aided diagnosis system applying NN, SVM, decision trees, and a fuzzy expert system whose rules were

Table 9.2 State of the art of ML for HF severity estimation.

HF Severity Estimation					
Study	**Target**	**Method**	**Features**	**Data Set**	**Evaluation Measures**
Pecchia et al. 2011	HF severity assessment Healthy vs. mild vs. severe HF	CART	HRV measures and ECG signals	29 subjects with HF 12 with mild HF 17 with severe HF 54 controls	Accuracy 79.30% Sensitivity 82.30% Specificity 75.00%
Guidi et al. 2012	NYHA stratification Mild vs. moderate vs. severe	NN, SVM, decision tree, fuzzy expert system	Anamnestic and instrumental data	136 patients 50 mild HF 39 moderate HF 47 severe HF	NN gives accuracy 86.10%
Melillo et al. 2013	NYHA stratification Mild vs. severe congestive HF	CART	HRV measures	44 subjects 12 subjects with mild HF 32 subjects with severe HF	Accuracy 85.40%, Sensitivity 93.30% Specificity 63.60%
Gladence et al. 2014	Mild vs. severe congestive HF	Bayesian belief network	HRV measures	303 subjects	Accuracy 74.44% Sensitivity 81.40% Specificity 71.70%
Shahbazi et al. 2015	NYHA stratification Mild vs. severe congestive HF	k-NN	HRV measures	44 subjects 12 with mild congestive HF 32 with severe congestive HF	Sensitivity 100% Specificity 100%
Guidi et al. 2015	Mild vs. moderate vs. severe congestive HF	RF	Demographics, physical examination features, BNP, medications, comorbidities, EF, ECG features	250 subjects 93 with mild HF 92 with moderate HF 65 with severe HF	Accuracy 81.30%

(Continued)

Table 9.2 (Continued)

HF Severity Estimation					
Study	**Target**	**Method**	**Features**	**Data Set**	**Evaluation Measures**
Aljaaf et al. 2015	Stratification of patient's current status in five levels. Healthy vs. low vs. moderate vs. high vs. extremely high.	C4.5	Demographics, chest pain, laboratory findings, ECG results, angina, weight, smoke, exercise	297 patients from the Cleveland heart disease database	Accuracy 86.53% Sensitivity 86.50% Specificity 95.50%
Chen et al. 2016	NYHA stratification Healthy vs. mild vs. moderate vs. severe	Decision-tree-based SVM	HRV measures	116 patients 44 with congestive HF 72 controls	HF prediction accuracy 89.83% Total accuracy 91.30%
Tripoliti et al. 2017	Identification of NYHA class as two-, three- and four-class classification problem	RF, random tree, logistic model trees, C4.5, ROT, SVM, radial basis function network, Bayesian network, Naive Bayes, multilayer perceptron, Simple CART.	102 features: grouped as demographics, allergies, medical condition, medications, biological data related with the HF disease, clinical examinations, adherence 76 features after feature selection	378 subjects 18 patients in NYHA class I, 125 patients in NYHA class II, 173 patients in NYHA class III, and 62 patients in NYHA class IV	The highest detection accuracy is 97.00% by applying RF and symmetrical uncertainty for the two-class problem, 87% ROT and Information Gain for the three-class problem and 67% by applying ROT and symmetrical uncertainty for the four-class problem
Zhang et al. 2017	Identification of NYHA class NYHA I vs. II vs. III vs. IV	NLP methods	Clinical notes	6174 clinical notes from 1370 subjects	SVM with n-gram features had the best accuracy (93.37%)

(Continued)

Table 9.2 (Continued)

HF Severity Estimation					
Study	**Target**	**Method**	**Features**	**Data Set**	**Evaluation Measures**
Ma et al. 2018	Class I vs. II or III, Class I vs. IV Classes II or III vs. IV	Ensemble tree classifier using fivefold cross-validation	EHR data: demographics, symptoms, medication, diagnosis, laboratory findings, cardiac vitals, angiogram, imaging, and stress test	461 patients	Class I vs. II or III with AUC 84.00%, Class I vs. IV with AUC 89.00% Class II or III vs. IV with AUC 88.00%
Groccia et al. 2018	Stratification of chronic HF patients current status into five levels, based on major cardiovascular worsening events.	Linear SVM, C4.5, NN, NB with six temporal weighting functions	Age, NYHA class, etiology, cardiovascular history, other diseases, vital parameters, major cardiovascular worsening events	50 chronic HF patients	Accuracy 71.00% AUC 91.00% Sensitivity 71.00% Specificity 100.00%

produced by a genetic algorithm. They measured the HF severity according to three levels (mild vs. moderate vs. severe), all assessments depending on NYHA classification. Their model was based on 136 patients (100 were used for training and 36 for testing). NN outperformed the other classifiers with 86.10% accuracy.

Both Melillo et al. in 2013 [66] and Shahbazi et al. in 2015 [67] analyzed standard long-term HRV measures from two public Holter databases. They used the data from 12 patients suffering from mild congestive HF (NYHA I and II), named as lower risk, and 32 suffering from severe congestive HF (NYHA III and IV), named as higher risk. The method proposed by Melillo et al. [66] achieved 85.40% accuracy, 93.30% sensitivity and 63.60% specificity employing the CART method, but was outperformed by Shahbazi et al. [67] that achieved 100.00% sensitivity and specificity. Shahbazi et al. applied generalized discriminant analysis (GDS) as a feature extraction method and the retained features were given as input to the k-NN classifier. Gladence et al. in 2014 [68] used also standard long-term HRV measures from 303 subjects. The Bayesian belief network classifier they used separated lower risk patients from higher risk ones, and reached 74.44% accuracy, 81.40% sensitivity, and 71.70% specificity.

Guidi et al. [69] designed another system in 2015 – a multilayer monitoring system for providing clinical assessment of HF severity to differentiate subjects according to three levels (mild vs moderate vs severe HF). They utilized a multisource data set (demographics, physical examination features, BNP, medications, comorbidities, EF, ECG features) from 250 subjects (93 with mild HF, 92 with moderate HF, and 65 with severe HF). By applying the RF classifier they achieved 81.30% accuracy. In 2015, Aljaaf et al. [70] classified HF patients into five categories: no risk, low risk, moderate risk, high risk, and extremely high risk. They used the Cleveland heart disease database (297 subjects, 137 with HF and 160 controls) and implemented the C4.5 classifier with 86.53% accuracy, 86.50% sensitivity, and 95.50% specificity.

In 2016, Chen et al. [71] classified congestive HF patients in four categories according to the NYHA class (healthy vs. mild vs. moderate vs. severe) by analyzing HRV measures and implementing a decision tree-based SVM with HF prediction accuracy of 89.83% and total accuracy of 91.30%. In 2017, Tripoliti et al. [72] estimated the severity of HF in terms of NYHA class. They addressed this problem as a two, three, and four class classification problem. They utilized 378 subjects (18 in NYHA class I, 125 in NYHA class II, 173 in NYHA class III and 62 patients in NYHA class IV) and 102 features grouped as demographics, allergies, medical condition, medications, biological data related to the HF disease, clinical examinations, and adherence. The highest detection accuracy was 97.00% by applying rotation forest (ROT) and symmetrical uncertainty for the two-class problem, 87.00% by applying ROT and Information Gain for the three-class problem, and 67.00% by applying ROT and symmetrical uncertainty for the four-class problem. In 2017, Zhang et al. [73] utilized 6174 clinical notes and applied natural language processing (NLP) methods to identify NYHA classification, achieving 93.70% accuracy with SVM.

A year later, Ma et al. [74] in their study examined whether NYHA classification can be estimated from EHR data, i.e. demographics, symptoms, medication, diagnosis, laboratory findings, cardiac vitals, angiogram, imaging, and stress tests, from 461 subjects. The ensemble tree classifier using fivefold cross-validation was able to discriminate between class I versus II or III with AUC 84.00%, between class I and IV with AUC 89.00%, and between classes II or III and IV with AUC 88.00%.

Groccia et al. in 2018 [75] developed a model for the early detection of worsening major cardiovascular events in patients with chronic HF. They utilized 50 chronic HF patients, applied various temporal weighting strategies, and analyzed their impact on the performance of predictive models. Finally, six temporal weighting functions were tested. The original data set was divided into a training (70.00%) and a test (30.00%) set. Linear SVM achieved the best accuracy (71.00%), AUC (91.00%), sensitivity (71.00%), and specificity (100.00%). An extended review of the literature is presented in Tripoliti et al. [72].

9.1.2.4 ML Applications in Clinical Prognosis

Predicting hospital readmissions or mortality in patients with HF is a huge challenge. Therefore, several studies have been conducted to evaluate the clinical prognosis of HF patients in terms of readmission to hospital and of mortality prediction. Accurate and early prediction can lead to adaptations in patient management in order to decrease the risk of adverse events.

9.1.2.5 ML Applications in Hospital Readmission Prediction

A large number of studies have focused on predicting the rate of readmission to hospital for HF patients (Table 9.3). In 2013, Vedomske et al. [76] applied the RF classifier to

Table 9.3 State of the art of ML for HF rehospitalization prediction.

Rehospitalization Prediction					
Study	**Target**	**Method**	**Features**	**Data Set**	**Evaluation Measures**
Vedomske et al. 2013	Prediction of 1-month readmission rate for congestive HF patients	RF	Administrative data, demographics	6904 visits 1441 readmissions	AUC 83.00%
Mortazavi et al. 2016	Prediction of 1-month and 6-month readmission rate for HF patients	RF, boosting, RF combined hierarchically with SVM or LR, and Poisson regression against traditional LR	Medical record data, laboratory results, physical examination information, quality of life, socioeconomic, and demographic data.	1004 patients for the 1-month readmissions 977 patients for the 6-month readmissions	For the 1-month prediction, boosting has 92.00% sensitivity and 79.00% specificity. For the 6-month prediction, RF has 94.00% sensitivity and 15.00% specificity.
Leong et al. 2017	1-month HF readmission Readmission risk was stratified into low risk (<10%), medium risk (10%-30%) and high risk (>30%)	Bivariate analysis and LR	Demographics, clinical information, NYHA class, Framingham criteria, echocardiographic and ECG features, laboratory values, psychosocial parameters, medications	1475 readmissions from 1098 patients 60% for training 40% for testing	AUC 76.00% Sensitivity 78.30% specificity 60.70%
Frizzell et al. 2017	Prediction of 1-month all-cause readmission rate for HF patients	Tree-augmented NB network, RF, gradient-boosted model, LR	Demographics, socioeconomic status, medical history, characterization of HF, medications, vital signs, weight, selected laboratories treatment, and discharge interventions.	56,477 patients 70.00% for training 30.00% for validation	C statistics for the validation sets were: 61.80%, 60.70%, 61.40%, 62.40% for the implemented models

(Continued)

Table 9.3 (Continued)

Rehospitalization Prediction					
Study	**Target**	**Method**	**Features**	**Data Set**	**Evaluation Measures**
Jamei et al. 2017	Prediction of 1-month all-cause readmission rate for HF patients	Artificial NN	EHR data	335,815 hospital visits 32,718 visits resulting in 1-month readmission	Sensitivity 60.00% Precision 24.00% AUC 78.00%
Golas et al. 2018	Prediction of 1-month readmission rate for HF patients	DUNs	EHR data	27,334 admissions from 11510 patients 6369 1-month readmissions for training	Accuracy 76.40% AUC 70.50%
Liu et al. 2019	Prediction of HF readmission rates	CNN	Clinical notes	58,000 hospital admissions of more than 46,000 patients	F1 score 75.60% in general readmission prediction F1 score of 73.30% in 1-month readmission prediction
Khayyat et al. 2019	CDSS to estimate and reduce the probability of readmission for congestive HF patients	Linear discriminant analysis	EHR data	822 readmissions	63% of the non-readmissions classified correctly 63% of the readmissions classified correctly
Ashfaq 2019	Prediction of 1-month hospital readmission rate for congestive HF patients	LSTM NN	Demographics, diagnoses, procedures, laboratory findings, physical examination, medications	7500 subjects	AUC 77.00%

(Continued)

Table 9.3 (Continued)

Rehospitalization Prediction					
Study	**Target**	**Method**	**Features**	**Data Set**	**Evaluation Measures**
Liu et al. 2020	Prediction of 1-month hospital readmission rate for congestive HF patients	Artificial NNs	EHR data	303,233 admissions from 2048 hospitals	AUC 64.00%
Kawai et al. 2020	Prediction of 1-month, 3-months and 12-months HF readmission rates.	Generalized linear model (GLM), boosted GLM, Bayesian GLM, Adaboost with bagging algorithm, Naive Bayes, RF and SVM.	EHR data	7413 patients 19% readmission rate at 30 day and 52% at 12 month. training 64% validation 16% independent test set 20%	Adaboost and RF achieved the best results HF readmission rates: AUC 61.00% for 1 month AUC 64.00% for 3 months AUC 71.00% for 12 months

administrative data and demographics to predict the 1-month readmission rate for congestive HF patients. The study showed that 20.90% of the patients followed 1-month readmission with AUC 83.00%. In 2016, Mortazavi et al. [77] compared the effectiveness of RF, boosting, RF combined hierarchically with SVM or LR, Poisson regression, and traditional LR to predict 1-month and 6-month all-cause readmissions and readmissions because of HF. For the 1-month prediction of readmission, boosting had 92.00% sensitivity and 79.00% specificity. For the 6-month prediction of readmission, RF had 94.00% sensitivity and 15.00% specificity.

In 2017, Frizzell et al. [78] and Jamei et al. [79] predicted the 1-month all-cause readmission rate for HF patients. Frizzell et al. [78] conducted a large-scale study in 56,477 patients, from which 70.00% were used for training and 30.00% for validation. They implemented ML algorithms (tree-augmented NB network, RF, gradient-boosted model, LR) on demographics, socioeconomic status, medical history, characterization of HF, medication, vital signs, selected laboratories treatment, and discharge interventions features. The C statistics for the validation sets were: 61.80%, 60.70%, 61.40%, 62.40% for the implemented models. Jamei et al. [79] implemented artificial NNs on 335,815 hospital visits, from which 32,718 visits resulted in 1-month readmission. Their model achieved 60.00% sensitivity, 24.00% precision, and 78.00% AUC. In the same year, Leong et al. [80] applied a bivariate analysis and LR in a multisource data set from 1475 readmissions from 1098 unique patients from which 60.00% were used for training and 40.00% for validation. The 1-month readmission risk was stratified into low, medium, and high risk with AUC 76.00%, sensitivity 78.30% and specificity 60.70%.

In 2018, Golas et al. [81] applied deep unified networks (DUNs), a DL network structure designed to avoid overfitting, with an accuracy of 76.40% and AUC 70.50% based on EHR data to predict the 1-month readmission rate for HF patients. Their model was trained on a large data set consisting of 27,334 admissions from 11,510 patients.

Ashfaq et al. [82] in 2019, applied the LSTM neural network on 7500 subjects with congestive HF with AUC 77.00% in predicting the 1-month readmission rate. This study targeted key elements of an EHR, i.e. demographics, diagnoses, procedures, laboratory findings, physical examination, and medications. Also in 2019, Liu et al. [83] utilized clinical notes using DL in order to predict HF readmission rates. Their model, based on a CNN, achieved F1 score 75.60% in general readmission prediction and 73.30% in 1-month readmission prediction. Khayyat et al. in 2019 [84] developed a clinical decision support system (CDSS) that would be able to estimate and reduce the probability of readmission for congestive HF patients. They used as input medical comorbidities and social factors of patients. The model they built achieved an accuracy of 63.00% for the non-readmissions and 63.00% for the readmissions.

In a 2020 study, Liu et al. [85] used the 2014 Nationwide Readmissions Database (NRD), that includes data from 2048 hospitals with nearly 15 million admissions. Their study cohort included 303,233 admissions for HF with 17.70% unplanned 1-month readmission rates. With AUC 64.00%, the artificial NN they implemented outperformed the hierarchical LR that was used as a baseline comparator. Also in 2020, Kawai et al. [86] compared several ML techniques to predict HF readmission rates with different prediction windows from 1-month to 12-months. In their study, 7413 patients were included, with 19% readmission rate at 1 month and 52.00% at 12 months. Adaboost with bagging algorithm and RF performed better with AUC 61.00%, 64.00%, and 71.00%, for the 1-month, 3-month, and 12-month prediction group, respectively,

9.1.2.6 ML Applications in Mortality Prediction

Other studies focus on developing a model to predict mortality among patients with HF (Table 9.4). In 2013, Pocock et al. [87] used the Meta-Analysis Global Group in Chronic Heart Failure (MAGGIC) international database with 39,372 patients from 30 studies, to create an easily used risk score for mortality in patients with HFrEF and HFpEF. They applied Poisson regression with forward stepwise feature selection and concluded to 13 independent features. All were highly significant $P < 0.002$, and most were overwhelmingly significant $P < 0.0001$.

In 2017, Miao et al. [88] utilized the public MIMIC II clinical database with 8059 patients and 32 features consisting of demographics, clinical variables, laboratory findings, and medications. They analyzed these features to develop a risk model for mortality prediction in patients with HF. They applied the improved random survival forest achieving C-statistic 0.821.

In 2019, Kwon et al. [89] applied a DL-based artificial intelligence algorithm for predicting mortality of patients with acute HF. The AUC of the model was 88.00% for predicting in-hospital mortality, 78.20% for predicting 12-month mortality, and 81.30% for 36-month mortality. They utilized 2165 patients with acute HF for training and 4759 patients with acute HF for testing. Their data set included demographic features, medications, laboratory results, and ECG and echocardiography findings.

Table 9.4 State of the art of ML for HF mortality prediction.

Mortality prediction					
Study	**Target**	**Method**	**Features**	**Data Set**	**Evaluation Measures**
Pocock et al. 2013	Mortality prediction in patients with HFrEF and HFpEF	Poisson regression models	Demographics, NYHA class, laboratory findings, medications, physical examination, lifestyle habits, comorbidities, EF	Used a large international database (39372 patients) from 30 studies	All were highly significant $P < 0.002$, and most were overwhelmingly significant $P < 0.0001$
Miao 2017	Mortality prediction in patients with HF	Improved random survival forest	Demographics, clinical variables, laboratory information, and medications	Public MIMIC II clinical database with 8059 patients	C-statistic 0.821
Kwon et al. 2019	Mortality prediction in patients with acute HF	DL-based artificial intelligence algorithm	Demographics, medications, laboratory results, ECG and echocardiographic features, final diagnosis	2165 subjects for training 4759 subjects for testing	88% AUC for predicting in-hospital mortality 78.2% AUC for predicting 12-month mortality 81.3% AUC for predicting 36-month mortality
Wang et al. 2020	Prediction for in-hospital mortality, 30-day and 1-year mortality after discharge.	Feature rearrangement-based convolution net	EHR data	10,203 records for in-hospital mortality with 539 death records 30-day mortality: 6260 records with 652 death records 1-year mortality: 4353 records with 1182 death records	In-hospital mortality: sensitivity 81.48%, AUC 90.37% 30-day mortality: sensitivity 80.01%, AUC 89.13% 1-year mortality: sensitivity 72.15%, AUC 89.13%

Yang 2020	All-cause mortality prediction in HF patients	RF	Demographics, ECG features, index of HF, echocardiographic features, and advanced laboratory biomarkers	506 patients	AUC 75.00%
Adler 2020	Mortality risk prediction Low vs. high	Boosted decision tree	Diastolic blood pressure, creatinine, blood urea nitrogen, haemoglobin, white blood cell count, platelets, albumin, and red blood cell distribution width	5822 subjects	AUC 88.00%
Jing 2020	1-year all-cause mortality prediction in HF patients	Nonlinear XGBoost	Demographics, laboratory test results, medications, ECG and echocardiographic features, vaccinations	26,971 patients with HF	AUC 77.00%

Wang et al. [90] proposed a feature rearrangement-based DL system for predicting in-hospital mortality, and 30-day and 1-year mortality after discharge. The data set used in this study was collected from the EHR system of a hospital in Shanghai. They utilized 10,203 records with 539 death records for in-hospital mortality, 6260 records with 652 death records for 1-month mortality, and 4353 records with 1182 death records for 1-year mortality. Their method scored 81.48% sensitivity and 90.37% AUC for in-hospital mortality, 80.01% sensitivity and 89.13% AUC for 1-month mortality, and 72.15% sensitivity and 89.13% AUC for 1-year mortality. Yang et al. [91] selected 506 HF patients, with more than 25,000 features, consisting of demographic information, electrocardiography measurements, index of HF, echocardiography, and advanced laboratory biomarkers. The RF model performed better on predicting all-cause mortality (AUC: 75.00%). Adler et al. [92] discriminated between low and high risk of death by identifying eight low-cost and commonly available features (diastolic blood pressure, blood urea nitrogen, creatinine, hemoglobin, white blood cell count, platelets, albumin, and red blood cell distribution width) from 5822 patients. A boosted decision tree achieved AUC 88.00%. Jing et al. [93] conducted a large-scale study on 26,971 subjects to predict 1-year all-cause mortality in patients with HF. They collected 26 clinical variables (demographic information, laboratory findings, medications), 90 diagnostic codes, 41 ECG features, 44 echocardiographic features, and eight evidence-based "care gaps," e.g. flu vaccine, blood pressure, and cardiac resynchronization therapy. They tested various ML models that achieved AUC 74.00% to 77.00%, with the nonlinear XGBoost model (AUC: 77.00%) outperforming the linear logistic regression (AUC: 74.00%).

9.1.2.7 ML Applications in Mortality or Readmission Prediction

Furthermore, a large number of studies focus on developing models for jointly predicting adverse events, i.e. mortality or rehospitalization in patients with HF (Table 9.5).

In 2013, Zhang et al. [94] utilized decision trees and LR to predict death risk or hospitalization due to worsening HF at one year. The mortality prediction had an accuracy of 89.20% for decision trees and 85.80% for LR and the composite outcome prediction had an accuracy of 79.70% for decision trees and 73.80% for the LR model. Their data set consisted of 284 patients for training and 160 patients for validation from the TEN-HMS (Trans-European Network Homecare Monitoring System) study, utilizing as input features demographics, physical examination, laboratory findings, medical history, quality of life, and EuroQol. NT-proBNP was the feature with the strongest prediction of mortality. In 2017, Tripoliti et al. [95] presented an ML based method for the prediction of adverse events (mortality and relapses) in patients with HF by analyzing breath and saliva biomarkers from 27 subjects. The prediction of adverse events achieved 77.00% accuracy using an ROT algorithm.

Awan et al. [96] in 2019, conducted a study on HF patients aged over 65 years and in hospital, where 23.60% of the patients were readmitted or died within 1 month of hospital discharge. They developed an MLP-based approach to predict 1-month HF readmission or death, achieving AUC 62.00%, sensitivity 48.00% and specificity 70.00%.

Table 9.5 State of the art of ML for HF prediction of adverse events.

Prediction of Adverse Events

Study	Target	Method	Features	Data Set	Evaluation Measures
Zhang et al. 2013	Prediction of death risk or hospitalization due to worsening HF at 12 months	Decision trees, LR	Demographics, physical examination, laboratory findings, medical history, quality of life, EuroQol	TEN-HMS study 284 patients for training 160 patients for validation	Accuracy 89.20% for mortality prediction with decision trees Accuracy 79.70% for adverse events prediction with decision trees
Tripoliti et al. 2017	Prediction of adverse events in patients with HF	ROT	Breath and saliva biomarkers	27 patients	77% accuracy, sensitivity, and specificity
Awan et al. 2019	Prediction of 1-month readmission or death rate for HF patients	MLP	Demographics, admission characteristics, medical history visits to emergency departments, medication, healthcare services out of hospital, death.	10,757 HF patients over 65 years old 23.6% were readmitted or died within 1 month of hospital discharge	AUC 62.00% Sensitivity 48.00% Specificity 70.00%
Angraal et al. 2020	Prediction of adverse events in patients with HFpEF through 3 years of observation	LR with a forward selection of variables, LR with a LASSO regularization for variable selection, RF, gradient descent boosting, SVM	Demographics, laboratory findings, ECG features, symptoms and quality of life score	1767 patients 50 years of age or older from the TOPCAT trial	RF classifier achieved the best result: 0.72 C-statistic for predicting mortality 0.76 C-statistic for hospitalization

(Continued)

Table 9.5 (Continued)

Prediction of Adverse Events					
Study	**Target**	**Method**	**Features**	**Data Set**	**Evaluation Measures**
Beecy 2020	Prediction of 1-month or 6-month readmission or all-cause mortality in patients with acute or chronic HF	Extreme gradient boosting	Socioeconomic features, clinical history, laboratory and radiologic findings, ECG and invasive coronary angiographic parameters	3774 patients with acute or chronic HF 3160 patients without unplanned death/readmission within 1 month after discharge 614 patients with unplanned death/readmission within 1 month after discharge	AUC 75.60%
Yang et al. 2020	Prediction of all-cause readmission or death at 1 month and 12 months for HF patients over 65 years of age	A Cox regression model was used to identify factors for the prediction of readmission or death at 1 month and 12 months. A nomogram was developed with bootstrap validation.	Demographics, echocardiographic and biochemical data, comorbidities, medications	854 patients 165 with 1-month readmission or death 212 with 12-month readmission or death 477 no events	The C-index of the 1-month and 12-month prediction model was 77.80% and 73.80% respectively
Zahavi et al. 2020	Prediction of 1-month and 12-month readmission or mortality	RF, LR, SVM, NN	EHR data	3838 patients	1-month readmission: RF AUC 12-month readmission: RF AUC 1-month mortality: RF AUC 1-month mortality: RF AUC

Angraal et al. in 2020 [97] utilized various classification algorithms to train the model for predicting the mortality and HF hospitalization through 3 years of follow-up in HFpEF patients. The RF classifier achieved the best result with a mean C-statistic of 0.72 for predicting mortality (Brier score: 0.17), and 0.76 for HF hospitalization (Brier score: 0.19). They used data from 1767 patients from the TOPCAT trial (Treatment of Preserved Cardiac Function Heart Failure with an Aldosterone Antagonist) and more specifically their data set consisted of demographic features, laboratory findings, electrocardiography data, symptoms, and quality of life score.

Also in 2020, Yang et al. [98] developed a method to predict all-cause readmission or mortality for HF patients over 65 years of age. The Cox regression model was used to identify the predictive features for adverse events at 1 month and 12 months. A nomogram was developed with bootstrap validation. The C-index of the 1-month and 12-month prediction model was 0.778 and 0.738, respectively. Zahavi et al. [99] compared various ML models (RF, LR, SVM, and NN) for 1-month and 12-month prediction of readmission and mortality. Their models were trained on 3838 patients during hospitalization for HF with 182 variables collected from EHR. RF achieved the best results in terms of AUC for all predictions.

Beecy et al. [100] also analyzed EHR data to predict the unplanned adverse events due to HF using a prediction window of 1 month or 6 months. In a total of 3774 subjects with acute or chronic HF, they implemented extreme gradient boosting with AUC 75.60%.

9.2 Two Prominent Applications

In this second part of the chapter, we demonstrate the results of two innovative studies: the first for HF diagnosis, and the second for HF severity estimation based on NYHA classification and the prediction of adverse events. The results for the HF diagnosis are part of the Kardiatool project [101], and the results for the severity estimation and the prediction of adverse events are part of the Hearten project [102].

9.2.1 HF Diagnosis

9.2.1.1 The Data Set

The data set for HF diagnosis consisted of 467 subjects (258 used as control subjects, 180 subjects with chronic HF, and 29 with acute HF). The HF diagnosis classification problem is defined as classifying the 258 control subjects versus the 209 HF subjects.

Data was provided by University College Dublin, National University of Ireland (409 patients), and the 2nd Department of Cardiology of the University Hospital of Ioannina (58 patients) as part of the Kardiatool project [101].

For each patient, data from different categories were recorded. More specifically, they were grouped into the following categories: general demographic information, personal history of cardiovascular disease, drugs, classical cardiovascular risk factors, laboratory findings, clinical examinations, symptoms, physical examination, and echocardiographic features (Figure 9.3).

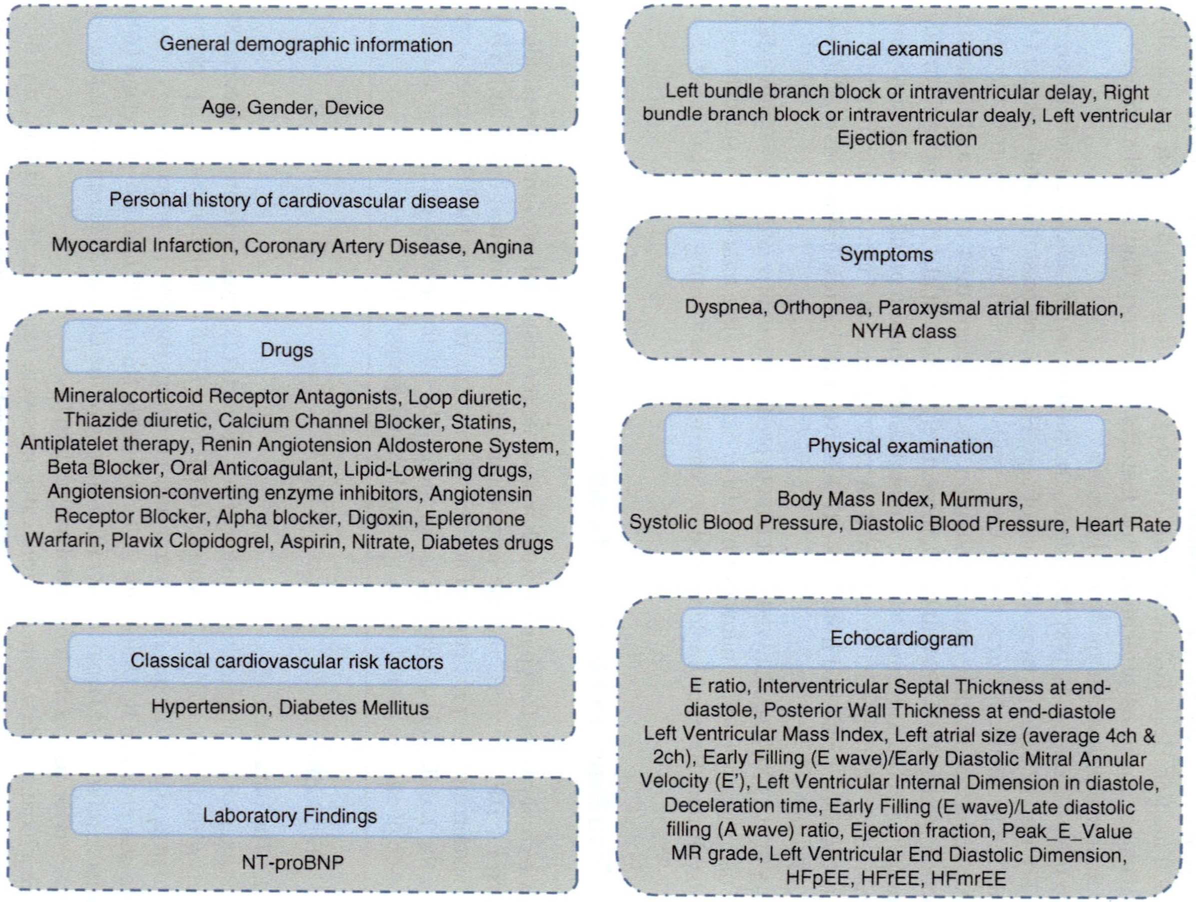

Figure 9.3 Data description for HF diagnosis.

9.2.1.2 Methodology

The proposed methodology consisted of three basic stages: preprocessing, feature selection, and classification. At the preprocessing stage features with more than (≥) 50% missing values and discrete features with unbalanced distribution of values were removed. Next, outliers and typos (e.g. 4,5 being recorded instead of 4.5) per feature were detected and corrected. A correlation-based feature selection method was used to assess the predictive ability of feature subsets and the degree of redundancy among them, preferring sets of features that were highly correlated with the class but with low intercorrelation [103]. In the classification stage, C4.5, RF, ROT, NB, k-NN, SVM, logistic model trees (LMT), and Bayes Network (BN) classifiers were applied. In order to achieve class balancing, the undersampling method was applied to the data set. The undersampling method is quite common for dealing with this problem [104]. It produces a random subsample with a given spread between class frequencies. The maximum spread between the rarest and most common class is specified. In our case, a random undersample of the majority class was followed, so that all classes have the same number of instances. The 10-fold cross-validation was applied in testing.

9.2.1.3 Results

After removing features with ≥ 50% missing values and deleting discrete features with unbalanced distribution of values, there were 30 remaining features (Figure 9.4). We also excluded from the data set NYHA classification that was recorded in all patients, since that would indicate a patient's condition. Finally, the classification of HF phenotype (HFpEF, HFrEF, HFmrEF) did not fit in our analysis since the models would be used for HF diagnosis in previously undiagnosed patients.

The results for the HF diagnosis problem, for the unbalanced class, are depicted in Table 9.6.

The results for HF diagnosis problem, for the balanced class, are depicted in Table 9.7.

The ROT classifier for the unbalanced class, without feature selection, gives the best result with an accuracy of 96.36%, sensitivity 96.50%, and specificity 96.20%.

9.2.2 Severity Estimation and Adverse Events Prediction

9.2.2.1 The Data Set

For both the severity estimation problem and the adverse event prediction, the data were collected retrospectively by three different clinical centers: Universita Di Pisa, Servicio Andaluz de Salud, and the 2nd Department of Cardiology of the University Hospital of Ioannina, as part of the HEARTEN project [102].

The recorded data can be grouped in the following categories: general information, medical condition, drugs, clinical examination, score information, biological data, allergies and drugs side-effects, sensor data, and biosensor data. More specifically, during hospitalization, for each patient the data shown in Figure 9.5 were collected.

Regarding the data retrieved from the sensor, the clinicians had to monitor the patient (starting from the day of admission) using a sensor device for 20 minutes every other day and at discharge.

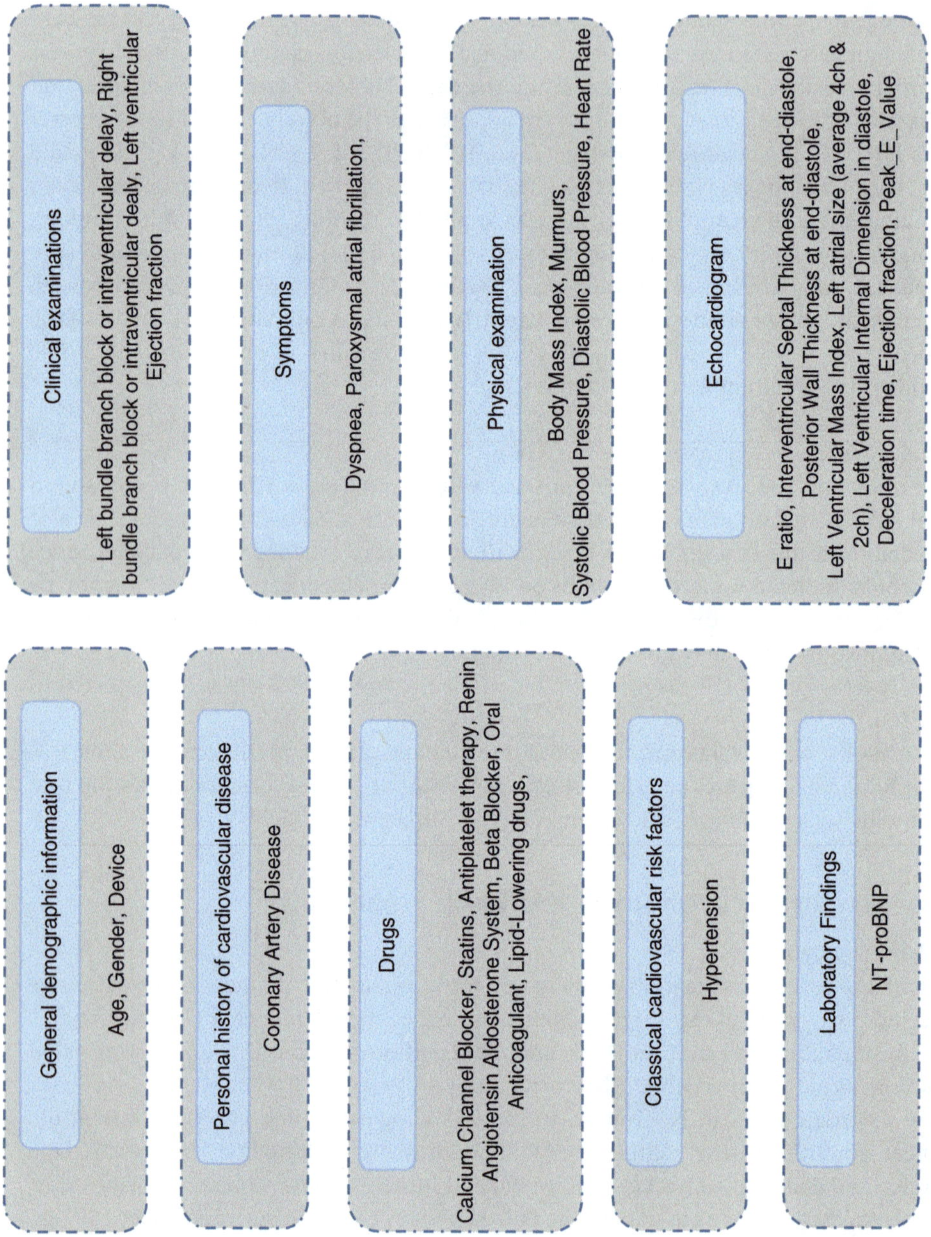

Figure 9.4 Features for HF diagnosis.

Table 9.6 HF diagnosis classification results, unbalanced class.

Classifier	Feature Selection	Accuracy%	Classifier	Feature Selection	Accuracy%
BN	No	91.86	**BN**	Yes	94.00
NB	No	92.72	**NB**	Yes	94.65
SVM	No	95.50	**SVM**	Yes	95.07
k-NN	No	88.87	**k-NN**	Yes	93.36
ROT	No	96.36	**ROT**	Yes	95.07
C4.5	No	91.43	**C4.5**	Yes	92.51
LMT	No	94.65	**LMT**	Yes	95.50
RF	No	95.29	**RF**	Yes	94.86

9.2.2.2 Methodology

The development of the model for the NYHA class detection module consisted of three basic stages: preprocessing, feature selection, and classification. During preprocessing, features with more than (≥) 60.00% missing values were removed. Furthermore, discrete features with unbalanced distribution of values were removed. In the second step, the wrapper approach and correlation-based feature selection algorithm were used. In the classification stage, RF, LMT, C4.5, ROT, SVM, radial basis function (RBF) Network, BN, Naive Bayes (NB), and Simple CART classifiers were applied. The classifiers were combined with resampling techniques (SMOTE algorithm), when the class was unbalanced. Resampling was performed only during the training of the model and not during the test for avoiding bias of classification results.

9.2.2.3 Results for HF Severity Estimation

The features removed after applying the preprocessing step are depicted in Figure 9.6.

The data set consisted of 92 patients' data. The model was trained to detect NYHA class II, NYHA class III, and NYHA class IV, since HF patients belonging only to one of

Table 9.7 HF diagnosis classification results, balanced class

Classifier	Feature Selection	Accuracy%	Classifier	Feature Selection	Accuracy%
BN	No	92.82	**BN**	Yes	93.78
NB	No	92.34	**NB**	Yes	94.50
SVM	No	94.98	**SVM**	Yes	94.74
k-NN	No	88.52	**k-NN**	Yes	93.30
ROT	No	95.22	**ROT**	Yes	95.22
C4.5	No	93.78	**C4.5**	Yes	92.82
LMT	No	95.22	**LMT**	Yes	94.98
RF	No	94.98	**RF**	Yes	94.50

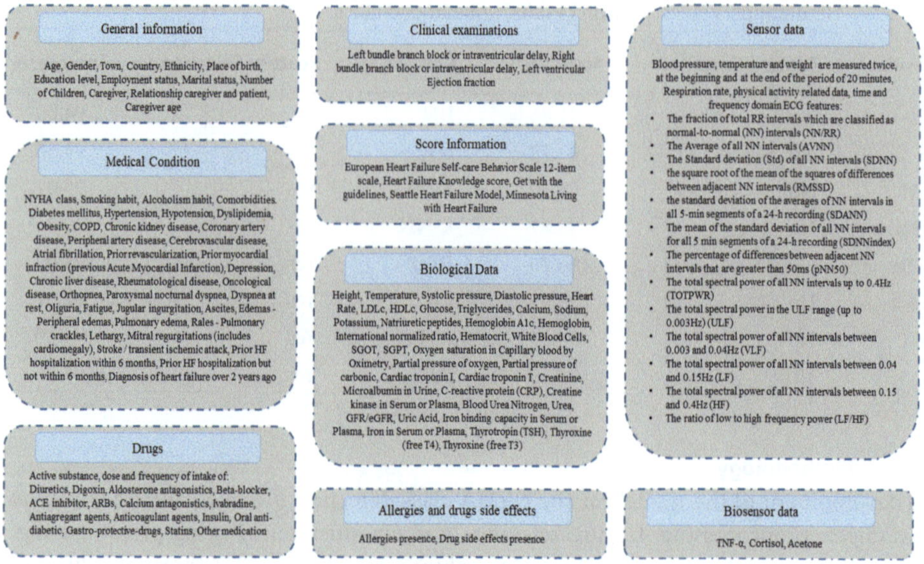

Figure 9.5 Data description for HF severity estimation and adverse events prediction.

these classes participated in the project. Different combinations of features were employed and the best results are presented in Table 9.8.

The RF classifier with 95% accuracy using the optimal set of features was selected. The features that remained following the feature selection were those shown in Figure 9.7.

9.2.2.4 Results for the Prediction of Adverse Events

The adverse events prediction model was built using the data from 82 patients. The results are presented in Table 9.9.

The classifier that produced the best results (in terms of accuracy) using the optimal set of features was selected. The classifier, according to Table 9.9, is ROT with 89.00% accuracy. The optimal set of features is the set of features remaining after the feature selection step (Figure 9.8).

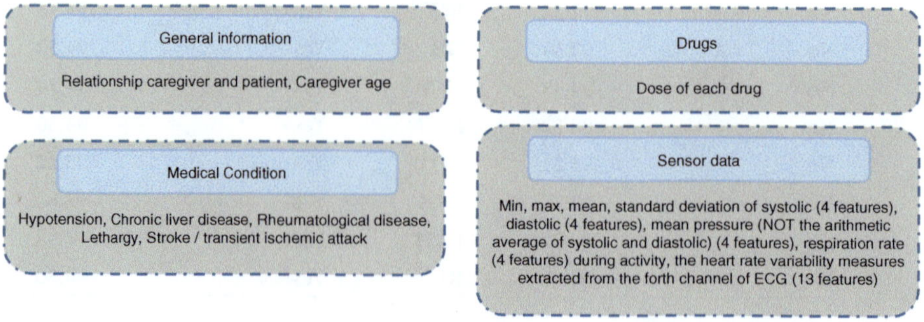

Figure 9.6 Removed features after the application of the preprocessing step.

Table 9.8 Results of the NYHA class detection model.

	Accuracy%	Classifier
Features only from sensors	86.00	RF
Features only from biomarkers	75.00	RF
Features from sensors and biomarkers	81.00	RF
All features without biomarkers	89.00	RF
All features without sensors	91.00	RF
Optimal set of features	95.00	RF

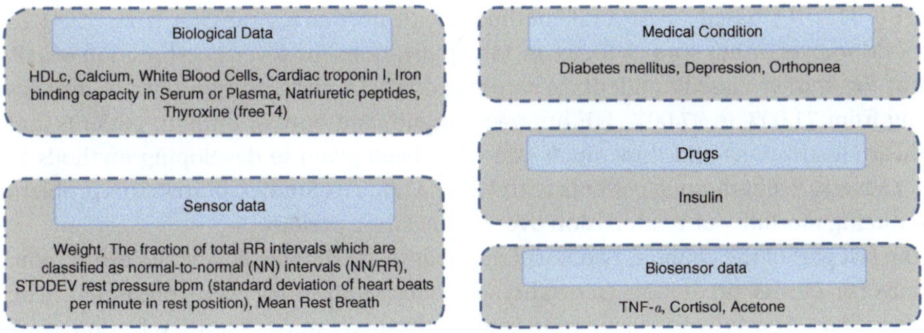

Figure 9.7 Optimal set of features for severity estimation.

Table 9.9 Results of the adverse events prediction model.

	Accuracy%	Classifier
Features only from sensors	78.00	RBF
Features only from biomarkers	81.00	LMT
Features from sensors and biomarkers	77.00	ROT
All features without biomarkers	80.00	ROT
All features without sensors	83.00	ROT
Optimal set of features	89.00	ROT

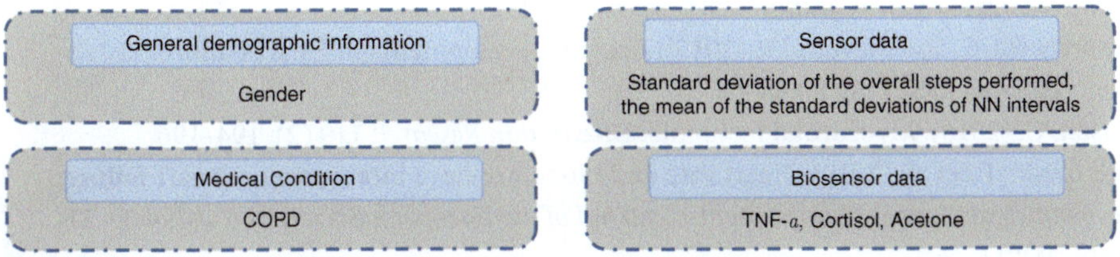

Figure 9.8 Optimal set of features for adverse events prediction.

9.3 Conclusions

In this chapter, after an introduction to HF, and HF classification, evaluation, and diagnosis methods we highlighted the importance and necessity of using ML techniques in medicine. Due to the increased incidence and the large financial costs required to diagnose HF, the diagnosis and treatment of the disease are extremely important.

An extensive review of the state of the art in the applications of ML in the management of HF was demonstrated, utilizing several types of features, HRV measurements, heart sound characteristics, ECG recorded signals, and EHR features – and studies using the Cleveland heart disease database or the EFFECT sudy data set.

As presented in the comparison Table 9.1 different approaches in the literature provide methods for detecting and diagnosing HF, acute HF, or the various types of HF (HFpEF, HFmrEF, HFrEF) based on several methods, with accuracies ranging from 72.41 to 99.93%. Moreover, other studies focus on ML applications for severity estimation of HF. Most of the studies classify patients according to NYHA classification with accuracies ranging from 71.00% to 97.00%. HF imposes a significant burden on both patients and healthcare institutions and thus much effort has been given to developing methods to predict adverse events among patients with HF or acute HF. Studies address this problem by predicting mortality or readmission over various time periods.

In the last part of the chapter, two novel methods of HF diagnosis, severity estimation, and adverse events prediction (mortality or rehospitalization) were presented. The models are based on ML approaches and consist of data cleaning, feature selection, class balancing, and classification steps. The results are high for all the addressed problems, while the innovation of the studies derives from the multiple data types that are utilized, especially the biomarkers and the data from the biosensors. Since these studies are based on the Kardiatool and Hearten projects, the demonstrated method for the HF diagnosis is integrated in a diagnostic tool in Kardiatool. In addition, the HF severity estimation and the adverse events prediction are embedded in the Hearten Knowledge Management System, which offers decision support in HF management. Through these tools, healthcare professionals can receive information related to a patient, detect the presence of HF, estimate the severity of a patient's condition, and predict the risk for adverse events; they can therefore adapt patient management accordingly.

References

1 Yancy, C., et al. (2013). 2013 ACCF/AHA guideline for the management of heart failure: executive summary. *Circulation* 128 (16): 1810–1852.

2 Dassanayaka, S. and Steven, J.P. (2015). Recent Developments in Heart Failure. *Circulation Research* 117 (7): 58–63.

3 Heusch, G. (2016). Myocardial Ischemia. *Circulation Research* 119 (2): 194–196.

4 Ponikowski, P., et al. (2019). Heart rate and blood pressure monitoring in heart failure. *European Heart Journal Supplements: Journal of the European Society of Cardiology* 21 (Suppl. M): 13–16.

5 Ponikowski, P., et al. (2016). 2016 ESC Guidelines for the diagnosis and treatment of acute and chronic heart failure: The task force for the diagnosis and treatment of acute and chronic heart failure of the European Society of Cardiology (ESC) Developed with the special contribution of the Heart Failure Association (HFA) of the ESC. *European Heart Journal* 37 (27): 2129–2200.
6 Pazos-López, P., et al. (2011). The causes, consequences, and treatment of left or right heart failure. *Vascular Health and Risk Management* 7: 237–254.
7 Reddy, Y.N.V. and Borlaug, B.A. (2019). Readmissions in heart failure: It's more than just in the medicine. *Mayo Clinic Proceedings* 94 (10): 1919–1921.
8 Mozaffarian, D., et al. (2015). Heart disease and stroke statistics—2015 update. *Circulation* 131 (4): e29–e322.
9 Lund., L.H. and Savarese, G. (2017). Global public health burden of heart failure. *Cardiac Failure Review* 3 (1): 7–11.
10 Groenewegen, A., et al. (2020). Epidemiology of heart failure. *European Journal of Heart Failure* 22 (8): 1342–1356.
11 Sabate, E. (2003). Adherence to long-term therapies: Evidence for action. World Health Organization.
12 Chen, J., et al. (2013). National trends in heart failure hospitalization after acute myocardial infarction for Medicare beneficiaries: 1998–2010. *Circulation* 128 (24): 2577–2584.
13 Alla, F., Zannad, F., and Filippatos, G. (2007). Epidemiology of acute heart failure syndromes. *Heart Failure Reviews* 12 (2): 91–95.
14 O'Connor, C.M. (2017). High heart failure readmission rates. *JACC. Heart Failure* 5 (5): 393.
15 Liu, L. and Eisen, H.J. (2014). Epidemiology of heart failure and scope of the problem. *Cardiology Clinics* 32 (1): 1–8.
16 Franzén, K., Saveman, B., and Blomqvist, K. (2006). Predictors for health related quality of life in persons 65 years or older with chronic heart failure. *European Journal of Cardiovascular Nursing* 6 (2): 112–120.
17 Van Riet, E.E., et al. (2016). Epidemiology of heart failure: The prevalence of heart failure and ventricular dysfunction in older adults over time. A systematic review. *European Journal of Heart Failure* 18 (3): 242–252.
18 Christiansen, M.N., et al. (2017). Age-specific trends in incidence, mortality, and comorbidities of heart failure in Denmark, 1995 to 2012. *Circulation* 135 (13): 1214–1223.
19 Barasa, A., et al. (2014). Heart failure in young adults: 20-year trends in hospitalization, aetiology, and case fatality in Sweden. *European Heart Journal* 35 (1): 25–32.
20 Wadhera, R.K., Yeh, R.W., and Maddox, K.E.J. (2019). The hospital readmissions reduction program — Time for a reboot. *The New England Journal of Medicine* 380 (24): 2289–2291.
21 Banerjee, D., et al. (2017). An informatics-based approach to reducing heart failure all-cause readmissions: The Stanford heart failure dashboard. *Journal of the American Medical Informatics Association* 24 (3): 550–555.

22 Singh, A. and Mehta, Y. (2018). Heart failure with preserved ejection fraction (HFpEF): Implications for the anesthesiologists. *Journal of Anaesthesiology, Clinical Pharmacology* 34 (2): 161–165.
23. Simmonds, S., et al. (2020). Cellular and molecular differences between HFpEF and HFrEF: A step ahead in an improved pathological understanding. *Cells* 9 (1): 242–264.
24 The Criteria Committee of the New York Heart Association. (1994). Nomenclature and Criteria for Diagnosis of Diseases of the Heart and Great Vessels, 9th edition. Boston: Little, Brown & Co.
25 Caraballo, C., et al. (2019). Clinical Implications of the New York Heart Association Classification. *Journal of the American Heart Association* 8 (23): e014240.
26 White, P. and Myers, M. (1921). The classification of cardiac diagnosis. *JAMA* 77: 1414–1415.
27 Farmakis, D., Papingiotis, G., and Parissis, J. (2017). Acute heart failure: Epidemiology and socioeconomic burden. *Continuing Cardiology Education* 3 (3): 88–92.
28 Inamdar, A.A. and Inamdar, A.C. (2016). Heart failure: Diagnosis, management and utilization. *Journal of Clinical Medicine* 5 (7): 62.
29 King, M., Kingery, J., and Casey, B. (2012). Diagnosis and evaluation of heart failure. *American Family Physician* 85 (12): 1161–1168.
30 Salerno, M., et al. (2017). Recent advances in cardiovascular magnetic resonance. *Circulation. Cardiovascular Imaging* 10 (6): e003951.
31 Sado, D.M., et al. (2011). CMR in heart failure. *Cardiology Research and Practice. https://doi.org/10.4061/2011/739157.*
32 Habib, G., et al. (2017). Multimodality Imaging in Restrictive Cardiomyopathies: An EACVI expert consensus document In collaboration with the "Working Group on myocardial and pericardial diseases" of the European Society of Cardiology Endorsed by The Indian Academy of Echocardiography. *European Heart Journal - Cardiovascular Imaging* 18 (10): 1090–1121.
33 Pereira, N.L., Grogan, M., and Dec, G.W. (2018). Spectrum of restrictive and infiltrative Cardiomyopathies: Part 1 of a 2-Part Series. *Journal of the American College of Cardiology* 71 (10): 1130–1148.
34 Madhok, V., et al. (2008). The accuracy of symptoms, signs and diagnostic tests in the diagnosis of left ventricular dysfunction in primary care: A diagnostic accuracy systematic review. *BMC Family Practice* 8 (9).
35 Obermeyer, Z. and Emanuel, E. (2016). Predicting the future - Big data, machine learning, and clinical medicine. *The New England Journal of Medicine* 375 (13): 1216–1219.
36 Deo, R.C. (2015). Machine learning in medicine. 132 (20): 1920–1930.
37 Sidey-Gibbons, J.A.M. and Sidey-Gibbons, C.J. (2019). Machine learning in medicine: A practical introduction. *BMC Medical Research Methodology* 19 (1): 64.
38 Yang, G., et al. (2010). A heart failure diagnosis model based on support vector machine. In: 3rd International Conference on Biomedical Engineering and Informatics, Yantai, China: 1105–1108.
39 Son, C.S., et al. (2012). Decision-making model for early diagnosis of congestive heart failure using rough set and decision tree approaches. *Journal of Biomedical Informatics* 45 (5): 999–1008.

40 Choi, E., et al. (2017). Using recurrent neural network models for early detection of heart failure onset. *Journal of the American Medical Informatics Association* 24 (2): 361–370.

41 Le, M.T., et *al.* (2020). Predicting heart failure using deep neural network. In: *2020 International Conference on Advanced Technologies for Communications (ATC)* 221–225.

42 Potter, E., et al. (2020). Machine learning applied to energy waveform ECG for prediction of Stage B heart failure in the community. *Journal of the American College of Cardiology* 75 (11): Suppl. 1 1894.

43 Pecchia, L., et al. (2011). Discrimination power of short-term heart rate variability measures for CHF assessment. *IEEE Transactions on Information Technology in Biomedicine* 15 (1): 40–46.

44 Walker, H.K., Hall, W.D., and Hurst, J.W. (1990). Clinical Methods: The History, Physical, and Laboratory Examinations, 3rd edition. Boston: Butterworths.

45 Zheng, Y., et al. (2015). Computer-assisted diagnosis for chronic heart failure by the analysis of their cardiac reserve and heart sound characteristics. *Computer Methods and Programs in Biomedicine* 122 (3): 372–383.

46 Gjoreski, M., et al. (2020). Machine learning and end-to-end deep learning for the detection of chronic heart failure from heart sounds. *IEEE Access* 8: 20313–20324.

47 Lal, H., et al. (2020). Detecting congestive heart failure by extracting multimodal features and employing machine learning techniques. *BioMed Research International* 6: 1–19.

48 Wang, L. and Zhou, X. (2019). Detection of congestive heart failure based on LSTM-based deep network via short-term RR intervals. *Sensors* 19 (7): 1502.

49 Chen, W., et al. (2017). A CHF detection method based on deep learning with RR intervals. In: *39th Annual International Conference of the IEEE Engineering in Medicine* 3369–3372.

50 Pires, I.M., et *al.* (2020). Machine learning for the evaluation of the presence of heart disease. *Procedia Computer Science* 177: 432–437.

51 Masetic, Z. and Subasi, A. (2016). Congestive heart failure detection using random forest classifier. *Computer Methods and Programs in Biomedicine* 130: 54–64.

52 Acharya, U.R., et *al.* (2019). Deep convolutional neural network for the automated diagnosis of congestive heart failure using ECG signals. *Applied Intelligence* 49 (1): 16–27.

53 Kim, K. and Kwon, J. (2019). Deep Learning for diagnosing heart failure from ECG signals. *The Journal of Heart and Lung Transplantation* 38 (4): Suppl. S375.

54 Kwon, J., et al. (2019). Development and validation of deep-learning algorithm for electrocardiography-based heart failure identification. *Korean Circulation Journal* 49 (7): 629–639.

55 Ning, W., et al. (2020). Automatic detection of congestive heart failure based on a hybrid deep learning algorithm in the internet of medical things. *IEEE Internet of Things Journal.*

56 Samuel, O., et al. (2017). An integrated decision support system based on ANN and Fuzzy_AHP for heart failure risk prediction. *Expert Systems with Applications* 68: 163–172.

57 Mohan, S., Thirumalai, C., and Srivastava, G. (2019). Effective heart disease prediction using hybrid machine learning techniques. *IEEE Access* 7: 81542–81554.

58 Ali, L., et al. (2019). An optimized stacked support vector machines based expert system for the effective prediction of heart failure. *IEEE Access* 7: 54007–54014.

59 Javeed, A., et al. (2019). An intelligent learning system based on random search algorithm and optimized random forest model for improved heart disease detection. *IEEE Access* 7: 180235–180243.

60 Reddy, Y.N.V., et al. (2018). A simple, evidence-based approach to help guide diagnosis of heart failure with preserved ejection fraction. *Circulation* 138 (9): 861–870.

61 Liu, Y., Guo, X., and Zheng, Y. (2019). An automatic approach using ELM classifier for HFpEF identification based on heart sound characteristics. *Journal of Medical Systems* 43 (9): 285.

62 Choi, D., et al. (2020). Artificial intelligence for the diagnosis of heart failure. *npj Digital Medicine* 3 (54).

63 Austin, P.C., et al. (2013). Using methods from the data-mining and machine-learning literature for disease classification and prediction: A case study examining classification of heart failure subtypes. *Journal of Clinical Epidemiology* 66 (4): 398–407.

64 Pecchia, L., Melillo, P., and Bracale, M. (2011). Remote health monitoring of heart failure with data mining via CART method on HRV features. *IEEE Transactions on Biomedical Engineering* 58 (3): 800–804.

65 Guidi, G., et al. (2012). Heart failure artificial intelligence-based computer aided diagnosis telecare system. In: Impact Analysis of Solutions for Chronic Disease Prevention and Management, Berlin, Heidelberg: Springer.

66 Melillo, P., et *al.* (2013). Classification tree for risk assessment in patients suffering from congestive heart failure via long-term heart rate variability. *IEEE Journal of Biomedical and Health Informatics* 17 (3): 727–733.

67 Shahbazi, F. and Asl, B. (2015). Generalized discriminant analysis for congestive heart failure risk assessment based on long-term heart rate variability. *Computer Methods and Programs in Biomedicine* 122 (2): 191–198.

68 Gladence, L.M., Ravi, T., and Karthi, M. (2014). An enhanced method for detecting congestive heart failure - Automatic Classifier. In: *IEEE International Conference on Advanced Communications, Control and Computing Technologies*, Ramanathapuram.

69 Guidi, G., et al. (2015). A multi-layer monitoring system for clinical management of congestive heart failure. *BMC Medical Informatics and Decision Making* 15 (3): S5.

70 Aljaaf, A.J., et al. (2015). Predicting the likelihood of heart failure with a multi level risk assessment using decision tree. In: *3rd International Conference on Technological Advances in Electrical, Electronics and Computer Engineering (TAEECE)*, Beirut: 101–106.

71 Chen, W., et al. (2016). A novel and effective method for congestive heart failure detection and quantification using dynamic heart rate variability measurement. *PLOS ONE* 11 (11).

72 Tripoliti, E.E., et al. (2017). Heart failure: Diagnosis, severity estimation and prediction of adverse events through machine learning techniques. *Computational and Structural Biotechnology Journal* 15: 26–47.

73 Zhang, R., et al. (2017). Automatic methods to extract New York Heart Association classification from clinical notes. In: *IEEE International Conference on Bioinformatics and Biomedicine (BIBM)*, Kansas City, MO, USA: 1296–1299.

74 Ma, S., et al. (2018). Estimating New York heart association classification for heart failure patients from information in the electronic health record. In: *2018 IEEE International Conference on Bioinformatics and Biomedicine (BIBM)* 1504–1507.

75 Groccia, M.C., et al. (2018). Predictive models for risk assessment of worsening events in chronic heart failure patients. In: *Computing in Cardiology Conference (CINC)*, Maastricht, Netherlands: 1–4.

76 Vedomske, M.A., Brown, D.E., and Harrison, J.H. (2013). Random forests on ubiquitous data for heart failure 30-Day readmissions prediction. In: *12th International Conference on Machine Learning and Applications*, 415–421. Miami, FL.

77 Mortazavi, B.J., et al. (2016). Analysis of machine learning techniques for heart failure readmissions. *Circulation. Cardiovascular Quality and Outcomes* 9 (6): 629–640.

78 Frizzell, J.D., et al. (2017). Prediction of 30-Day all-cause readmissions in patients hospitalized for heart failure: Comparison of machine learning and other statistical approaches. *JAMA Cardiology* 2 (2): 204–209.

79 Jamei, M., et al. (2017). Predicting all-cause risk of 30-day hospital readmission using artificial neural networks. *PLOS ONE* 12 (7): e0181173.

80 Leong, K.T., et al. (2017). Risk stratification model for 30-day heart failure readmission in a multiethnic South East Asian Community. *The American Journal of Cardiology* 119 (9): 1428–1432.

81 Golas, S.B., et al. (2018). A machine learning model to predict the risk of 30-day readmissions in patients with heart failure: A retrospective analysis of electronic medical records data. *BMC Medical Informatics and Decision Making* 18: 44.

82 Ashfaq, A., et al. (2019). Readmission prediction using deep learning on electronic health records. *Journal of Biomedical Informatics* 97: 103256.

83 Liu, X., et al. (2019). Predicting heart failure readmission from clinical notes using deep learning. In: IEEE International Conference on Bioinformatics and Biomedicine (BIBM), San Diego, CA, USA: 2642–2648.

84 Khayyat, A., et al. (2019). Decision support tool to estimate and reduce the probability of readmission for congestive heart failure patients. In: Systems and Information Engineering Design Symposium (SIEDS), Charlottesville, VA: 1–6. doi: 10.1109/SIEDS.2019.8735596.

85 Liu, W., et al. (2020). Predicting 30-day hospital readmissions using artificial neural networks with medical code embedding. *PLOS ONE* 15 (4): e0221606.

86 Kawai, A., et al. (2020). Machine learning prediction tools for all-cause readmissions in patients hospitalised for heart failure using routinely collected medical record data. *Heart, Lung & Circulation* 29: 382.

87 Pocock, S.J., et al. (2013). Predicting survival in heart failure: A risk score based on 39,372 patients from 30 studies. *European Heart Journal* 34 (19): 1404–1413.

88 Miao, F., et al. (2018). Predictive modeling of hospital mortality for patients with heart failure by using an improved random survival forest. *IEEE Access* 6: 7244–7253.

89 Kwon, J., et al. (2019). Artificial intelligence algorithm for predicting mortality of patients with acute heart failure. *PLOS ONE* 14 (7): e0219302.

90 Wang, Z., et al. (2020) Feature rearrangement based deep learning system for predicting heart failure mortality. *Computer Methods and Programs in Biomedicine* 191.

91 Yang, S. and Hua, W. (2020). Machine learning with biomarkers improves the prediction of long-term outcomes in heart failure patients treated with cardiac resynchronization therapy. *Journal of the American College of Cardiology* 75 (11): Suppl. 1, 390.

92 Adler, E.D., et al. (2020). Improving risk prediction in heart failure using machine learning. *European Journal of Heart Failure* 22 (1): 139–147.

93 Jing, L., et al. (2020). A machine learning approach to management of heart failure populations. *JACC. Heart Failure* 8 (7): 578–587.

94 Zhang, J., et al. (2013). Identifying patients at risk of death or hospitalization due to worsening heart failure using decision tree analysis: Evidence from the Trans-European Network-Home-Care Management System (TEN-HMS) study. *International Journal of Cardiology* 163 (2): 149–156.

95 Tripoliti, E.E., et al. (2017). Predicting heart failure patient events by exploiting saliva and breath biomarkers information. In: *2017 IEEE 17th International Conference on Bioinformatics and Bioengineering (BIBE)*. (Oct. 2017), Herndon, VA, 285–290,

96 Awan, S.E., et al. (2019). Machine learning-based prediction of heart failure readmission or death: Implications of choosing the right model and the right metrics. *ESC Heart Failure* 6: no. 428–435.

97 Angraal, S., et al. (2020). Machine learning prediction of mortality and hospitalization in heart failure with preserved ejection fraction. *JACC. Heart Failure* 8 (1): 12–21.

98 Yang, M., et al. (2020). A novel nomogram to predict all-cause readmission or death risk in Chinese elderly patients with heart failure. *ESC Heart Failure* 7 (3): 1015–1024.

99 Zahavi, G., et al. (2020). Machine learning models predict 30-day and 1-year mortality in Heart Failure. *Journal of the American College of Cardiology* 75 (11): Suppl. 1, 858–858.

100 Beecy, A.N., et al. (2020). Utilizing electronic health data and machine learning for the prediction of 30-day unplanned readmission or all-cause mortality in heart failure. *Cardiovascular Digital Health Journal* 1 (2): 71–79.

101 Tripoliti, E.E., et al. (2018). KardiaTool: An integrated POC solution for Non-invasive diagnosis and therapy monitoring of heart failure patients. In: *2018 40th Annual International Conference of the IEEE Engineering in Medicine and Biology Society (EMBC)*. 3878–3881. doi:10.1109/EMBC.2018.8513298.

102 Tripoliti, E.E., et al. (2019). HEARTEN KMS – A knowledge management system targeting the management of patients with heart failure. *Journal of Biomedical Informatics* 94: 103203.

103 Hall, M. (1998). Correlation-based Feature Selection for Machine Learning. New Zealand: University of Waikato.

104 Luengo, J., et al. (2011). Addressing data complexity for imbalanced data sets. *Applied Software Computing* 15: 1909–1936.

10

Clinical Applications of Artificial Intelligence in Early and Accurate Detection of Low-Concentration CVD Biomarkers

Meena Laad, Sajna M.S, Kishor Kumar Sadasivuni, and Sadiya Waseem

10.1 Introduction

Cardiovascular diseases (CVDs) are a mix of several types of disorders affecting the heart and blood vessels (Figure 10.1). Mainly, a plaque is formed in the artery walls and narrows the arteries, giving rise to a severe condition called atherosclerosis. This narrowing of arteries obstructs the blood flow and makes the free flow of blood difficult, leading to a heart attack or stroke. CVDs are one of the leading causes of death globally and a major obstacle to sustainable human growth and wellbeing [1]. A study reported that the occurrence of the majority of CVDs was observed in industrialized countries having high incomes [2]. But in the last few decades, the absolute burden of CVDs is seen more in developing countries and is expected to grow more in the twenty-first century [2, 3]. To assess the CVD associated risk factors, several health examination surveys have been conducted in some of the countries with low and middle income [4]. A systematic evaluation of data collected through various resources can reduce the CVD mortality rate to a great extent.

10.2 Risk Assessment and Early Detection of CVDs Using Biosensors

Traditionally, CVD prevention begins with identifying potential risk factors. Treatment cost and healthcare expenditures are escalating; therefore, there is a crucial requirement for early detection followed by proper treatment of asymptomatic CVD [5]. Also, many individuals indicating low-risk levels have shown early evidence of CVD. There is an important need to understand the factors responsible for the initiation, associated symptoms, and early and accurate detection of CVD, thereby reducing the high risk of unexpected death. The early and fast diagnosis of CVDs is essential not only to save patient's life but also to save huge hospitalization costs and time in successful prognosis of the disease.

Present CVD detection methods rely greatly on conducting laboratory tests and take several hours or sometimes days to produce the results. According to the World Health

Predicting Heart Failure: Invasive, Non-Invasive, Machine Learning, and Artificial Intelligence Based Methods, First Edition. Edited by Kishor Kumar Sadasivuni, Hassen M. Ouakad, Somaya Al-Maadeed, Huseyin C. Yalcin, and Issam Bait Bahadur.

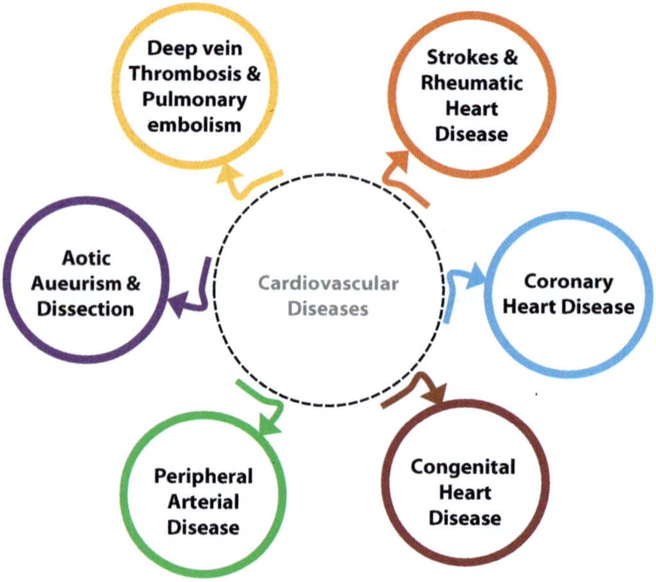

Figure 10.1 Various types of CVD and their origin.

Organization, the criteria for diagnosing CVD are that patients should show characteristic conditions such as severe pain in the chest, changes in diagnostic ECG, and elevated levels of biomarkers in blood sample [6].

A biosensor is considered as a very effective analytical tool in medical diagnostics for rapid detection of CVD disease at an early stage. Biosensors have revolutionized CVD diagnosis and prognosis. A biosensing device is made to detect and measure specific target molecules. The underlying principle used in the design of biosensors is to immobilize a biological receptor material on an appropriate transducer's surface, which further transforms this biochemical signal into measurable electronic signals such as optical, piezoelectric, electrochemical, magnetic, or acoustic signals [7–11].

A variety of CVD detection sensors is available, which are very accurate, quick in detection, easy to carry, and don't cause any damage to the environment. Recent research studies in microfluidics and advanced nanomaterials have led to the development of more efficient diagnostics requiring little analysis time. They incorporate several clinical assays into a compact, single portable unit. The nanotechnology industry is rapidly growing and creating highly efficient tools based on multidisciplinary research involving nanofluids, drug delivery, microelectronics, and analytical chemistry [12–16].

Current CVD diagnostic techniques require blood tests to assess relevant biomarker levels. A biomarker is measured on a biosample such as a blood, urine, or tissue test. It can also be the data recording obtained from a person's blood pressure, ECG, etc., and includes imaging tests like an echocardiogram or CT scan.

Different imaging techniques, such as electrocardiograms, computed tomography (CT), and angiograms, are also used for CVD detection. These clinical methods provide vital information about cardiovascular health, but they consume periods of time. They also require sample preparation and depend on the skill and experience of the physician to interpret the results correctly, which delays the treatment. This long time period during diagnosis sometimes results in the deterioration of the condition of the patient.

Sensor platforms are required for early and accurate diagnosis of CVD. There are various sensor platforms based on the optical and mechanical properties of the biosensing materials. Electrochemical-based detection techniques are preferred due to their high sensitivity, reduced cost, and faster detection; electrochemical impedance spectroscopy (EIS) has exhibited excellent results in detecting low concentrations of many clinically important biomarkers used to diagnose CVDs. The application of biomarkers that can be recognized in blood has attracted many researchers' interest recently in this area [17].

The vascular wall discharges molecules into the blood, gives necessary information about the relevant pathological processes happening in the human system. The concentrations of the released molecules provide potential information of different pathological processes and can act as biomarkers.

An ideal cardiac biomarker has some characteristic features, such as strong clinical sensitivity, which are very specific in marking the target molecules. It is quickly released in the blood, leading to fast diagnosis, maintains a high elevation level for a longer duration in the blood, and is able to assay quantitatively.

A wide range of potential biomarkers need simultaneous analysis for the correct diagnosis of CVD [18–20]. One research study reported a set of 177 plasma markers for the detection of CVDs [20].

The quantification of biomarkers is required to detect CVD quickly and accurately to plan a proper strategy for the care of cardiac patients. Quick and reliable detection of these biomarkers helps physicians to distinguish between diseases that show similar symptoms. As the clinically significant sensing ranges of some important biomarkers have very low concentrations, they need highly sensitive assay methods.

10.3 Different Types of Cardiac Biosensors

There are various types of biosensor, as shown in Figure 10.2.

10.3.1 Optical Biosensors

Optical biosensors are very sensitive and efficient biosensors. They detect biomarkers by observing the variation in frequency, phase, amplitude, and state of polarization of the input light responding to the biorecognition processes. Optical biosensors make use of material properties for detection of CVD, such as colorimetry, fluorescence, luminescence, fibre optics, etc. [21]. ELISA (enzyme-linked immunosorbent assay) based biomarkers use optical properties of chromogenic reporters (Figure 10.3). These biomarkers give signals which are colorimetric, fluorogenic, or luminescent in nature. ELISA has been extensively used for cardiac marker detection [22–25]. Research continues into further miniaturization of the sensor platform without compromising on detection ability.

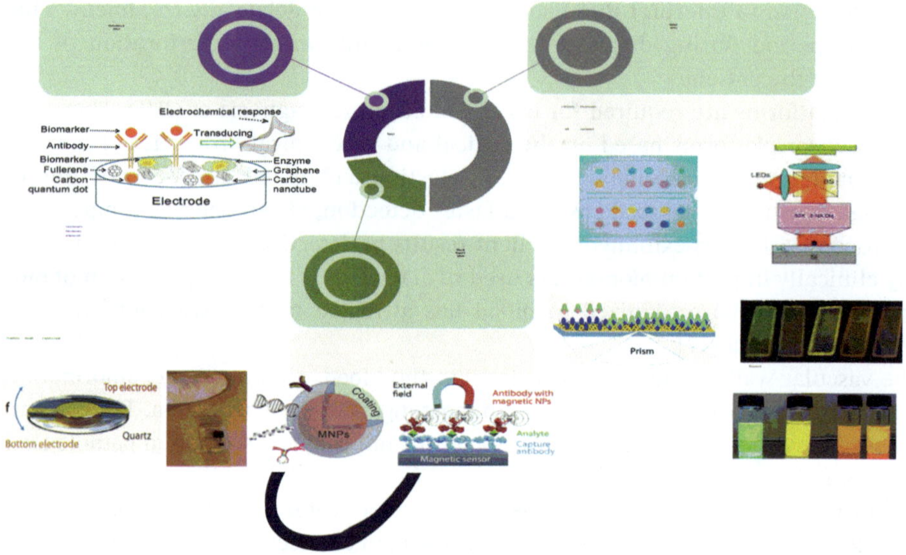

Figure 10.2 Various types of sensing mechanism for CVD.

Surface plasmon resonance (SPR) is an effective and widely used optical transduction sensing technique used in most of the commercial optical biosensors. These biosensors work on special electromagnetic waves that are surface plasmon and identify variation in the refractive index (RI) on the surface of metal [20]. Surface plasmons are surface electromagnetic waves that propagate in a direction parallel to the metal interface.

10.3.2 Electrochemical Biosensors

In electrochemical biosensors, an immobilized detecting probe holds together the target molecules selectively. The detection of target molecules is based on observing the variations in current or voltage at a local surface. The potentiometric (Figure 10.4), amperometric, and impedimetric transducers used in these biosensors convert vital chemical information into a measurable amperometric signal. These biosensors are low cost and easy to manufacture [27].

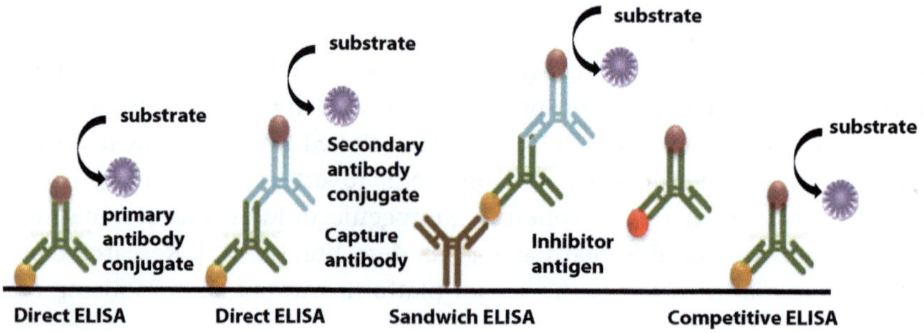

Figure 10.3 Different types of ELISA techniques.

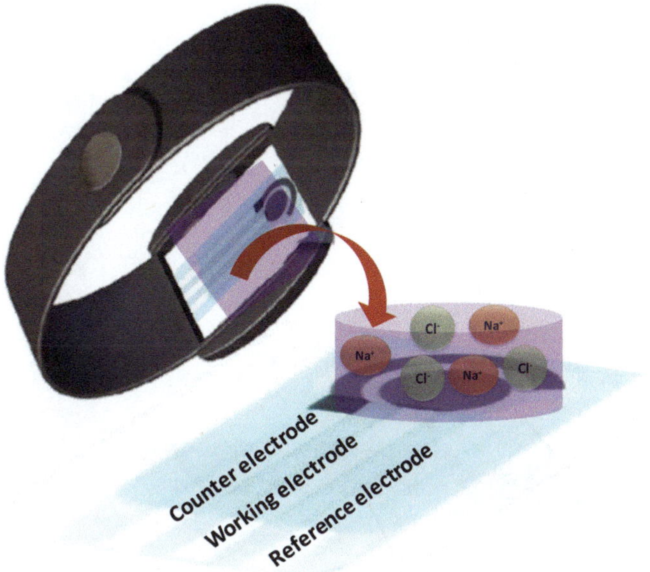

Figure 10.4 Wearable potentiometric ion sensor.

10.3.2.1 Application of Nanomaterials in Electrochemical Biosensors

Nanotechnology has demonstrated new and unique detection platforms for biomarker detection for cardiac diseases with the applications of different types of nanomaterials like nanoparticles, nanowires, nanotubes, and nanocomposites. Nanotechnology offers a lot of flexibility in the choice of nano-size materials to quantify the signal, which in turn measures the concentration of the analyte.

A group of researchers used micro- and nano-polystyrene polymer structures to design electrochemical biosensors. The study concluded that reducing the surface texture to nano-size improved the detection sensitivity for C-reactive protein biomarkers [28].

10.3.3 Magnetic Biosensors

In life sciences, magnetic particles or magnetic beads have been in use in establishing biological assays. Biological cells, pathogens, toxins antibodies, toxins, proteins, etc. can be categorized by connecting them to microbeads which are superparamagnetic in nature. The size of these particles ranges from a few nanometers to micrometers. The structure of magnetic beads comprises tiny magnetite crystallites encapsulated in ceramic or plastic spheres. Biological species like DNA or antibodies are coated on these beads which selectively bind to the target analyte (Figures 10.2, 10.5) [29].

10.4 Limitations of Biosensor Technology in the Detection of CVDs

The number of patients suffering from CVDs is growing at an alarming rate in the world. Precious lives can be saved if CVDs are diagnosed at an early stage of their progression, as physicians will be able to give proper treatment and allow faster recovery in patients.

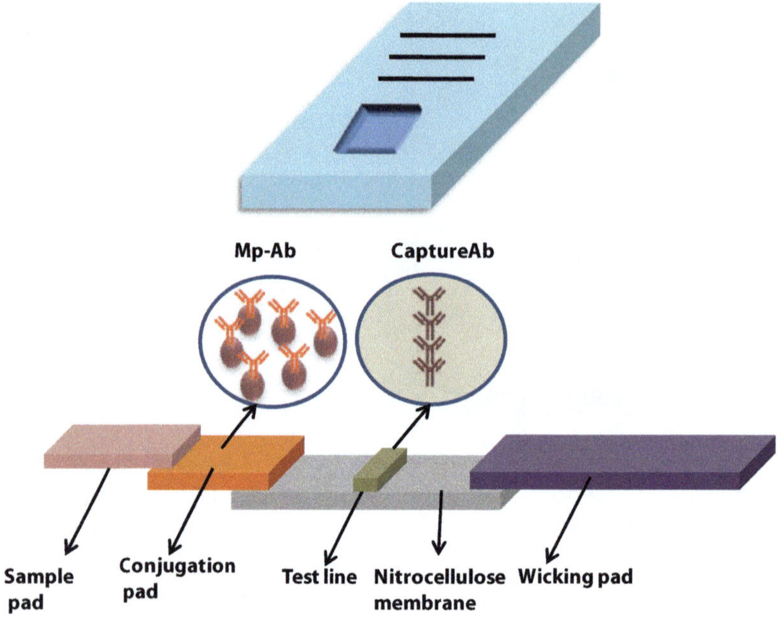

Figure 10.5 DNA based magnetic biosensor.

It is critical to fabricate simple and efficient CVD diagnostic devices, which can quickly detect multiple cardiac biomarkers in biological fluids in very low volume. Accurate detection using biomarkers is challenging, as most cardiac biomarkers also mark common inflammation. Hence, it becomes very difficult to differentiate cardiovascular risks. A patient may have an inflammatory process and no CVD at all, and biomarkers can report false positives.

Therefore, there is an urgent need to explore new techniques and tools to enable fast and accurate detection of cardiovascular risks, helping physicians to make correct clinical decisions. It has become essential to identify new and non-inflammatory biomarkers for CVD, developing biorecognition elements, exploring biomarkers that can directly detect CVD in biological fluids, and developing miniature, portable electronic transducers.

It's a big challenge to achieve CVD diagnostic tools with rapid, high sensitivity, specificity, low-cost, and accurate biosensors. Artificial intelligence (AI) provides excellent tools for the discovery of new biosensing materials for the early and precise detection of CVDs. New materials that are more functional can be discovered with a multidisciplinary approach that brings together researchers from diversified fields such as science, engineering, biomedical, and design backgrounds. This demands a radical shift away from traditional methods for the synthesis of new materials. There are several stages involved in materials discovery, such as conception, synthesis, and characterization. The entire process is carried out in the same sequence. As a result, only a limited number of materials can be tested at a time. AI has great potential for faster and more efficient material development for specific applications but AI tools, large computational data sets, and automated robotic systems have not yet been widely used for this purpose.

Computational techniques combined with AI can transform the understanding of vital information from available medical data. These techniques interpret the data in the form of structured, optimized, and meaningful information, which is readily available for the physicians for timely and accurate diagnosis.

Rapidly evolving technologies based on AI are non-invasively illuminating the fundamental processes contributing to CVDs. New insights into CVDs and strokes have important therapeutic implications for an expanding population of patients. Digitized medical data combined with information and telecommunication techniques are revolutionizing the diagnosis and treatment of complex cardiovascular abnormalities.

In making their clinical decisions, medical practitioners need to learn and keep up with rapidly evolving AI tools and techniques, and to apply them in interpreting health-related data received from different sources. AI applications in cardiac care are opening a range of possibilities to provide new personalized healthcare services. Personalized new contacts between patients and medical practitioners are being established, with health data and telemedicine moving healthcare from a passive to a pervasive activity. Physicians, scientists are integrating AI for faster, accurate, and effective diagnosis and treatment.

10.5 Application of AI in CVD Detection

In cardiology, AI technologies are being used in cardiac precision medicine, clinical assessment, cardiac imaging analysis, and automated robotic systems (Figure 10.6). They bring faster and accurate results in detecting CVDs, which previously would take hours or days to get detected with traditional methods.

In improving and optimizing CVD outcomes, AI techniques can drastically transform the way cardiology is practiced today. Specifically, the image techniques have offered innovative tools to effectively interpret data and arrive at a correct clinical assessment.

Machine learning (ML) and deep learning (DL) techniques of AI not only assist medical practitioners with faster and accurate clinical decisions, but also significantly improve medical knowledge by handling huge volumes of complex health data and revealing clinically significant information about CVDs.

The application of information and communication technology (ICT) is becoming central to the creation of a personalized and efficient healthcare service. It not only helps elderly and chronically ill cardiovascular patients to receive good medical care in the comfort of their homes, but also significantly reduces hospitalization costs and improves patients' quality of life [30]. Early and accurate diagnosis and prognosis assessment are crucial to enhance CVD outcomes. The focus, however, rests on imaging when AI is used in cardiovascular medicine.

ML, DL, and cognitive computing are AI techniques that can be effectively applied in early and accurate diagnosis, prediction of CVD outcome, and prognosis assessment of CVD.

A vast number of quantitative, qualitative, and transactional data sets are generated from electronic health records and other resources, and these need AI techniques to be effectively and meaningfully interpreted [31]. Some of the AI techniques used in cardiovascular medicine and digital healthcare applications are described below:

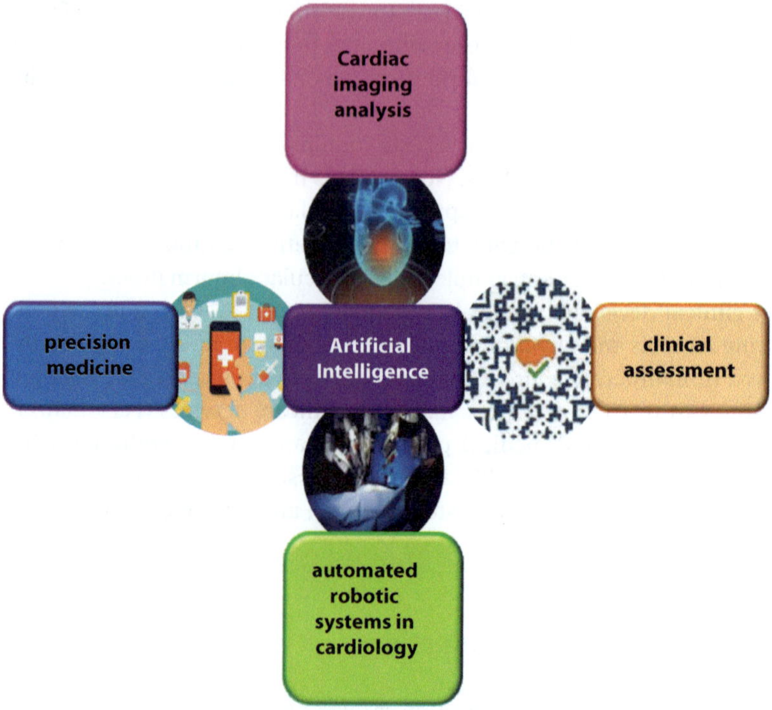

Figure 10.6 Role of AI in CVD treatment.

10.5.1 Telemedicine and Mobile Health

Telemedicine and mobile health (mHealth) are gaining popularity and playing a significant role in the deterrence of CVDs and overall upgrading of cardiac care services. mHealth forms an integral part of eHealth and ICT such as computers, smartphones, mHealth applications, and patient monitoring services. AI is beneficial for remote follow-up of patients, medication reminders, real-time medical counselling, and early warnings of symptoms. This vital generated information can be used to access the healthcare information and lead to general improvement in healthcare services [32]. mHealth supports individuals in maintaining their health under the monitoring of physicians while allowing them to continue their daily activities. From a clinician's perspective, AI can prove to be extremely effective in collecting voice medical data and connecting electronic medical records, thereby significantly reducing the work of clinicians [33]. Mobile devices have shown great promise in preventing CVDs, with self-monitoring apps and their use in activities such as diet monitoring, physical activity, blood pressure (BP) and sleep monitoring. These applications help patients to maintain a healthy exercise routine and proper weight, controlling blood glucose and normal BP and lipid profile [34–37]. A study reported by Apple and Stanford Medicine [38] assessed whether the Apple heart study app, used for the analysis of pulse rate data collected from the Apple Watch, could identify irregular heart rhythms.

10.5.2 Internet of Things

The internet of things (IoT) comprises a network of physical devices, buildings, vehicles, and other objects embedded with electronic components, software, sensors, and network connections to collect and exchange data. IoT can drastically transform the way health-care services are provided today and can provide fast medical services in remote areas where there is no immediate medical help available. In the case of CVDs, where timely medical help is highly essential to save patients' lives, IoT can be a great benefit, effectively sending data received from the patient to remote physicians who can access it and can monitor patient's physical status in real time.

In cardiovascular medicine, collected data related to blood pressure, ECG, and SpO_2 can help the physician to diagnose and prescribe the necessary treatment. It will reduce hospital visits as well as hospitalization costs. IoT techniques along with real-time analytical algorithms can be instrumental in sending pre-warnings to patients about possible cardiac attacks.

Wearable sensors combined with ML analytics can improve clinical outcomes and significantly reduce hospitalizations in cases of heart failure [39–41].

10.5.3 DL and ML

ML offers a set of new algorithms and tools for the construction of inferential and predictive models which are driven by data [34, 42]. Figure 10.7 gives an overview of the ML

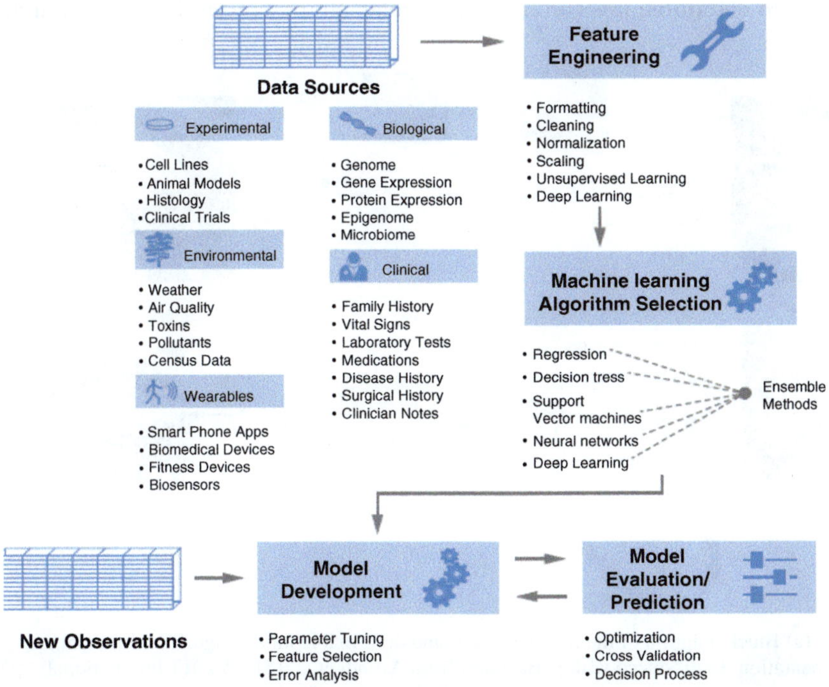

Figure 10.7 Overview of the ML workflow. Reproduced with permission from Johnson et al. [33].

workflow. DL uses neural networks and is characterized by automated algorithms which can extract meaningful patterns from the collected data [43]. It imitates the complexity of a human brain, making hierarchical representations from data that has multiple levels of abstraction [43, 44].

Physicians diagnose the disease according to their training, knowledge, experience, and clinical results. DL could prove to be extremely beneficial in expanding and improving their medical knowledge and understanding. ML models and DL can provide great help in clinical practice in a wide range of CVDs. Echocardiographic data and clinical factors combined with AI tools can diagnose, classify, estimate the severity, and predict the adverse events in CVDs [45–48]. Ouyang et al. [49] successfully designed an innovative video-based DL algorithm: EchoNet-Dynamic. This model can evaluate cardiac functions with accuracy better than human experts can from echocardiogram videos alone.

10.5.4 Magnetic Resonance Imaging

Magnetic resonance imaging (MRI) is emerging as a strong option for assessing several cardiovascular pathological entities. It is a very effective tool for the non-invasive measurement of left and right ventricular volumes and ejection fraction (EF) [50].

In cardiac MRI, ventricular segmentation is an important application for implementing ML models (Figure 10.8). It not only quantifies the volumetric but also increases the efficiency and reproducibility of clinical assessments [51–53]. It helps in the detailed tissue characterization essential to diagnose and manage the treatment of CVD [54]. It has the ability to determine myocardial and vascular injuries precisely. One research

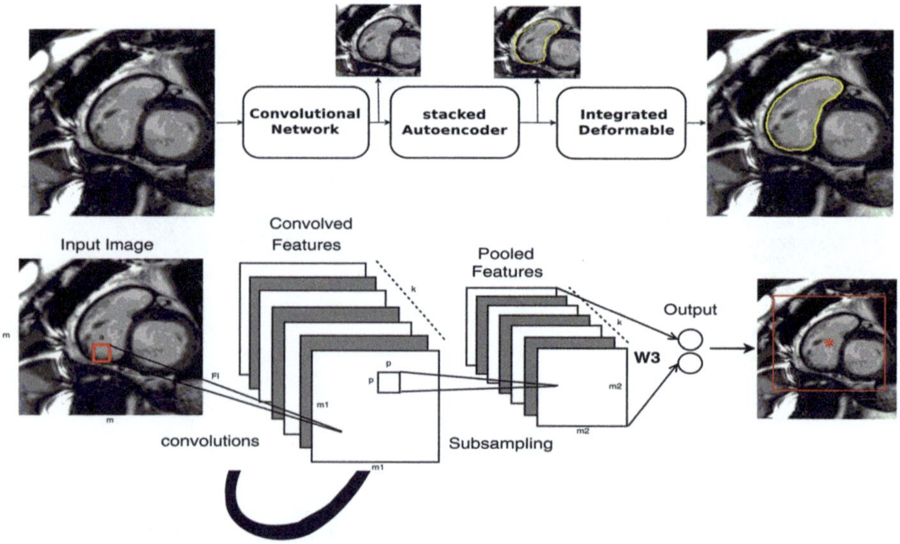

Figure 10.8 (a) Block diagram of the integrated DL and deformable model algorithm for right ventricle segmentation. Reproduced with permission from Avendi et al. [51] © 2017 International society of magnetic resonance in medicine, Publisher Wiley online library. (b) Block diagram of the convolutional network for automatic localization. Reproduced with permission from Avendi et al. [51] © 2017 International society of magnetic resonance in medicine, Publisher Wiley online library License Elsevier.

study used DL algorithms for the segmentation of the right ventricular chamber [55]. Another important application of ML was observed in the recognition of subacute or chronic myocardial scar [56].

10.5.5 Echocardiography

Echocardiography has a crucial role in the diagnosis and treatment of CVDs and correct quantitative evaluation of cardiovascular functions and structures. AI is successfully applied in automated measurement features including left ventricular EF, chamber dimensions, wall thickness, etc. (Figure 10.9) [57, 58].

AI tools, specifically ML, offer new possibilities of better accuracy in interpreting the image in clinical echocardiography practice. ML models reveal different features in an image, identifying a range of disease patterns by considering each pixel in the image and its connections [59]. These models interpret the unused data generated by multidimensional imaging techniques like 3D echocardiography and speckle tracking, thereby significantly reducing the analysis time and improving reproducibility [43].

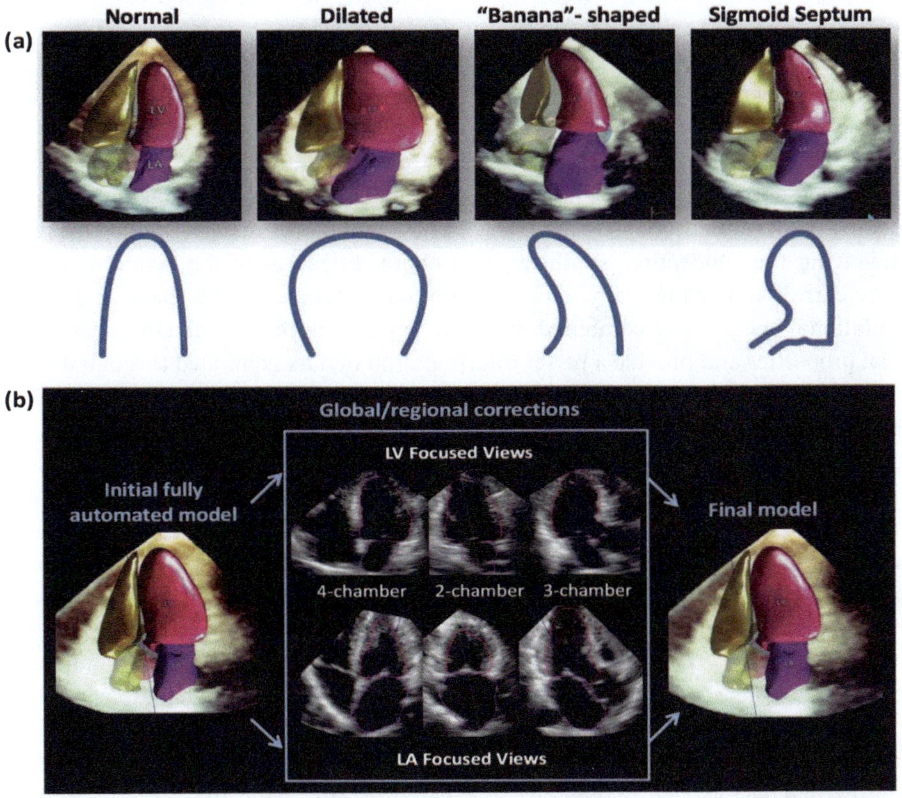

Figure 10.9 (a) Different left ventricular shapes that the automated software was trained to recognize [58]. (b) An automated technique for left heart 3D chamber quantification. Following initial fully automated detection of left ventricular and left atrial endocardial surfaces (left), the software allows the user to perform manual corrections of the endocardial boundaries when needed (center), resulting in final 3D casts of the cardiac chambers [58].

10.5.6 Cardiac CT

CT is a non-invasive imaging technique that is gaining in popularity for diagnosing and monitoring coronary artery disease (CAD). CT provides excellent visualization of the coronary arteries with high spatial resolution [60–61]. ML models are effectively using image analysis for quick and accurate diagnosis and cardiac risk assessment.

10.6 Conclusions and Future Perspectives

Despite significant development in diagnosis and risk assessment techniques, CVDs remain one of the leading causes of morbidity and mortality worldwide. The medical records indicate that CVDs begin with the progression of risk factors that turn into the development of subclinical atherosclerosis and finally end in overt CVD. Biomarkers are used to diagnose the disease, identify high-risk individuals, and enable physicians to make effective CVD treatment strategies. Though clinical assessment results form the basis for patient management, they have their own constraints in terms of time, accuracy, portability, etc.

Along with the fast spread of several diseases affecting heart and blood vessels, cases of CVDs are also on the rise, making diagnosis and prognosis both very complex and challenging. As a result, the need for new biomarkers will continue to grow. The expanding research in the discovery of new biomarkers demands a systematic organization with fast and accurate interpretation of data.

Accelerating the discovery of new biomarkers requires multidisciplinary research. It has become essential to radically shift from traditional methods of material discovery to AI-enabled modern methods. The discovery of new biomarker materials follows a process involving the conception, synthesis, and characterization of the material. These steps are carried out sequentially, and only limited materials can be tested at a time. Computational techniques combined with AI transform the understanding of the material properties and provide a better interpretation of data generated through different material characterization techniques. The faster discovery of materials enables researchers to develop new biomarkers for the accurate and quick detection of diseases.

Technological advancements in AI have opened new areas and tools in the creation of novel modeling and predictive techniques for clinical applications in CVDs and have begun to infuse and reform cardiovascular medicine. AI tools can significantly change the way cardiology is practiced today. Cardiac imaging, ML, and cognitive computing can provide the opportunity to develop efficient and accurate tools for the interpretation of data and making correct clinical decisions.

Rapidly emerging AI techniques are non-invasively revealing the fundamental processes underlying CVDs. Digitalization of healthcare practices is remarkably proving to be an effective diagnostic tool that rectifies complex heart related abnormalities.

Multimodality images, electronic health records, and mHealth devices safely store underutilized data for each patient. AI is capable of improving the status quo, and learning from these voluminous data in order to create new knowledge and understanding and enabling physicians to apply them in specific situations. Each heartbeat contains significant information, and cardiovascular medicine is one area which, when combined with AI, can march toward personalized and precise cardiocare.

The design and development of biosensors enabled with AI can be called the next-generation biosensors, and are a promising solution to the current problems in the detection and treatment of CVD. Moreover, AI also shows great potential in designing and crafting efficient wearable medical devices for the real-time checking of heart rate, rhythm, and thoracic fluid. Though there are currently several challenges to adopting AI in clinical practice, with consistent efforts in this direction, AI can bring a new dimension to more personalized and precise cardiac healthcare services in the next few years. The general understanding of AI techniques by physicians and clinicians will bring a drastic change in cardiovascular diagnosis and prognosis.

References

1 Roth, G.A., Abate, D., Abate, K.H., et al. (2018). Global, regional, and national age-sex-specific mortality for 282 causes of death in 195 countries and territories, 1980–2017: A systematic analysis for the global burden of disease study 2017. *The Lancet* 392 (10159): 1736–1788.

2 Murray, C.J. and Lopez, A. (1996). The global burden of disease. Harvard School of Public Health. *Harvard University Press* 1: 201–246.

3 Yao, C., Wu, Z., and Wu, Y. (1993). The changing pattern of cardiovascular diseases in China. *World Health Statistics Quarterly. Rapport Trimestriel De Statistiquessanitairesmondiales* 46 (2): 113–118.

4 World Bank. (1993). World Development Report: Investing in Health. New York: Oxford University Press.

5 Kwan, G.F., Mayosi, B.M., Mocumbi, et al. (2016). Endemic cardiovascular diseases of the poorest billion. *Circulation* 133 (24): 2561–2575.

6 Duprez, D. (2006). Early detection of cardiovascular disease-the future of cardiology. *EJ ESC Counc. CardiolPract* 4 (19): 1.

7 Yusuf, S., Pearson, M., Sterry, H., et al. (1984). The entry ECG in the early diagnosis and prognostic stratification of patients with suspected acute myocardial infarction. *European Heart Journal* 5 (9): 690–696.

8 Daniels, J.S. and Pourmand, N. (2007). Label-free impedance biosensors: Opportunities and challenges. *Electroanalysis: An International Journal Devoted to Fundamental and Practical Aspects of Electroanalysis* 19 (12): 1239–1257.

9 Kwon, Y.C., Kim, M.G., Kim, E.M., et al. (2011). Development of a surface plasmon resonance-based immunosensor for the rapid detection of cardiac troponin I. *Biotechnology Letters* 33 (5): 921–927.

10 Krishnamoorthy, S., Iliadis, A.A., Bei, T., et al. (2008). An interleukin-6 ZnO/SiO2/Si surface acoustic wave biosensor. *Biosensors and Bioelectronics* 24 (2): 313–318.

11 Lorencova, L., Sadasivuni, K.K., Kasak, P., and Tkac, J. (2020). Ti 3 C 2 MXene-based nanobiosensors for detection of cancer biomarkers. In *Novel Nanomaterials*. IntechOpen.

12 Prabakaran, S., Jeyaraj, M., Nagaraj, A., Sadasivuni, K.K., and Rajan, M. (2019). Polymethyl methacrylate–ovalbumin@ graphene oxide drug carrier system for high anti-proliferative cancer drug delivery. *Applied Nanoscience* 9 (7): 1487–1500.

13 Vinothini, K., Jeyaraj, M., Kumar, S.K., and Rajan, M. (2019). Dual role of lanthanum oxide nanoparticles functionalized co-polymeric micelle for extended anti-cancer drug delivery. *ChemistrySelect* 4 (18): 5206–5213.

14 Koppala, S., Swamiappan, S., Gangarajula, Y., Xu, L., Sadasivuni, K.K., Ponnamma, D., and Rajagopalan, V. (2018). Calcium deficiency in hydroxyapatite and its drug delivery applications. *Micro & Nano Letters* 13 (4): 562–564.

15 Praphakar, R.A., Jeyaraj, M., Mehnath, S., Higuchi, A., Ponnamma, D., Sadasivuni, K.K., and Rajan, M. (2018). A pH-sensitive guar gum-grafted-lysine-β-cyclodextrin drug carrier for the controlled release of 5-flourouracil into cancer cells. *Journal of Materials Chemistry B* 6 (10): 1519–1530.

16 Monson, C.F., Driscoll, L.N., Bennion, E., et al. (2009). Antibody–antigen exchange equilibria in a field of an external force: Design of reagentless biosensors. *Analytical Chemistry* 81 (17): 7510–7514.

17 Altintas, Z., Fakanya, W.M., and Tothill, I.E. (2014). Cardiovascular disease detection using bio-sensing techniques. *Talanta* 128: 177–186.

18 Honikel, M.M., Lin, C.E., Probst, D., et al. (2018). Facilitating earlier diagnosis of cardiovascular disease through point-of-care biosensors: A review. *Critical Reviews in Biomedical Engineering* 46 (1).

19 McDonnell, B., Hearty, S., Leonard, P., et al. (2009). Cardiac biomarkers and the case for point-of-care testing. *Clinical Biochemistry* 42 (7–8): 549–561.

20 Vasan, R.S. (2006). Biomarkers of cardiovascular disease: Molecular basis and practical considerations. *Circulation* 113 (19): 2335–2362.

21 Anderson, L. (2005). Candidate-based proteomics in the search for biomarkers of cardiovascular disease. *The Journal of Physiology* 563 (1): 23–60.

22 Fan, X., White, I.M., Shopova, S.I., et al. (2008). Sensitive optical biosensors for unlabeled targets: A review. *Analytica Chimica Acta* 620 (1–2): 8–26.

23 Leung, W., Chan, C.P., Leung, M., et al. (2005). Novel "digital-style" rapid test simultaneously detecting heart attack and predicting cardiovascular disease risk. *Analytical Letters* 38 (3): 423–439.

24 Cho, I.H., Paek, E.H., Kim, Y.K., et al. (2009). Chemiluminometric enzyme-linked immunosorbent assays (ELISA)-on-a-chip biosensor based on cross-flow chromatography. *Analyticachimicaacta* 632 (2): 247–255.

25 Darain, F., Yager, P., Gan, K.L., and Tjin, S.C. (2009). On-chip detection of myoglobin based on fluorescence. *Biosensors and Bioelectronics* 24 (6): 1744–1750.

26 Park, J.P., Cropek, D.M., and Banta, S. (2010). High affinity peptides for the recognition of the heart disease biomarker troponin I identified using phage display. *Biotechnology and Bioengineering* 105 (4): 678–686

27 Homola, J. and Piliarik, M. (2006). Surface plasmon resonance (SPR) sensors. In: Surface Plasmon Resonance Based Sensors Homola, J., 45–67. Berlin, Heidelberg: Springer.

28 Tweedie, M., Subramanian, R., Lemoine, P., et al. (2006, August). Fabrication of impedimetric sensors for label-free point-of-care immunoassay cardiac marker systems, with passive microfluidic delivery. In: *2006 International Conference of the IEEE Engineering in Medicine and Biology Society*, 4610–4614. IEEE.

29 Kunduru, V., Bothara, M., Grosch, J., et al. (2010). Nanostructured surfaces for enhanced protein detection toward clinical diagnostics. *Nanomedicine: Nanotechnology, Biology and Medicine* 6 (5): 642–650.

30 Arakaki, A., Hideshima, S., Nakagawa, T., et al. (2004). Detection of biomolecular interaction between biotin and streptavidin on a self-assembled monolayer using magnetic nanoparticles. *Biotechnology and Bioengineering* 88 (4): 543–546.

31 Romiti, S., Vinciguerra, M., Saade, W., et al. (2020). Artificial intelligence (AI) and cardiovascular diseases: An unexpected alliance. *Cardiology Research and Practice* 2020 https://doi.org/10.1155/2020/4972346.

32 Murdoch, T.B. and Detsky, A.S. (2013). The inevitable application of big data to health care. *Jama* 309 (13): 1351–1352.

33 World Health Organization. (2017). WHO | EHealth at WHO. [10 Apr 2017]. Available from: http://www.who.int/ehealth/about/en/.

34 Johnson, K.W., Torres Soto, J., Glicksberg, B.S., et al. (2018). Artificial intelligence in cardiology. *Journal of the American College of Cardiology* 71 (23): 2668–2679.

35 Rivera, J., McPherson, A., Hamilton, J., et al. (2016). Mobile apps for weight management: A scoping review. *JMIR mHealth and uHealth* 4 (3): e87.

36 Neve, M., Morgan, P.J., Jones, P.R., et al. (2010). Effectiveness of web-based interventions in achieving weight loss and weight loss maintenance in overweight and obese adults: A systematic review with meta-analysis. *Obesity Reviews* 11 (4): 306–321.

37 Walsh III, J.A., Topol, E.J., and Steinhubl, S.R. (2014). Novel wireless devices for cardiac monitoring. *Circulation* 130 (7): 573–581.

38 Azar, K.M., Lesser, L.I., Laing, B.Y., et al. (2013). Mobile applications for weight management: Theory-based content analysis. *American Journal of Preventive Medicine* 45 (5): 583–589.

39 Perez, M.V., Mahaffey, K.W., Hedlin, H., et al. (2019). Large-scale assessment of a smartwatch to identify atrial fibrillation. *New England Journal of Medicine* 381 (20): 1909–1917.

40 Kulkarni, A. and Vijaykumar, S. (2016). Application of Internet of Things in artificial heart pacemakers and its impact on security. *International Journal of Current Trends in Engineering & Research (IJCTER)* 2 (5): 604–610.

41 Stehlik, J., Schmalfuss, C., Bozkurt, B., et al. (2020). Continuous wearable monitoring analytics predict heart failure hospitalization: The LINK-HF multicenter study. *Circulation. Heart Failure* 13 (3): e006513.

42 Perl, L., Soifer, E., Bartunek, J., et al. (2019). A novel wireless left atrial pressure monitoring system for patients with heart failure, first ex-vivo and animal experience. *Journal of Cardiovascular Translational Research* 12 (4): 290–298.

43 Al'Aref, S.J., Anchouche, K., Singh, G., and Slomka, P. (2018). Clinical applications of machine learning in cardiovascular disease and its relevance to cardiac imaging. *European Heart Journal* 40 (24): 10.1093/eurheartj/ehy404.

44 Miotto, R., Wang, F., Wang, S., et al. (2018). Deep learning for healthcare: Review, opportunities and challenges. *Briefings in Bioinformatics* 19 (6): 1236–1246.

45 Al'Aref, S.J., Anchouche, K., Singh, G., et al. (2019). Clinical applications of machine learning in cardiovascular disease and its relevance to cardiac imaging. *European Heart Journal* 40 (24): 1975–1986.

46 Cikes, M., Sanchez-Martinez, S., Claggett, B., et al. (2019). Machine learning-based phenogrouping in heart failure to identify responders to cardiac resynchronization therapy. *European Journal of Heart Failure* 21 (1): 74–85.

47 Lancaster, M.C., Salem Omar, A.M., Narula, S., et al. (2019). Phenotypic clustering of left ventricular diastolic function parameters: Patterns and prognostic relevance. *JACC. Cardiovascular Imaging* 12 (7Part 1): 1149–1161.

48 Horiuchi, Y., Tanimoto, S., Latif, A.M., et al. (2018). Identifying novel phenotypes of acute heart failure using cluster analysis of clinical variables. *International Journal of Cardiology* 262: 57–63.

49 Ouyang, D., He, B., Ghorbani, A., et al. (2020). Video-based AI for beat-to-beat assessment of cardiac function. *Nature* 580 (7802): 252–256.

50 Demirkiran, A., Everaars, H., Amier, R.P., et al. (2019). Cardiovascular magnetic resonance techniques for tissue characterization after acute myocardial injury. *European Heart Journal-Cardiovascular Imaging* 20 (7): 723–734.

51 Winther, H.B., Hundt, C., Schmidt, B., et al. (2018). ν-net: Deep learning for generalized biventricular mass and function parameters using multicenter cardiac MRI data. *JACC. Cardiovascular Imaging* 11 (7): 1036–1038.

52 Avendi, M.R., Kheradvar, A., and Jafarkhani, H. (2017). Automatic segmentation of the right ventricle from cardiac MRI using a learning-based approach. *Magnetic Resonance in Medicine* 78 (6): 2439–2448.

53 Tan, L.K., McLaughlin, R.A., Lim, E., et al. (2018). Fully automated segmentation of the left ventricle in cine cardiac MRI using neural network regression. *Journal of Magnetic Resonance Imaging* 48 (1): 140–152.

54 Reinstadler, S.J., Thiele, H., and Eitel, I. (2015). Risk stratification by cardiac magnetic resonance imaging after ST-elevation myocardial infarction. *Current Opinion in Cardiology* 30 (6): 681–689.

55 Avendi, M.R., Kheradvar, A., and Jafarkhani, H. (2017). Automatic segmentation of the right ventricle from cardiac MRI using a learning-based approach. *Magnetic Resonance in Medicine* 78 (6): 2439–2448.

56 Baessler, B., Mannil, M., Oebel, S., et al. (2018). Subacute and chronic left ventricular myocardial scar: Accuracy of texture analysis on nonenhanced cine MR images. *Radiology* 286 (1): 103–112.

57 Medvedofsky, D., Mor-Avi, V., Amzulescu, M., et al. (2018). Three-dimensional echocardiographic quantification of the left-heart chambers using an automated adaptive analytics algorithm: Multicentre validation study. *European Heart Journal-Cardiovascular Imaging* 19 (1): 47–58.

58 Cheema, B., Hsieh, C., Adams, D., et al. (2019). Automated guidance and image capture of echocardiographic views using a deep learning-derived technology. *Circulation* 140 (Suppl. 1): A15694–A15694.

59 Alsharqi, M., Woodward, W.J., Mumith, J.A., et al. (2018). Artificial intelligence and echocardiography. *Echo Research and Practice* 5 (4): R115–R125.

60 Levin, D.C., Parker, L., Halpern, E.J., et al. (2019). Coronary CT angiography: Reversal of earlier utilization trends. *Journal of the American College of Radiology* 16 (2): 147–155.

61 Coenen, A., Kim, Y.H., Kruk, M., et al. (2018). Diagnostic accuracy of a machine-learning approach to coronary computed tomographic angiography–based fractional flow reserve: Result from the MACHINE consortium. *Circulation. Cardiovascular Imaging* 11 (6): e007217.

11

Commercial Non-Invasive and Invasive Devices for Heart Failure Prediction

A Review

Jayakanth Kunhoth, Nandhini Subramanian, and Ahmed Bouridane

11.1 Introduction

According to statistics provided in Roth et al. [1], the total number of cardiovascular cases has doubled, and death-related cardiovascular diseases have increased by 50% globally in the last three decades. Heart failure is a chronic condition where the heart fails to pump sufficient blood and oxygen for the body. A report from the American Heart Association reveals that one in five people is prone to heart failure and 50% of these patients will live a maximum of 5 years after experiencing heart failure [2]. The different risks which can lead to heart failures are high systolic blood pressure (hypertension), high fasting plasma glucose, high low-density lipoprotein cholesterol, high body mass index (BMI), impaired kidney function, ambient and household air pollution, tobacco, dietary risks, low physical activity, sedentary behavior, alcohol, chronic stress, adverse childhood experiences, and excess body/abdominal fat (obesity) [1, 3]. Age, ethnicity, family history/genetics, and gender are some of the non-modifiable factors leading to heart failure [3]. Fatigue, breathlessness, elevated jugular venous pressure, peripheral edema, etc. are the common symptoms of heart failure. Chronic heart failures (CHFs) have become a burden to current healthcare systems, mainly because of the increased hospital admissions. Not only do the admissions themselves increase for acute diseases, but frequent visits to the outpatient clinic are also required to monitor the status of the patient. Furthermore, during the current pandemic, in-person monitoring and frequent hospital visits are not possible, as they are highly risky. Frequent testing and analysis of physiological values, as well as the electronic health records of individuals, aid in assessing the condition of heart failure patients. These health records include various readings such as heartbeats per minute, the fluid level in the lungs, the oxygen level in the blood, ejection fraction levels, etc.

Current technological advancements in electronic health record data acquirement and management allow the recording of laboratory testing reports, medical imaging data, and personal health information into an electronic format with the help of multiple sensors. These recorded health data can be further processed to predict and monitoring of various conditions and stages of heart failure using mathematical models, data mining techniques, and machine learning methods. Numerous efforts have been taken over the

Predicting Heart Failure: Invasive, Non-Invasive, Machine Learning, and Artificial Intelligence Based Methods, First Edition. Edited by Kishor Kumar Sadasivuni, Hassen M. Ouakad, Somaya Al-Maadeed, Huseyin C. Yalcin, and Issam Bait Bahadur.

last decades to improve the quality of service to patients using invasive and non-invasive remote monitoring techniques for heart failure. Invasive devices are implanted inside the patient's body. They collect physiological readings from the human body and assist the patient with or without remote communication from an external source. On the other hand, non-invasive devices include various wearables or bands that are externally attached to an individual's body and record important physiological data for predicting heart failure. Currently available non-invasive methods for heart failure monitoring include monitoring of the heartbeat using electrocardiography, monitoring blood pressure (BP) daily using BP sensor devices, bioimpedance monitoring, wearables like smartwatches, pocket devices and Fitbits, and mobile health apps for telemonitoring. Invasive devices are effective and precise but can be used for limited cases only. Non-invasive methods do not need to be implanted and can be used easily with reduced risk, precision [4], and other performance metrics. Non-invasive devices are cost-effective and safe compared to invasive devices [5].

In the literature, researchers have proposed several devices [6–9] for monitoring and predicting heart failure conditions by measuring various physiological signals including heart rate, BP, pulmonary artery pressure, electrocardiogram (ECG), etc. This chapter briefly reviews the current invasive and non-invasive devices that are commercially available for monitoring the risk and health status of heart failure patients.

11.2 Non-Invasive Devices for Monitoring Heart Failure Patients

Recent advancements in sensor technology have made the development of high-performance, low-cost microsensors easier. This has positively impacted the development of various non-invasive devices or external devices for assisting heart failure patients. External devices for heart failure monitoring include various wearables, such as activity bands, smartwatches, ECG patches, and vests that can estimate heart rate, BP, and pulmonary fluid levels as well as tracking the activity of the users. This section discusses various available external devices for monitoring and predicting the risk, hospital readmission, and mortality of heart failure patients.

11.2.1 Electrocardiography

Electrocardiography is the process of generating an ECG to detect the problems in the rhythm of the heart and, by extension, for early prediction of a heart attack as well as heart failure. The results of the study conducted by James et al. [10] showed that ECG is a simple and useful test for predicting heart failure in its early stages. The findings of the study are based on the fact that, unlike non-heart failure patients, heart failure patients have "significantly prolonged QRS duration, prolonged QT duration, prolonged QTc, and more rightward T wave axis." Moreover, ECG features have been extensively used in the literature to detect heart failure. Several artificial intelligence technology-based heart failure prediction systems developed in the literature are based on ECG features [11]. These systems utilize traditional machine learning [12] as well as deep learning methodologies [13] for automated prediction of various heart failure conditions using patients' ECG features.

A few existing deep learning-based systems [14–18] have achieved acceptable performance for predicting heart failure with preserved ejection fraction. The findings of this research show the efficacy of detecting heart failure using electrocardiography.

11.2.1.1 Electrocardiography-Based Monitoring Systems

There are many types of external electrocardiography-based systems available, one of them being the Holter monitor. Holter monitors are small, wearable electrocardiography devices that contain multiple electrodes and data recording devices. A general diagram of a Holter monitor is given in Figure 11.1.

The purpose of a Holter monitor is to record the ECGs of an individual over a period of time (24–72 hours). Atrial fibrillation [19] is a type of arrhythmia predominantly found in patients with heart failure. The recordings from Holter monitors enable doctors or physicians to detect arrhythmias, which helps in the early diagnosis of heart failure. In certain cases, resting ECG conducted in clinics fails to detect heart rhythm abnormalities in patients experiencing early symptoms of heart disease. In this scenario, the physician or cardiologist might suggest using a Holter monitor for 24–48 hours. Furthermore, patients with a history of heart disease or recovered from heart-related surgeries are also advised to use Holter monitors for a couple of days. There is very little risk associated with wearing a Holter monitors, the only possible risks being associated with having electrodes attached to the skin, as the attached electrodes can often cause skin irritations. However, the Holter monitor is not water-resistant and patients are advised to not bathe or swim while the device is attached to their body for recording the physiological values. Moreover, the patients are advised to stay outside the proximity of metal detectors, microwaves, or other devices that can break off the signals from the electrodes attached to the body. After fitting a Holter monitor on a patient's body, the cardiologist provides the patient with a diary to record their activities and symptoms. The patients have to write down all the activities they do while wearing the Holter monitor, noting also the exact time when they do them. They also have to note in the dairy if they

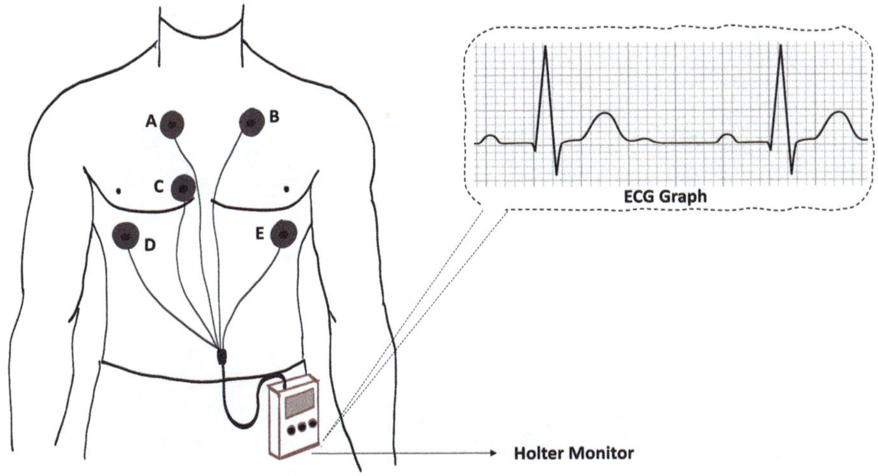

Figure 11.1 ECG reading using a Holter monitor (A, B, C, D, and E are electrodes).

experience any symptoms such as fluttering or skipped heartbeats, chest pain, shortness of breath, etc., and the time of occurrence. Once the monitoring period is over, the cardiologist will go through the continuous ECG recorded in the device over the monitoring period, and carry out a detailed analysis. During the analysis, the cardiologist goes through the patient dairy and, for each recorded activity as well as a symptom, the ECG recorded in the device at that particular time is investigated with the help of computers preloaded with algorithms to discover any abnormalities in the heartbeat. So the precise recording of activities and symptoms in patient dairy is essential in Holter monitoring and any mistake in the recordings can severely affect the result analysis procedure. Medtronic, GE Healthcare, and Abbot are the major producers of commercially available Holter monitoring devices, with recent devices including many functionalities such the ability to communicate directly with patients' Bluetooth-enabled smartphones or PCs.

Another type of portable ECG-based device is the event monitor. Event monitors are similar to the Holter monitors responsible for recording heart signals. However, while Holter monitors are configured to record the heart rhythm continuously for 24 or 48 hours, event monitors are used to record the heartbeats when the patient activates them. Some of the event monitors available on the market can automatically turn on the heartbeat recording when an abnormal heart rhythm is identified. Event monitors are available in many types, with symptom event monitors and memory looping event monitors being the most common. Symptom monitors record the heart's electrical signal after activation, while memory looping monitors record data from a few minutes before the activation. This feature of memory looping monitors provides additional information for doctors to analyze the heart condition. Mobile cardiac telemetry (MCT) devices are similar to Holter monitors and event monitors, but they are equipped with more advanced features to provide real-time assistance for patients. The general workflow of MCT devices is shown in Figure 11.2.

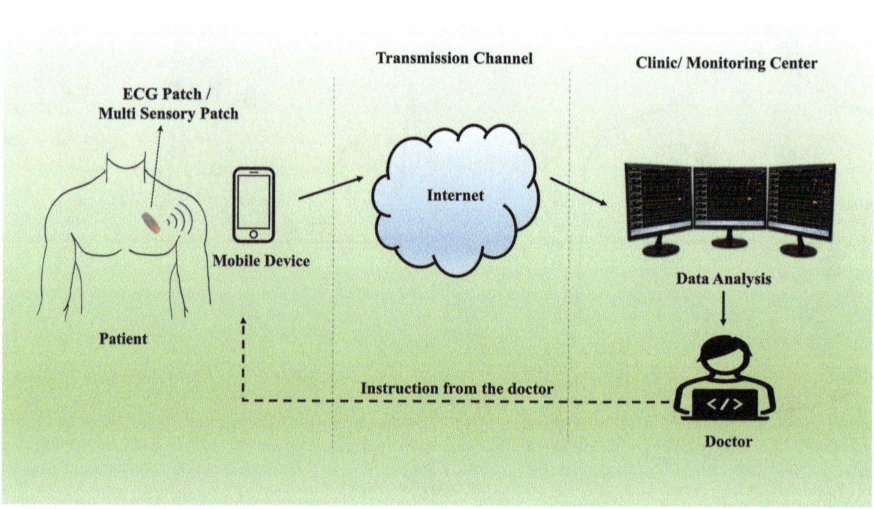

Figure 11.2 General workflow of MCT devices.

The ECG patch or multisensory patch attached to the patient's body will record multiple sensors' data or ECG data and send it to the mobile device installed with a software application via Bluetooth or WiFi. The mobile device software is configured to transmit the data to the monitoring center via the internet. The monitor center will receive the data and analyze it to ensure that there is no abnormal event. If any abnormal events are detected, the monitor center will provide emergency instructions to the patient with the help of a qualified doctor. Unlike Holter monitors, MCT devices can be attached to the body of the patient for recording the heart rhythm for up to 30 days. Several research studies have been conducted to demonstrate the benefits of MCT devices over event monitors and Holter monitors. The comparative study conducted by Tsang and Mohan [20] shows that the diagnostic yield of arrhythmia is significantly higher in patients monitored with MCT devices compared to the patients monitored with event monitors and Holter monitors. The study was conducted on a total of more than 200,000 patients over a 5-year period.

Both MCT devices and Holter monitors are designed to assist the cardiologist in monitoring patients with heart diseases. However, there are distinctive differences between them in terms of the monitoring period, recording method, data storage, data analysis, size of devices, etc. In the case of the monitoring period, usually, the Holter monitors are configured to monitor the heart activity for a maximum of 72 hours while MCT devices are assigned for 30 days. There are exceptions in the Holter monitor's monitoring period. In a few cases, the Holter monitors are prescribed for 7–14 days. Compared with MCT devices, the limited wear time of the Holter monitor reduces the inconvenience to patients caused by monitoring devices. However, the extended wear time of MCT devices is beneficial for asymptotic patients in certain cases, for example detecting arrhythmia that may not occur during the short period in which a Holter monitor is being worn. Generally, the Holter monitoring is conducted in a manner where the device is assigned to record the heart activities for a given period and the data recorded in the device are analyzed once the monitoring period is over. In Holter monitors assigned for 7–14 days, any abnormalities recorded during the monitoring period will not be addressed and analyzed till the monitoring period is over and the device is returned to the clinic. On the other hand, the MCT devices are configured to continuously record the heart activity and send the recorded data to the server or remote analysis center for instantaneous analysis. The instantaneous recording and monitoring capability of MCT devices enable immediate assistance for the patient if any abnormalities are detected. In this context, MCT devices are more beneficial than Holter monitors for patients with a history of heart failure symptoms as well as for patients suffering from acute heart failure conditions.

In traditional Holter monitors, the data are stored locally using an internal chip. Local storage is enough for the Holter monitor due to the short monitoring period. In old devices, cassettes were used to store the recorded data. Some of the latest Holter monitors have the functionality to backup and store the recorded data in the cloud. The MCT devices allow both local and cloud storage. Usually, the data are sent to the cloud for immediate analysis. However, certain conditions, such as the absence of internet connectivity, affect the cloud storage process. In this case, the data is stored locally and transferred to the cloud once internet connectivity is restored. Moreover, the latest devices are equipped with the functionality to transmit the data to personal computers and smartphones. The Holter monitors are bulkier compared with MCT devices and require more wires as well as leads;the latest MCT devices are very small and devoid of wires.

Many companies like ACS Diagnostics, Biotelemetry, and Medicomp are producing different commercial MCT monitoring systems according to the needs of the patients. Further, the recent systems can provide real-time analysis and assistance to patients. In addition, multifunctioning MCT systems which have multiple functionalities, such as MCT monitoring, Holter monitoring, event monitoring, etc., are currently available on the market. ACS Diagnostics, the leading MCT developer in the US has released a multi-functional MCT device named Core^{12}. The company reports that it is the first of its kind of multifunctional device to be approved by the US Food and Drug Administration (FDA). The single device ACS Core^{12} provides a resting 12-lead ECG test, 24 hours Holter monitoring, event monitoring, and MCT monitoring.

11.2.2 BP and Heart Failure

Hypertension is one of the main causes of cardiovascular disease and its associated risks, including death. Many previous research studies have shown that hypertension will worsen the condition of heart failure patients and it is essential to maintain an optimum BP value [21]. In this context, the daily BP measurement of an individual diagnosed with heart failure is required. Frequent BP readings and reporting them to the doctor help to reduce the impact and risk of hypertension in patients with heart failure. Many home-based and clinical-based BP sensing devices are currently available. Most of the home-based BP sensing devices are small in size, portable, and affordable. An individual with minimal technical knowledge can operate these devices to measure BP. However, the accuracy of home-based BP systems is still a concern. A cross-sectional study was conducted by Ruzicka et al. [22], analyzing the accuracy of home BP devices. The result of the study suggests that home BP monitoring can aid in the early detection of hypertension. But the inaccurate readings of several of the available devices can adversely affect hypertension management and cause risks related to hypertension.

BP can be controlled naturally in many ways. Overweight is one of the main causes of raised BP. Reducing body weight lowers BP, as can increased activity and daily exercise. Increased activity and daily exercise will increase the heart rate and breathing rates which make the heart stronger and thereby less effort is required by the heart to pump. Proper diet can have a big impact on lowering BP. Controlling sodium intake can lower BP in healthy individuals, while increased potassium intake can reduce the effect of sodium in the body and lowers BP. Individuals with high BP are advised to have potassium-rich foods like low-fat dairy products, fish, fruits, and vegetables such as avocado, orange, banana, tomato, greens, etc. Smoking can cause sudden fluctuations in BP and continuous use of tobacco products can cause damage to the lining of artery walls and increase BP. Stopping smoking can reduce BP as well as increasing overall health. Excess stress control and restful sleep for at least 8 hours per day can also lower BP to an extent.

11.2.3 Body Weight Monitoring and Heart Failure

Body weight is considered to be one of the factors for predicting whether a heart failure condition is getting worse or not. It is based on the fact that heart failure leads to the accumulation of fluid (edema) in the body followed by rapid weight gain [23]. The rapid weight gain due to edema can lead to urgent hospitalization and, in the worst case, to death. Usually, diuretic therapy is recommended for hospitalized heart failure patients due to fluid retention and rapid weight gain [24]. The Heart Failure Society of America advises heart failure patients to monitor their body weight daily and report to the doctor if any abnormality is found [25]. The body weight measurement tool is an invasive device that can be used to measure fluctuations in body weight. Advanced body weight measurement tools are equipped with innovative features to aid body weight data collection and the ability to share the data across multiple mobile devices.

Even though edema is a symptom of heart failure, monitoring body weight alone will not aid in managing heart failure patients. A research study conducted in 2009 by Zhang et al. [23] examined the effect of body weight alone in monitoring heart failure patients. The study focused on analyzing how well weight gain algorithms can predict hospitalization in patients with worsening heart failure conditions. Three algorithms were compared in the study, with two of the algorithms being very simple and triggering an alert when the weight gain was, respectively, over 1.4 kg or 2.2 kg in a day. The third algorithm analysed the short-term weight gain average and long-term weight gain average to trigger the alert. The 168 patients who participated in the study were advised to measure their body weight twice a day: before breakfast and before the evening meal, after emptying the bladder, while wearing light clothes and no shoes. Among the analyzed algorithms, the third one, based on the average of short-term weight and long-term weight, displayed better performance. In that context, body weight alone is not beneficial for telemonitoring heart failure patients. However, integrating body weight along with other physiological readings, such as ECG or heart rate, can improve the precision of the telemonitoring systems.

Body mass index (BMI) is one of the crucial indirect indicators for heart disease. BMI and BP values are closely related. Higher BMI values are demonstrated as an independent risk factor for hypertension, and hypertension is one of the important risk factors for heart diseases. The relation between BMI value ranges and their associated disease risks for adults older than 20 years is given in Table 11.1.

Table 11.1 BMI value ranges and associated health risks.

BMI Range	Category	Associated Health Risks
< 18.5	Underweight	Osteoporosis, anemia, skin, hair problems
18.5–24.9	Normal weight	Low risk for heart disease (but there is a higher risk if there is a bad cholesterol level and triglyceride levels are high), diabetes
25–29.9	Overweight	High risk for heart disease, hypertension, diabetes
30 <	Obese	Very high risk for heart disease, hypertension, diabetes, kidney disease

It is clear from Table 11.1 that individuals falling into the overweight and obese categories have a high risk for heart diseases. However, individuals with normal weight categories also have a risk for heart disease if their cholesterol levels are not normal. Moreover, the risk of heart disease depends not only on BMI, but also on other factors such as lifestyle, smoking, sleeping hours, etc.

11.2.4 Bioimpedance Monitoring and Heart Failure

Bioimpedance analysis is a leading and economically feasible method utilized for estimating body composition as well as health monitoring. Bioimpedance analysis estimates the total body fluid and aids in monitoring the fluid levels in the human body. Heart failure patients can benefit from the application of bioimpedance analysis, which is based on the electrical properties of the human body. It measures how well the body resists the flow of electrical signals when a small electric current is passed through the it. The fats in the body have a high resistance against an electric current, while the water has low resistance. There are multiple types of bioimpedance analysis systems available, including systems which are focused on estimating the body composition of the lower body alone (leg-to-leg bioimpedance analysis), upper body alone (hand-held bioimpedance analysis), and the whole body (hand-to-foot bioimpedance analysis). The general workflow of a hand-to-foot bioimpedance analysis system is shown in Figure 11.3. The system comprises multiple electrodes, with some placed under the feet and the rest attached to the hand. A weak or small electric current is transmitted from the electrodes in the feet to the abdominal region via the leg. In addition, the electrodes in the hand are used to send weak electric signals from the hand to the abdomen and leg via the arm. The resistance induced by the body is estimated by evaluating the voltage drop observed

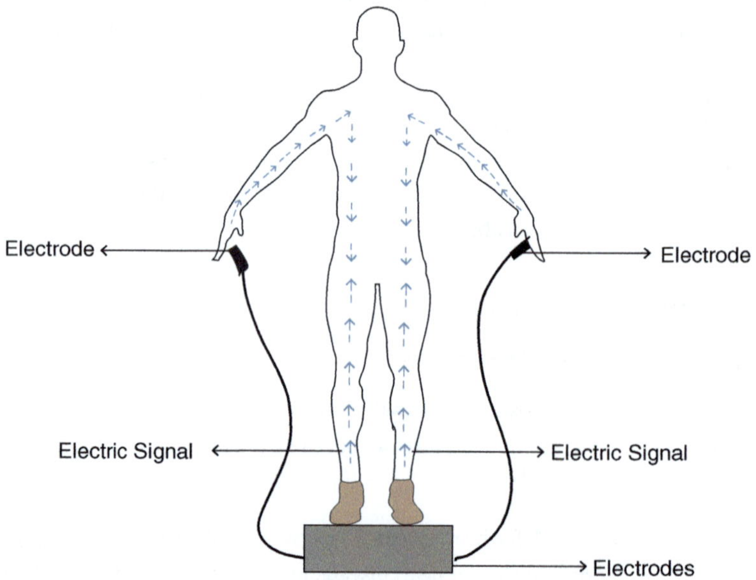

Figure 11.3 Hand-to-leg bioimpedance analysis system.

while the weak electric current is passed through the body. The observed voltage drop, as well as frequency values, are further processed by the incorporated algorithm to estimate the body composition.

Numerous studies have proved the positive effect of bioimpedance analysis for monitoring heart failure patients. Initially, bioimpedance analysis was conducted invasively by transmitting a weak current from the wires of pacemakers and defibrillators [26]. Now, however, non-invasive devices are pervasively used for bioimpedance analysis and heart failure monitoring. Whole-body impedance, as well as transthoracic impedance measurements, are utilized in the literature to predict the risk in heart failure patients [27, 28]. Kataoka [29] proposed a novel non-invasive method for integrating a bioimpedance index along with body weight for managing the health conditions of heart failure patients. The proposed method showed that the bioimpedance index and body weight combination have significantly increased the predictive accuracy for detecting the worsening of heart failure conditions. However, the method was evaluated in only a few subjects. A study by Gyllensten et al. [30] compared the performance of traditional algorithms based on body weight and bioimpedance measurement for early prediction of risk heart failure patients. In the study, 91 patients with CHF were made to wear a transthoracic bioimpedance vest containing textile electrodes on both sides to transmit current at variable frequencies to the body. Along with the bioimpedance measurement, body weight was also monitored for a period of 10 months. Compared with body weight, the bioimpedance measurement provided a more accurate prediction for early indication of risk in heart failure patients.

In Anand et al.'s MUSIC study [9], a non-randomized study for evaluating the efficacy of a multisensory device for monitoring patients suffering from congestive heart failure utilized the body composition measurement along with other physiological values. Another study examined the efficacy of a fluid accumulation vest (transthoracic bioimpedance vest) for monitoring heart failure patients [31]. The selected subjects of the study were made to wear the vest and take the body composition measurement. The body composition measurements were sent to the clinic using smartphones and internet connectivity. The observed output of the study in 180 patients showed that monitoring the body composition measurement using the fluid accumulation vest can predict the risk, including that of hospitalization, of the patient in advance.

11.2.5 Smart Wearable and Pocket-Sized Devices for Monitoring of the Heart

US FDA-approved smart wearables that are equipped with multiple sensors, including smartwatches, smart bands, vests or socks embedded with sensors, ECG patches, etc., are currently available for monitoring heart conditions. Current generation smartwatches and smart bands are equipped with activity recognition sensors and with heart rate and heart rhythm sensors. The readings from these sensors can be utilized for monitoring of and predicting risk in patients with heart failure. Triaxial accelerometers, global positioning systems, and barometers are included in the smartwatches and bands to accurately estimate the physical activity of an individual. A recent research study [32] found that the data from a pedometer is suitable for detecting the risk and severity of heart failure conditions. All the participants of the study were equipped with a smartphone and a first-generation Apple smartwatch. In one of the experiments, the participants had to do a 6-minute walk while wearing a pedometer built-in to the smartwatch. The study showed that results from the 6-minute walking test are sufficient for the risk assessment of heart failure patients. Smart wearables, including smartwatches, utilize photoplethysmography and ECG techniques to estimate heart rate and the rhythm of heartbeats. Various studies [33, 34] have shown that a high resting heart rate and heart rate variability are risk factors for heart failure patients. In this context, the heart rate variability measure from smart wearables can be utilized for early prediction in heart failure patients. However, the accuracy of smart wearables' heart rate estimation impacts the overall precision of the prediction system. Multiple studies have been conducted to assess the accuracy of photoplethysmography sensors in smartwatches for heart rate estimation. The third generation Apple Watch and Fitbit Charge 2 have shown acceptable heart rate estimation accuracy in a study [35].

A comparative study conducted by Etiwy et al. [36] evaluated the heart rate estimation accuracy of multiple smartwatches, including Apple Watch, Garmin Forerunner, etc., and of one chest strap, Polar H7. The results obtained showed that the chest strap was more accurate than smartwatches for heart rate monitoring. The accuracy of the Apple Watch for measuring heart rate variability in heart failure patients during admission to the hospital and after discharge is currently being evaluated in a clinical trial (NCT04510779). Generally, the electrode in Apple Watches can be used to obtain a 1-lead electrocardiogram. The available ECG feature in the Apple Watch can be extended to obtain a 3-lead [37], 6-lead, or 12-lead ECG [38] by keeping the watch in various regions of the body. Zoll Medical Corporation has developed the μCor™ patch for managing heart failure as well as arrhythmia. The FDA-approved patch is equipped with a radio frequency sensor, an ECG monitor for early detection of adverse heart conditions. The radio frequency sensor is responsible for monitoring the pulmonary fluid levels and the pulmonary fluid level is utilized for assessing heart failure decompensation. μCor™ is currently under clinical trials (NCT03476187) for predicting heart failures. The general components of various smart wearables for monitoring heart failure patients are shown in Figure 11.4.

11.2.6 Telemonitoring of Heart Failure Using Multiple Commercially Available Non-Invasive Devices

Several studies have been conducted to examine and analyze the effect of telemonitoring heart failure patients remotely using multiple non-invasive devices. Chaudhary et al. [39] conducted a study across 1653 patients for analyzing the effect of telemonitoring in heart failure patients. In the study, 826 patients were monitored via telemonitoring and the rest were given usual care. The study utilized the telephone and a body weight scale for monitoring the patients. The daily body weight and symptoms experienced by the patients were recorded by an interactive voice response system via the telephone. The obtained results show that telemonitoring did not improve the prediction. Moreover, there were no beneficial effects while using body weight as the primary metric for heart failure condition assessment. Another study utilized a BP monitor along with a telephone and body weight scale for monitoring heart failure patients and observed

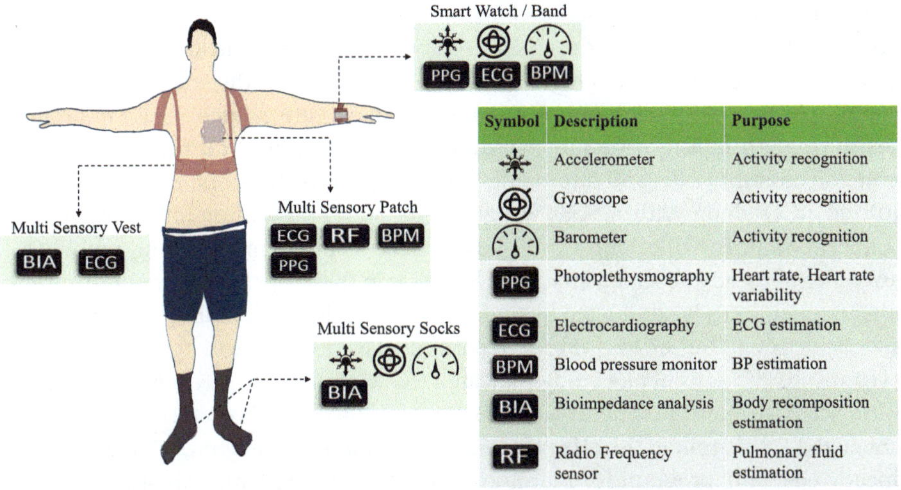

Figure 11.4 General components of smart wearable devices for heart failure monitoring.

beneficial effects such as low mortality rate as well as low hospitalization rate [8]. MUSIC, a multisensor randomized study for monitoring heart failure utilized a multi-sensor device adhered to the chest of 543 patients to acquire the physiological readings [9]. The system achieved a sensitivity of 65% for detecting the worsening of heart failure.

Some recent works have used multiple devices including telephone, mobile phone, body weight scale, pulse oximeter, video monitors, ECG, BP monitor, etc. in their studies for monitoring heart failure patients. The brief details of non-invasive devices used in research studies conducted in the last 5 years for telemonitoring heart failure patients are given in Table 11.2.

Table 11.2 Non-invasive devices used in recent research studies for monitoring heart failure patients.

		Devices Used for Recording Physiological Values			
Study	**Number of Patients**	**ECG**	**BP Monitor**	**Pulse Oximeter**	**Body Weight Scale**
Koehler et al. [40]	710	✓	✓	✗	✓
Galiner et al. [41]	937	✗	✗	✗	✓
Gingele et al. [6]	382	✓	✗	✓	✓
Koehler et al. [7]	1571	✓	✓	✓	✓
Ware et al. [42]	98	✗	✓	✗	✓
Pekmezaris et al. [43]	89	✗	✓	✓	✓
Inglis et al. [44]	9332	✓	✓	✗	✓
Ong et al. [45]	1437	✓	✓	✗	✓
Chaudhary et al. [39]	1653	✗	✗	✗	✓
Ferrante et al. [8]	1518	✗	✓	✗	✓

It is clear from Table 11.2 that a significant number of studies have utilized physiological data from multiple non-invasive devices for remote monitoring of heart failure patients. Except for Gingele et al. [6] and Ong et al. [45], it is observed in the studies that utilization of multiple devices for telemonitoring has generated positive outcomes for improving the health of heart failure patients, including reducing the hospital readmission rate, reducing the mortality rate, and improving the lifestyle of the patients, etc. Gingele et al. [6] utilized ECG along with a body weight scale and BP monitor for recording the physiological values, while Ong et al. [45] utilized a pulse meter along with ECG. However, neither study observed any positive effects in the subjects after monitoring. On the other hand, the study conducted by Inglis et al. [44] utilized the same combination of invasive devices as Ong et al. [45] for recording the physiological readings, but the observed results of Inglis et al.'s study indicated the telemonitoring system having positively impacted the lifestyle of heart failure patients and reduced hospital admission rate. Galiner et al. [41] examined the effectiveness of a telemonitoring approach along with a therapeutic coaching program for monitoring heart failure patients. All of the subjects were provided with a body weight scale and a questionnaire consisting of eight questions related to the systems. The body weight, as well as answers to the questionnaire, were uploaded to a server for automatic assessment. However, after 3 years, it was observed that the telemonitoring method that was implemented had not lowered the rate of hospitalization or death.

11.2.7 Role of Mobile Health Apps in Heart Failure Self-Care

According to the statistics provided by Forbes in 2017 [46], there exist more than 50,000 mobile health (mHealth) apps on the market that are focused on ameliorating the mental and physical fitness of individuals. Some of the available apps have been developed for general well-being while the rest are for specific purposes such as maternal care, childcare, chronic disease management, etc. Numerous studies have analyzed the role of mHealth apps for self-care in heart failure patients [47–49]. Among these, a few mHealth apps are focused on educating heart failure patients. Most of the mHealth apps that focus on therapeutic education rely on text messaging. Multiple automated messages are sent to patients to educate them on the diet to be followed, symptoms, and how to differentiate these symptoms from other diseases which have similar symptoms. Furthermore, the apps provide questionnaires that are related to heart failure symptoms, which the patients must complete. Some of the apps have integrated the physiological values from home-based devices such as body weight scales and BP monitors to provide additional care to heart failure patients. The observed results of the studies have shown that mHealth apps have improved the knowledge about heart failure and its associated issues in heart failure patients as well as increasing their involvement in self-care. However, most of the mHealth apps in the literature have conducted only a pilot study in a few subjects to analyze the usability and effects of self-care.

There are several commercially available mHealth apps for heart failure self-care. The majority of theses are available free in popular application stores such as Google's Play Store and Apple's AppStore. A systematic app search was conducted in Wali et al. [50] to examine various commercially available heart failure apps. They found that more than 70 apps were currently available in the market for heart failure self-care. Among these, only about 25 apps have sufficient features to help heart failure patients. Moreover, more than half of the available apps did not even have a basic weight management feature, which is one of the fundamental attributes considered necessary for evaluating the health of heart failure patients. According to the study, existing mHealth apps lack patient-centered design and require advanced features based on the user's need to guarantee the usability of the app. Among the commercially available apps, a few have been introduced by scientific societies such as the American Heart Association, Swiss Federation of Cardiology, Heart Failure Society of America, etc., but the rest have been developed by private technology companies. The app search conducted by Wali et al. [50] found that the app Heart Failure Storylines, developed by the Heart Failure Society of America, has better functionalities than other commercially available apps. The latest analysis of commercially available heart failure apps conducted by Mortara et al. [51] also rated the Heart Failure Storylines app as the better one for heart failure patients along with the HF Path app introduced by American Heart Association.

11.3 Invasive Devices for Monitoring Heart Failure Patients

This section briefly discusses the available invasive techniques and commercially available invasive devices and sensors. The available invasive devices for remote monitoring of heart failures are classified into right ventricle (RV) pressure monitoring, pulmonary artery (PA) pressure sensors, left atrial (LA) pressure sensors, and intrathoracic impedance monitoring. The commercial devices falling under each category and the corresponding clinical trials are given in detail. The overall working of invasive devices with remote monitoring is shown in Figure 11.5. Patients with invasive pressure sensors

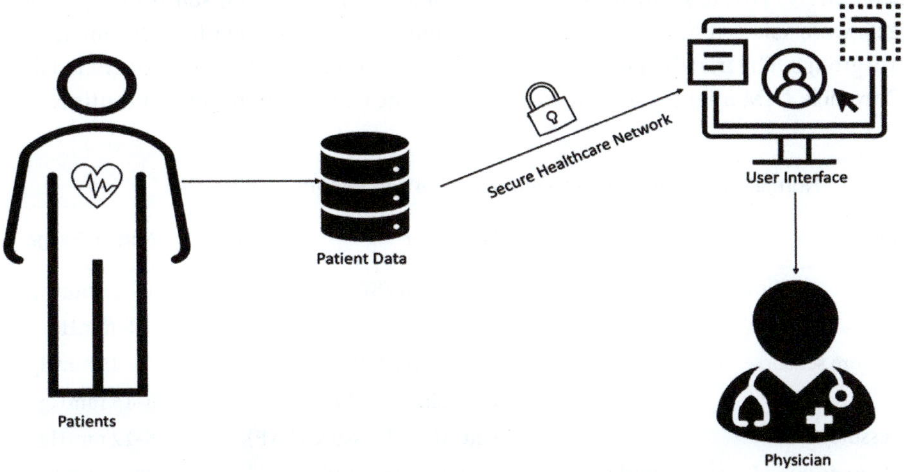

Figure 11.5 Overall working of remotely monitored invasive devices.

like CardioMEMS and HeartPOD collect the data that can help in monitoring heart failure. The data is transferred to the user interface through a secure healthcare network. Physicians can access the patient's data via the user interface.

The expected normal range values of different pressure parameters considered in each category of invasive devices are given in Table 11.3.

11.3.1 RV Pressure Monitoring

RV pressure sensors are used in measuring the diastolic and systolic pressure of the right ventricle. During the opening of the pulmonary valve, the diastolic pressure of the PA is measured, which is helpful in calculating the left ventricle diastolic pressure and pulmonary capillary wedge pressure, and thereby arriving at the intracardiac filling pressures. A strong relationship between the RV pressure and the PA pressure is observed during invasive catheterization [52–54]. Recording and reporting of ventricular pressure are performed at end-systole and end-diastole. The normal range of the RV systolic pressure is 25–30-mmHg and the RV end-diastolic pressure is 5–7 mmHg. The left ventricle systolic pressure is normally equal to the systolic arterial pressure and the left ventricular end-diastolic pressure is less than 10 mmHg. With the increase in age, the left ventricle systolic pressure also increases [55].

With these findings as the base, the Chronicle implantable hemodynamic monitor (Chronicle IHM) was developed by Medtronic, Inc., Minneapolis, Minnesota. The Chronicle IHM consists of two parts – a device that is placed in the pectoral area like a pacemaker, and a pressure sensor on the tip (like a transvenous lead) placed in the RV outflow tract or septum. This device is not compatible with MRI scanning, cardiac resynchronization therapy (CRT), or atrial pacing devices, which is a disadvantage in using this device.

A study on 32 heart failure patients was initially undertaken and the results showed a decrease of 57% in hospital admissions. From this result, a clinical trial – the COMPASS-HF (Chronicle Offers Management to Patients with Advanced Signs and Symptoms of Heart Failure) – was conducted on advanced heart failure patients from the New York Heart Association (NYHA) to study the effectiveness of the Chronicle IHM sensors [56]. Varied subjects were selected for the study (274 patients) and were divided into Chronicle and control groups. The trial did not show significant result changes and it was concluded that the Chronicle IHM might add value in addition to the existing management routine.

Table 11.3 Normal range values of different pressure parameters.

Category	Parameter	Normal Range
RV pressure monitoring	Systolic (RVSP)	15–25 mmHg
	Diastolic (RVDP)	0–8 mmHg
PA pressure sensors	Systolic (PASP)	15–25 mmHg
	Diastolic (PADP)	8–15 mmHg
LA pressure sensor	Left Atrial Pressure (LAP)	6–12 mmHg
Intrathoracic impedance monitoring	Thoracic Resistance	200–5000 Ω cm

11.3.2 PA Pressure Sensors

Unlike the RV pressure monitoring sensor (the Chronicle IHM), PA pressure sensors measure the diastolic PA pressure directly. The CardioMEMS (Cardio-Microelectromechanical) HF System developed by Abbott, Sylmar, CA, is a PA pressure sensor that is placed in any branch of the pulmonary artery. This sensor measures the diastolic, systolic, and mean pulmonary artery pressures every day. The collected data is then transferred over a secure network. The increase in the PA pressure is an indication of the onset of the decompensation and happens in advance of other clinical symptoms. The sensor is placed on the femoral vein during right heart catheterization and is powered externally. Unlike Chronicle IHM, CardioMEMS is MRI- and CRT-compatible with increased longevity.

The CHAMPIONS (CardioMEMS Heart Sensor Allows Monitoring of Pressure to Improve Outcomes in NYHA Class III Heart Failure Patients) trial was conducted in the US in 2011 to study the CardioMEMS sensor [57, 58]. The initial study included 550 patients who were NYHA class III, had had previous hospitalization, and had guideline-recommended HF therapy. The study group was divided into control and treatment groups. The pressure information is only available for the treatment group and not for the control group. Two studies – MEMS-HF (CardioMEMS European Monitoring Study for Heart Failure) and the US Post-Approval Study (PAS) – confirmed that CardioMEMS reduced the number of hospitalizations and improved the quality of life of the patients. CardioMEMS is the only FDA-approved invasive sensor for monitoring PA pressure with a European Conformity (CE) mark.

Yet another PA pressure sensor, the Cordella Pulmonary Artery Pressure Sensor System, has been developed by Endotronix, Inc., Chicago. Cordella is like CardioMEMS with additional benefits provided by the Corella HF system. Some vital parameters, such as BP, oxygen saturation, weight, and heart rate are recorded in addition to the diastolic PA pressure. The studies are ongoing, with two clinical studies currently being carried out. The first is the SIRONA trial being conducted on 15 NYHA class III patients [59]. The trial did not show any complications or system-related failures. The values measured by the PAP sensors matched with the right heart catheterization at the end of the 90-day trial period. The second study, the European SIRONA II CE Mark Trial was conducted on 60 patients from the NYHA class II with compromised ventricle ejection. The PROACTIVE-HF IDE Trial is a similar trial being conducted in the US. Cordella is not FDA approved, does not possess the European Conformity mark, and is not available for commercial use.

11.3.3 LA Pressure Sensors

PA pressures may not be useful in all cases of heart failure. For example, it is difficult to manage patients with advanced CHF with only the knowledge of PA pressure. In this case, the LA pressure or pulmonary capillary wedge pressure has proved to be helpful. Abbott, formerly St. Jude Medical/Savacor, Inc., Abbott Park, IL, developed the HeartPOD LA pressure sensor. This sensor consists of a lead with an antenna coil and is implanted through the femoral vein in the left atrium. The antenna is then connected to the lead through subclavian or auxiliary veins. This device is compatible with CRT devices and is powered externally by a hand-held computer modified for this purpose. MRI compatibility and longevity are still unknown. A patient advisory module (PAM) is placed on the antenna which reminds patients to measure the pressure and take their medication. The collected data is made available to the physicians through secured networks.

A small clinical study with eight patients concluded that HeartPOD is safe, secure, and practical to use [60]. Another trial, called Hemodynamically Guided Home Self-Therapy in Severe Heart Failure Patients (HOMEOSTASIS), with 40 patients conducted a further study by isolating patients and not monitoring them for 3 months [61]. Later, the LAP data was used to optimize the treatment course. Another trial, the Left Atrial Pressure Monitoring to Optimize Heart Failure Therapy (LAPTOP-HF) trial, was based on the results from the HOMEOSTASIS trial.

Vectorious Medical Technologies, Tel Aviv, Israel developed a more advanced LAP sensor based on the findings of the LAPTOP-HF trial, named V-LAP system. The V-LAP Left Atrium Monitoring System for Patients With Chronic Systolic and Diastolic Congestive Heart Failure (VECTOR-HF) trial is currently being performed to study the V-LAP system.

Biosensors are used to measure a chemical or biological reaction by generating signals proportional to the amount and concentration of the analyte. Portable biosensors take the blood or serum to analyze different factors for analyzing and monitoring patients' care. The detection of pregnancy by human chorionic gonadotropin (hCG) using colorimetric pregnancy tests is the best example of portable biosensors. Wearable biosensors can be used to detect heart rate, BP, respiration rate, skin temperature, and brain activity. The accuracy and stability of the wearable biosensors are questionable. The privacy, security, and storage of the data collected by the biosensors is another factor to be considered. Invasive devices like pressure sensors have better accuracy and longer-term reliability compared with biosensors [62].

11.3.4 Intrathoracic Impedance Monitoring

Fluid overload is a common problem faced by heart failure patients and in severe cases can lead to hospitalization. Intrathoracic impedance monitoring can be correlated with fluid overload and can help in preventing hospitalization. The intrathoracic impedance is inverse to the pulmonary capillary wedge pressure and fluid balance. A decreased value of intrathoracic impedance indicates the onset of decompensation [63].

The OptiVol Fluid Status Monitor developed by Medtronic Inc. is used to monitor intrathoracic impedance. The impedance is measured over a period of 14 months to help the physician make informed decisions. A coil to the Can pathway is implanted in the thoracic cavity using the Consulta™ CRT-P. After measuring the impedance values for the entire day, the average impedance value is calculated. From all the available values, a reference impedance value is decided. The following clinical trials have been conducted to study the practical utility of OptiVol: MID-HeFT Trial [63], PARTNERS HF [64], OFISSER [65], FAST [66], and CONNECT [67]. The St. Jude Medical (SJM)

CorVue^{TM} congestion monitor is another advanced intrathoracic impedance monitor. Table 11.4 gives brief details about each of the categories and some of their characteristics.

11.3.5 Commercially Available Devices for Heart Failure Treatment

Invasive devices which can help in reducing the risks in severe heart failure patients and reduce the chances of open-heart surgery are available on the market. Some of the newly FDA-approved devices that can help extensively in repairing heart failures are given in this section. First, is the LV assist device, HeartMate3, introduced by Abbott and approved by the FDA in October 2018. HeartMate3 has shown its effectiveness in multiple studies – a feasibility study and ELEVATE. Abbott's MitraClip can be used for advanced heart failure and mitral regurgitation also. The Impulse Dynamics Optimizer Smart System is used to strengthen the heart to beat on its own. Shunts are common in treating CHFs. Two shunts – Corvia's InterAtrial Shunt Device (IASD) and V-Wave InterAtrial Shunt Device are currently being considered by the FDA and clinical studies are ongoing.

11.4 Discussion

Early detection of the onset of CHF is crucial to reduce the number of hospitalizations, which in turn may become a burden to the healthcare system. Heart failure affects not only the healthcare system but also the life quality of patients. Many research studies conducted in the literature have displayed the effectiveness of non-invasive methods for monitoring heart failure patients. Among these, body weight measurement using a weighing scale seems to be the cheapest solution. However, body weight measurement for detecting fluid retention alone is not sufficient to differentiate the health conditions of heart failure patients. Instead of relying on body weight measurement, recent studies have examined the possibility of bioimpedance sensors for measuring body recomposition and detecting water retention. Furthermore, radio frequency sensors have also shown their effectiveness in estimating pulmonary fluid levels.

Most non-invasive monitoring devices rely on internet services for data transmission and patient monitoring. Even though existing devices are equipped with the capability to store the data locally in the absence of the internet and transmit it to the remote server once the internet connection is restored, steady internet service is required in the patient's premises for the uninterrupted working of the monitoring system. The lack of uninterrupted internet services in rural areas hinders the usage of these devices. Various physiological values, including BP, heart rate variability, ECG, etc., are combined in multiple research works to remotely monitor heart failure patients and obtained results have shown the monitoring effectiveness. Currently, smartwatches and smart wearables have sensors for measuring pressure, heart rate variability, ECG, etc. Some studies have found that the sensors embedded in smartwatches have acceptable accuracy. However, more studies about these embedded sensors are required to show their efficacy for heart failure monitoring tasks.

Table 11.4 Categories, device, company name, clinical trials, and additional characteristics of invasive devices for heart failure monitoring.

						Compatibility	
Category	**Device**	**Company**	**Trial**	**No. of Patients**	**Parameter**	**CRT**	**MRI**
RV pressure monitoring	Chronicle IHM	Medtronic	COMPASS-HF	274	Systolic and diastolic RV pressure	X	X
PA pressure sensors	CardioMEMS	Abbott	CHAMPIONS	550	Diastolic, systolic and mean PA pressures	✓	✓
	Cordella	Endotronix	SIRONA	15	PA pressure with vitals	✓	✓
LA pressure sensors	HeartPOD	Abbott	HOMEOSTASIS	40	LA pressure	✓	✓
	V-LAP	VMT, Israel	VECTOR-HF	45		✓	✓
Intrathoracic impedance monitoring	OptiVol	Medtronic	HeFT, PARTNERS HF, OFISSER, FAST, CONNECT	Ongoing	Intrathoracic impedance	-	-

Another serious concern while using smart wearables is that of data privacy and regulation policies. Smart wearables record a heavy amount of data including location data as well as physiological data. These recorded data are valuable for commercial firms they can be utilized for analyzing customer behavior to extend the firms' market. Various countries around the world have strict rules to ensure that commercial medical devices maintain fair data usage and regulation policies. However, these rules are applicable only for the devices which are developed for medical examination alone. Although non-invasive methods can help to reduce the overall health risk of heart failure patients to an acceptable extent, they are not as effective as invasive devices. Nevertheless, a substantial number of patients worldwide prefer non-invasive devices over invasive devices, because the former are economically feasible and devoid of the safety issues that are associated with internal implantation.

Apart from non-invasive devices, commercially available invasive devices that are currently used for monitoring CHFs have been described in this chapter. Each of the categories discussed is used for different applications and the physicians must choose which device to implant based on the patient's details and severity of the condition. There are three factors to consider before deciding on the best-suited device. First is safety. The Chronicle IHM had better safety and fewer complications. However, it did not show significant results in reducing the number of hospitalizations in HF patients. The second factor is efficacy, and HeartPOD had better efficacy in preventing the number of hospitalizations, but safety was compromised as the implant led to increased complications. In other words, safety and efficacy are inversely correlated. Cost-effectiveness is the third important factor to be considered. Many devices discussed are not cost-effective and their longevity is still being tested. Overall, the CardioMEMS has proved to have better safety and efficacy, and is cost-effective as well. It must be reiterated that CardioMEMS is the only device that is FDA approved, has a European Conformity (CE) mark, and is available for commercial use.

11.5 Future Outlook

This section provides a brief future insight on non-invasive and invasive systems for heart failure monitoring and proposes how the evolving technology can contribute to the future development of heart failure monitoring systems.

- Currently available non-invasive devices, as well as invasive devices equipped with remote monitoring functionality, are providing treatment or advice feedback to patients with the help of a physician or cardiologist. They can focus on implementing treatment algorithms that are based on the latest artificial intelligence methods such as deep learning or machine learning prediction models trained with a large amount of data including various attributes such as laboratory values, pulmonary pressure, symptoms, etc. This will enable the development of fully automated systems for heart failure monitoring.
- This review discussed various smartwatches and smart wearables which are equipped with multiple sensors for recording physiological values. In this context, developing

smartphone applications to record and analyze those values from those sensors has the potential to monitor heart failure patients non-invasively.

- The role of mHealth apps for the self-care of heart failure patients was discussed in this review and it was found that the mHealth apps have the potential to educate the heart failure patients about the disease, symptoms, precautions, etc. However, most of the existing apps lack user-centered design. In the future, developers can focus on developing apps with improved user-centric design. Furthermore, they can focus on developing apps for patients who have less knowledge about smartphone operations.
- The existing commercially available devices or proposed devices in the literature have not addressed the security of patients' data during transfer as well as storage for better privacy and security of the patients' latest information, where security techniques like encryption and steganography can be employed.
- A mix of invasive and non-invasive devices can be employed in the future to get the benefit from both. A hybrid model which combines both invasive and non-invasive techniques can be developed.
- An effective, efficient, and interdisciplinary collaboration between doctors and engineers is required to develop safe, reliable, and long-term devices to effectively monitor heart failure.

11.6 Conclusion

Heart failure is causing an economic burden on the hospital system, due to constant admission and readmission of the patients. It also affects the patients' quality of life. Currently, heart failure is detected using the symptoms and signs which appear late and are not reliable. Non-invasive and invasive methods are available to detect heart failure at early stages. In recent years, the number of research activities in the field of remote monitoring techniques for heart failure monitoring is increasing rapidly. Non-invasive methods are easy to use and safe, but accuracy and reliability are compromised. Invasive methods are accurate and reliable, but the safety is questionable. Invasive methods are available only in a limited number of cases. In this chapter, the commercially available invasive and non-invasive devices for heart failure monitoring are discussed. Discussion of the advantages and disadvantages of these devices was included. Finally, a future outlook section was added to mention possible future directions in this field.

References

1 Roth, G.A., Mensah, G.A., Johnson, C.O., Addolorato, G., Ammirati, E., Baddour, L.M., Barengo, N.C., Beaton, A.Z., Benjamin, E.J., Benziger, C.P., Bonny, A., Brauer, M., Brodmann, M., Cahill, T.J., Carapetis, J., Catapano, A.L., Chugh, S.S., Cooper, L.T., Coresh, J., and Murray, C.J.L. (2020). Global burden of cardiovascular diseases and risk factors, 1990–2019: Update from the GBD 2019 study. *Journal of the American College of Cardiology* 76 (25). https://doi.org/10.1016/j.jacc.2020.11.010.

2 Virani, S.S., Alonso, A., Benjamin, E.J., Bittencourt, M.S., Callaway, C.W., Carson, A.P., Chamberlain, A.M., Chang, A.R., Cheng, S., Delling, F.N., Djousse, L., Elkind, M.S.V., Ferguson, J.F., Fornage, M., Khan, S.S., Kissela, B.M., Knutson, K.L., Kwan, T.W., Lackland, D.T., and Heard, D.G. (2020). Heart disease and stroke statistics—2020 update: A report from the American Heart Association. *Circulation*. https://doi.org/10.1161/CIR.0000000000000757.

3 Priorities for Health Promotion and Public Health. (2021). Priorities for Health Promotion and Public Health (ed. S. Robinson). Routledge. https://doi.org/10.4324/9780367823689.

4 Nguyen, L.S. and Squara, P. (2017). Non-invasive monitoring of cardiac output in critical care medicine. *Frontiers in Medicine* 4 (NOV). https://doi.org/10.3389/fmed.2017.00200.

5 Veenis, J.F. and Brugts, J.J. (2020). Remote monitoring of chronic heart failure patients: Invasive versus non-invasive tools for optimising patient management. *Netherlands Heart Journal* 28 (1). https://doi.org/10.1007/s12471-019-01342-8.

6 Gingele, A.J., Ramaekers, B., Brunner-La Rocca, H.P., De Weerd, G., Kragten, J., Van Empel, V., Van Der Weg, K., Vrijhoef, H.J.M., Gorgels, A., Cleuren, G., Boyne, J.J.J., and Knackstedt, C. (2019). Effects of tailored telemonitoring on functional status and health-related quality of life in patients with heart failure. *Netherlands Heart Journal* 27 (11). https://doi.org/10.1007/s12471-019-01323-x.

7 Koehler, F., Koehler, K., Deckwart, O., Prescher, S., Wegscheider, K., Winkler, S., Vettorazzi, E., Polze, A., Stangl, K., Hartmann, O., Marx, A., Neuhaus, P., Scherf, M., Kirwan, B.A., and Anker, S.D. (2018). Telemedical Interventional Management in Heart Failure II (TIM-HF2), a randomised, controlled trial investigating the impact of telemedicine on unplanned cardiovascular hospitalisations and mortality in heart failure patients: Study design and description of the intervention. *European Journal of Heart Failure* 20 (10). https://doi.org/10.1002/ejhf.1300.

8 Ferrante, D., Varini, S., MacChia, A., Soifer, S., Badra, R., Nul, D., Grancelli, H., and Doval, H. (2010). Long-term results after a telephone intervention in chronic heart failure: DIAL (Randomized trial of phone intervention in chronic heart failure) follow-up. *Journal of the American College of Cardiology* 56 (5). https://doi.org/10.1016/j.jacc.2010.03.049.

9 Anand, I.S., Tang, W.H.W., Greenberg, B.H., Chakravarthy, N., Libbus, I., and Katra, R.P. (2012). Design and performance of a multisensor heart failure monitoring algorithm: Results from the multisensor monitoring in Congestive Heart Failure (MUSIC) study. *Journal of Cardiac Failure* 18 (4). https://doi.org/10.1016/j.cardfail.2012.01.009.

10 James, S., Murphy, T., Waterhouse, D., Gallagher, J., O'Connell, E., Barton, D., and McDonald, K. (2015). 22 Role of 12-lead electrocardiography in predicting heart failure in the community. *Heart* 101 (5). https://doi.org/10.1136/heartjnl-2015-308621.22.

11 Lih, O.S., Jahmunah, V., San, T.R., Ciaccio, E.J., Yamakawa, T., Tanabe, M., Kobayashi, M., Faust, O., and Acharya, U.R. (2020). Comprehensive electrocardiographic diagnosis based on deep learning. *Artificial Intelligence in Medicine* 103. https://doi.org/10.1016/j.artmed.2019.101789.

12 Masetic, Z. and Subasi, A. (2016). Congestive heart failure detection using random forest classifier. *Computer Methods and Programs in Biomedicine* 130. https://doi.org/10.1016/j.cmpb.2016.03.020.

13 Hannun, A.Y., Rajpurkar, P., Haghpanahi, M., Tison, G.H., Bourn, C., Turakhia, M.P., and Ng, A.Y. (2019). Cardiologist-level arrhythmia detection and classification in ambulatory electrocardiograms using a deep neural network. *Nature Medicine* 25 (1). https://doi.org/10.1038/s41591-018-0268-3.

14 Chen, W., Liu, G., Su, S., Jiang, Q., and Hung, N. (2017). A CHF detection method based on deep learning with RR intervals. *Proceedings of the Annual International Conference of the IEEE Engineering in Medicine and Biology Society, EMBS*. https://doi.org/10.1109/EMBC.2017.8037578.

15 Chen, W., Zheng, L., Li, K., Wang, Q., Liu, G., and Jiang, Q. (2016). A novel and effective method for congestive heart failure detection and quantification using dynamic heart rate variability measurement. *PLoS ONE* 11 (11). https://doi.org/10.1371/journal.pone.0165304.

16 Acharya, U.R., Fujita, H., Oh, S.L., Hagiwara, Y., Tan, J.H., Adam, M., and Tan, R.S. (2019). Deep convolutional neural network for the automated diagnosis of congestive heart failure using ECG signals. *Applied Intelligence* 49 (1). https://doi.org/10.1007/s10489-018-1179-1.

17 Wang, L. and Zhou, X. (2019). Detection of congestive heart failure based on LSTM-based deep network via short-term RR intervals. *Sensors (Switzerland)* 19 (7). https://doi.org/10.3390/s19071502.

18 Attia, Z.I., Kapa, S., Lopez-Jimenez, F., McKie, P.M., Ladewig, D.J., Satam, G., Pellikka, P.A., Enriquez-Sarano, M., Noseworthy, P.A., Munger, T.M., Asirvatham, S.J., Scott, C.G., Carter, R.E., and Friedman, P.A. (2019). Screening for cardiac contractile dysfunction using an artificial intelligence–enabled electrocardiogram. *Nature Medicine* 25 (1). https://doi.org/10.1038/s41591-018-0240-2.

19 Lubitz, S.A., Benjamin, E.J., and Ellinor, P.T. (2010). Atrial fibrillation in congestive heart failure. *Heart Failure Clinics* 6 (2). https://doi.org/10.1016/j.hfc.2009.11.001.

20 Tsang, J.P. and Mohan, S. (2013). Benefits of monitoring patients with mobile cardiac telemetry (MCT) compared with the Event or Holter monitors. *Medical Devices: Evidence and Research* 7 (1). https://doi.org/10.2147/MDER.S54038.

21 Oh, G.C. and Cho, H.-J. (2020). Blood pressure and heart failure. *Clinical Hypertension* 26 (1). https://doi.org/10.1186/s40885-019-0132-x.

22 Ruzicka, M., Akbari, A., Bruketa, E., Kayibanda, J.F., Baril, C., and Hiremath, S. (2016). How accurate are home blood pressure devices in use? A cross-sectional study. *PLoS ONE* 11 (6). https://doi.org/10.1371/journal.pone.0155677.

23 Zhang, J., Goode, K.M., Cuddihy, P.E., and Cleland, J.G.F. (2009). Predicting hospitalization due to worsening heart failure using daily weight measurement: Analysis of the Trans-European Network-Home-Care Management System (TEN-HMS) study. *European Journal of Heart Failure* 11 (4). https://doi.org/10.1093/eurjhf/hfp033.

24 Gronda, E., Vanoli, E., Sacchi, S., Grassi, G., Ambrosio, G., and Napoli, C. (2020). Risk of heart failure progression in patients with reduced ejection fraction: Mechanisms and therapeutic options. *Heart Failure Reviews* 25 (2). https://doi.org/10.1007/s10741-019-09823-z.

25 Heart Failure Society of America and others. (2006). Self-care: Following Your Treatment Plan and Dealing with Your Symptoms. St Paul, Minn, USA: Heart Failure Society of America.

26 Wang, L., Lahtinen, S., Lentz, L., Rakow, N., Kaszas, C., Ruetz, L., Stylos, L., and Olson, W.H. (2005). Feasibility of using an implantable system to measure thoracic congestion in an ambulatory chronic heart failure canine model. *PACE - Pacing and Clinical Electrophysiology* 28 (5). https://doi.org/10.1111/j.1540-8159.2005.40009.x.

27 Cotter, G., Moshkovitz, Y., Kaluski, E., Cohen, A.J., Miller, H., Goor, D., and Vered, Z. (2004). Accurate, noninvasive continuous monitoring of cardiac output by whole-body electrical bioimpedance. *Chest* 125 (4). https://doi.org/10.1378/chest.125.4.1431.

28 Lyons, K.J., Bischoff, M.K., Fonarow, G.C., and Horwich, T.B. (2017). Noninvasive bioelectrical impedance for predicting clinical outcomes in outpatients with heart failure. *Critical Pathways in Cardiology* 16 (1). https://doi.org/10.1097/HPC.0000000000000105.

29 Kataoka, H. (2009). Novel monitoring method for the management of heart failure: Combined measurement of body weight and bioimpedance index of body fat percentage. *Future Cardiology* 5 (6). https://doi.org/10.2217/fca.09.47.

30 Gyllensten, I.C., Bonomi, A.G., Goode, K.M., Reiter, H., Habetha, J., Amft, O., and Cleland, J.G.F. (2016). Early indication of decompensated heart failure in patients on home-telemonitoring: A comparison of prediction algorithms based on daily weight and noninvasive transthoracic bioimpedance. *JMIR Medical Informatics* 4 (1). https://doi.org/10.2196/medinform.4842.

31 Dovancescu, S., Saczynski, J.S., Darling, C.E., Riistama, J., Sert Kuniyoshi, F., Meyer, T., Goldberg, R., and McManus, D.D. (2015). Detecting heart failure decompensation by measuring transthoracic bioimpedance in the outpatient setting: Rationale and design of the SENTINEL-HF study. *JMIR Research Protocols* 4 (4). https://doi.org/10.2196/resprot.4899.

32 Werhahn, S.M., Dathe, H., Rottmann, T., Franke, T., Vahdat, D., Hasenfuß, G., and Seidler, T. (2019). Designing meaningful outcome parameters using mobile technology: A new mobile application for telemonitoring of patients with heart failure. *ESC Heart Failure* 6 (3). https://doi.org/10.1002/ehf2.12425.

33 Fox, K., Ford, I., Steg, P.G., Tendera, M., Robertson, M., and Ferrari, R. (2008). Heart rate as a prognostic risk factor in patients with coronary artery disease and left-ventricular systolic dysfunction (BEAUTIFUL): A subgroup analysis of a randomised controlled trial. *The Lancet* 372 (9641). https://doi.org/10.1016/S0140-6736(08)61171-X.

34 Singh, N., Moneghetti, K.J., Christle, J.W., Hadley, D., Froelicher, V., and Plews, D. (2018). Heart rate variability: An old metric with new meaning in the era of using mHealth technologies for health and exercise training guidance. Part two: Prognosis and training. *Arrhythmia and Electrophysiology Review* 7 (4). https://doi.org/10.15420/aer.2018.30.2.

35 Nelson, B.W. and Allen, N.B. (2019). Accuracy of consumer wearable heart rate measurement during an ecologically valid 24-hour period: Intraindividual validation study. *JMIR MHealth and UHealth* 7 (3). https://doi.org/10.2196/10828.

36 Etiwy, M., Akhrass, Z., Gillinov, L., Alashi, A., Wang, R., Blackburn, G., Gillinov, S.M., Phelan, D., Marc Gillinov, A., Houghtaling, P.L., Javadikasgari, H., and Desai, M.Y. (2019). Accuracy of wearable heart rate monitors in cardiac rehabilitation. *Cardiovascular Diagnosis and Therapy* 9 (3). https://doi.org/10.21037/cdt.2019.04.08.

37 Avila, C.O. (2019). Novel use of Apple Watch 4 to obtain 3-lead electrocardiogram and detect cardiac ischemia. *The Permanente Journal* 23. https://doi.org/10.7812/TPP/19-025.

38 Singhal, A. and Cowie, M.R. (2020). The role of wearables in heart failure. *Current Heart Failure Reports* 17 (Issue 4). https://doi.org/10.1007/s11897-020-00467-x.

39 Chaudhry, S.I., Mattera, J.A., Curtis, J.P., Spertus, J.A., Herrin, J., Lin, Z., Phillips, C.O., Hodshon, B.V., Cooper, L.S., and Krumholz, H.M. (2010). Telemonitoring in patients with heart failure. *New England Journal of Medicine* 363 (24). https://doi.org/10.1056/nejmoa1010029.

40 Koehler, J., Stengel, A., Hofmann, T., Wegscheider, K., Koehler, K., Sehner, S., Rose, M., Deckwart, O., Anker, S.D., Koehler, F., and Laufs, U. (2021). Telemonitoring in patients with chronic heart failure and moderate depressed symptoms: Results of the Telemedical Interventional Monitoring in Heart Failure (TIM-HF) study. *European Journal of Heart Failure* 23 (1). https://doi.org/10.1002/ejhf.2025.

41 Galinier, M., Roubille, F., Berdague, P., Brierre, G., Cantie, P., Dary, P., Ferradou, J.M., Fondard, O., Labarre, J.P., Mansourati, J., Picard, F., Ricci, J.E., Salvat, M., Tartière, L., Ruidavets, J.B., Bongard, V., Delval, C., Lancman, G., Pasche, H., and Pathak, A. (2020). Telemonitoring versus standard care in heart failure: A randomised multicentre trial. *European Journal of Heart Failure* 22 (6). https://doi.org/10.1002/ejhf.1906.

42 Ware, P., Ross, H.J., Cafazzo, J.A., Laporte, A., Gordon, K., and Seto, E. (2018). Evaluating the implementation of a mobile phone–based telemonitoring program: Longitudinal study guided by the consolidated framework for implementation research. *JMIR MHealth and UHealth* 6 (7). https://doi.org/10.2196/10768.

43 Pekmezaris, R., Nouryan, C.N., Schwartz, R., Castillo, S., Makaryus, A.N., Ahern, D., Akerman, M.B., Lesser, M.L., Bauer, L., Murray, L., Pecinka, K., Zeltser, R., Zhang, M., and Dimarzio, P. (2019). A randomized controlled trial comparing telehealth self-management to standard outpatient management in underserved black and hispanic patients living with heart failure. *Telemedicine and E-Health* 25 (10). https://doi.org/10.1089/tmj.2018.0219.

44 Inglis, S.C., Clark, R.A., Dierckx, R., Prieto-Merino, D., and Cleland, J.G.F. (2017). Structured telephone support or non-invasive telemonitoring for patients with heart failure. *Heart* 103 (4). https://doi.org/10.1136/heartjnl-2015-309191.

45 Ong, M.K., Romano, P.S., Edgington, S., Aronow, H.U., Auerbach, A.D., Black, J.T., De Marco, T., Escarce, J.J., Evangelista, L.S., Hanna, B., Ganiats, T.G., Greenberg, B.H., Greenfield, S., Kaplan, S.H., Kimchi, A., Liu, H., Lombardo, D., Mangione, C.M., Sadeghi, B., and Yan, T. (2016). Effectiveness of remote patient monitoring after discharge of hospitalized patients with heart failure the better effectiveness after transition-heart failure (BEAT-HF) randomized clinical trial. *JAMA Internal Medicine* 176 (3). https://doi.org/10.1001/jamainternmed.2015.7712.

46 Bell, L. (2017). Best Health and Fitness Apps You Should Download Right Now. Forbes.

47 Bartlett, Y.K., Haywood, A., Bentley, C.L., Parker, J., Hawley, M.S., Mountain, G.A., and Mawson, S. (2014). The SMART personalised self-management system for congestive heart failure: Results of a realist evaluation. *BMC Medical Informatics and Decision Making* 14 (1). https://doi.org/10.1186/s12911-014-0109-3.

48 Nundy, S., Razi, R.R., Dick, J.J., Smith, B., Mayo, A., O'Connor, A., and Meltzer, D.O. (2013). A text messaging intervention to improve heart failure self-management after hospital discharge in a largely African-American population: Before-After study. *Journal of Medical Internet Research* 15 (3). https://doi.org/10.2196/jmir.2317.

49 Portz, J.D., Vehovec, A., Dolansky, M.A., Levin, J.B., Bull, S., and Boxer, R. (2018). The development and acceptability of a mobile application for tracking symptoms of heart failure among older adults. *Telemedicine and E-Health* 24 (2). https://doi.org/10.1089/tmj.2017.0036.

50 Wali, S., Demers, C., Shah, H., Wali, H., Lim, D., Naik, N., Ghany, A., Vispute, A., Wali, M., and Keshavjee, K. (2019). Evaluation of heart failure apps to promote self-care: Systematic app search. *JMIR MHealth and UHealth* 7 (11). https://doi.org/10.2196/13173.

51 Mortara, A., Vaira, L., Palmieri, V., Iacoviello, M., Battistoni, I., Iacovoni, A., Macera, F., Pasqualucci, D., Bochicchio, M., and De Maria, R. (2020). Would you prescribe mobile health apps for heart failure self-care? An integrated review of commercially available mobile technology for heart failure patients. *Cardiac Failure Review* 6. https://doi.org/10.15420/cfr.2019.11.

52 Reynolds, D.W., Bartelt, N., Taepke, R., and Bennett, T.D. (1995). Measurement of pulmonary artery diastolic pressure from the right ventricle. *Journal of the American College of Cardiology* 25 (5). https://doi.org/10.1016/0735-1097%2894%2900510-W.

53 Chuang, P.P., Wilson, R.F., Romans, D.C., Stone, K., Bergman, T., Bennett, T.D., and Kubo, S.H. (1996). Measurement of pulmonary artery diastolic pressure from a right ventricular pressure transducer in patients with heart failure. *Journal of Cardiac Failure* 2 (1). https://doi.org/10.1016/S1071-9164(96)80008-X.

54 Ohlsson, Å., Bennett, T., Nordlander, R., Rydén, J., Åström, H., and Rydén, L. (1995). Monitoring of pulmonary arterial diastolic pressure through a right ventricular pressure transducer. *Journal of Cardiac Failure* 1 (2). https://doi.org/10.1016/1071-9164(95)90018-7.

55 Miller-Hance, W.C. and Gertler, R. (2019). Essentials of cardiology. In: A Practice of Anesthesia for Infants and Children. https://doi.org/10.1016/B978-0-323-42974-0.00016-1.

56 Bourge, R.C., Abraham, W.T., Adamson, P.B., Aaron, M.F., Aranda, J.M., Magalski, A., Zile, M.R., Smith, A.L., Smart, F.W., O'Shaughnessy, M.A., Jessup, M.L., Sparks, B., Naftel, D.L., and Stevenson, L.W. (2008). Randomized controlled trial of an implantable continuous hemodynamic monitor in patients with advanced heart failure. The COMPASS-HF study. *Journal of the American College of Cardiology* 51 (11). https://doi.org/10.1016/j.jacc.2007.10.061.

57 Abraham, W.T., Adamson, P.B., Bourge, R.C., Aaron, M.F., Costanzo, M.R., Stevenson, L.W., Strickland, W., Neelagaru, S., Raval, N., Krueger, S., Weiner, S., Shavelle, D., Jeffries, B., and Yadav, J.S. (2011). Wireless pulmonary artery haemodynamic monitoring in chronic heart failure: A randomised controlled trial. *The Lancet* 377 (9766). https://doi.org/10.1016/S0140-6736(11)60101-3.

58 Abraham, W.T., Stevenson, L.W., Bourge, R.C., Lindenfeld, J.A., Bauman, J.G., and Adamson, P.B. (2016). Sustained efficacy of pulmonary artery pressure to guide adjustment of chronic heart failure therapy: Complete follow-up results from the CHAMPION randomised trial. *The Lancet* 387 (10017). https://doi.org/10.1016/S0140-6736(15)00723-0.

59 Mullens, W., Sharif, F., Dupont, M., Rothman, A.M.K., and Wijns, W. (2020). Digital health care solution for proactive heart failure management with the Cordella Heart

Failure System: Results of the SIRONA first-in-human study. *European Journal of Heart Failure* 22 (10). https://doi.org/10.1002/ejhf.1870.

60 Ritzema, J., Melton, I.C., Richards, A.M., Crozier, I.G., Frampton, C., Doughty, R.N., Whiting, J., Kar, S., Eigler, N., Krum, H., Abraham, W.T., and Troughton, R.W. (2007). Direct left atrial pressure monitoring in ambulatory heart failure patients: Initial experience with a new permanent implantable device. *Circulation* 116 (25). https://doi.org/10.1161/CIRCULATIONAHA.107.702191.

61 Ritzema, J., Troughton, R., Melton, I., Crozier, I., Doughty, R., Krum, H., Walton, A., Adamson, P., Kar, S., Shah, P.K., Richards, M., Eigler, N.L., Whiting, J.S., Haas, G.J., Heywood, J.T., Frampton, C.M., and Abraham, W.T. (2010). Physician-directed patient self-management of left atrial pressure in advanced chronic heart failure. *Circulation* 121 (9). https://doi.org/10.1161/CIRCULATIONAHA.108.800490.

62 Li, P., Lee, G.H., Kim, S.Y., Kwon, S.Y., Kim, H.R., and Park, S. (2021). From diagnosis to treatment: Recent advances in patient-friendly biosensors and implantable devices. *ACS Nano* 15 (2). https://doi.org/10.1021/acsnano.0c06688.

63 Yu, C.M., Wang, L., Chau, E., Chan, R.H.W., Kong, S.L., Tang, M.O., Christensen, J., Stadler, R.W., and Lau, C.P. (2005). Intrathoracic impedance monitoring in patients with heart failure: Correlation with fluid status and feasibility of early warning preceding hospitalization. *Circulation* 112 (6). https://doi.org/10.1161/CIRCULATIONAHA.104.492207.

64 Whellan, D.J., Ousdigian, K.T., Al-Khatib, S.M., Pu, W., Sarkar, S., Porter, C.B., Pavri, B.B., and O'Connor, C.M. (2010). Combined heart failure device diagnostics identify patients at higher risk of subsequent heart failure hospitalizations. Results from PARTNERS HF (Program to access and review trending information and evaluate correlation to symptoms in patients with heart failure) study. *Journal of the American College of Cardiology* 55 (17). https://doi.org/10.1016/j.jacc.2009.11.089.

65 Small, R.S., Wickemeyer, W., Germany, R., Hoppe, B., Andrulli, J., Brady, P.A., Labeau, M., Koehler, J., Sarkar, S., Hettrick, D.A., and Tang, W.H.W. (2009). Changes in intrathoracic impedance are associated with subsequent risk of hospitalizations for acute decompensated heart failure: Clinical utility of implanted device monitoring without a patient alert. *Journal of Cardiac Failure* 15 (6). https://doi.org/10.1016/j.cardfail.2009.01.012.

66 Abraham, W.T., Compton, S., Haas, G., Foreman, B., Canby, R.C., Fishel, R., Mcrae, S., Toledo, G.B., Sarkar, S., and Hettrick, D.A. (2011). Intrathoracic impedance vs daily weight monitoring for predicting worsening heart failure events: Results of the fluid accumulation status trial (FAST). *Congestive Heart Failure* 17 (2). https://doi.org/10.1111/j.1751-7133.2011.00220.x.

67 Crossley, G.H., Boyle, A., Vitense, H., Chang, Y., and Mead, R.H. (2011). The CONNECT (Clinical evaluation of remote notification to reduce time to clinical decision) trial: The value of wireless remote monitoring with automatic clinician alerts. *Journal of the American College of Cardiology* 57 (10). https://doi.org/10.1016/j.jacc.2010.12.012.

12

Artificial Intelligence Based Commercial Non-Invasive and Invasive Devices for Heart Failure Diagnosis and Prediction

Kanchan Kulkarni, Eric M. Isselbacher, and Antonis A. Armoundas

12.1 Introduction

Heart failure (HF) is a highly morbid disease affecting over 26 million people worldwide [1, 2] and accounting for about 20% of all hospitalizations among the elderly population [3]. Despite many efforts, the financial burden of this chronic disease in the US remains unacceptably high [4] and HF readmissions alone constitute a significant healthcare expenditure [5]. Efforts to reduce the rehospitalization burden using conventional markers have been largely ineffective [6], primarily since efficient interventions in the ambulatory setting remain elusive.

Clinically, HF is characterized by reduced cardiac output and high intracardiac pressures resulting in pulmonary edema, peripheral edema, and increased jugular venous pressure and usually accompanied by symptoms of breathlessness and fatigue. However, patients can present with asymptomatic structural or functional cardiac abnormalities such as left ventricular dysfunction, which are known precursors of acute HF or decompensated HF (Figure 12.1). As demonstrated by Figure 12.1, prior to clinical manifestations of symptoms of decompensated HF that necessitate hospitalization, there is a progressive development of changes in cardiac function manifested by changes in intracardiac pressure, autonomic balance, and intrathoracic impedance. Hence, recognition of these precursors, which are related to poor outcomes, can play a vital role in reducing mortality in patients with asymptomatic ventricular dysfunction [8].

Multiple invasive devices that monitor the right ventricular, left atrial, and pulmonary artery pressure [6, 9–12] have been investigated as a means to reduce HF readmissions. Furthermore, with the recent upsurge in telemedicine, use of virtual communication has become commonplace in healthcare institutions across the US, paving the way for remote monitoring tools that can provide healthcare and clinical decision support to people that do not have direct access to in-hospital services.

As there are several different underlying pathologies that can cause HF, identification of these diverse pathologies for predicting the onset of HF constitutes an integral part of the diagnostic process. Artificial intelligence (AI) based methods offer a promising approach for the prediction, early detection, and risk assessment for individuals prone to

Predicting Heart Failure: Invasive, Non-Invasive, Machine Learning, and Artificial Intelligence Based Methods, First Edition. Edited by Kishor Kumar Sadasivuni, Hassen M. Ouakad, Somaya Al-Maadeed, Huseyin C. Yalcin, and Issam Bait Bahadur.

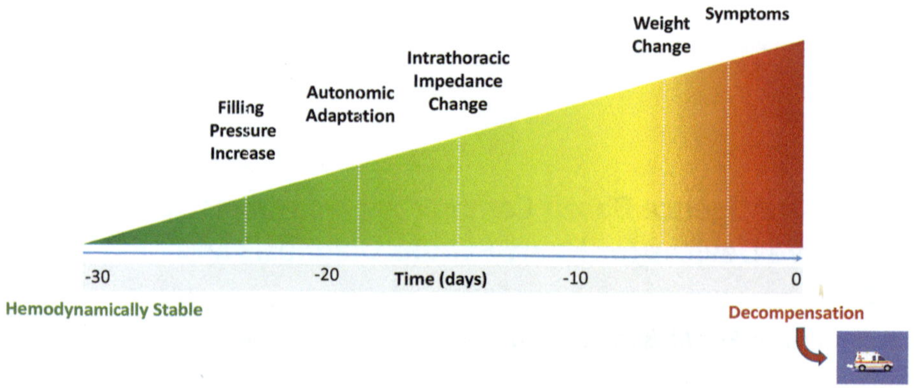

Figure 12.1 Schematic representation of the pathophysiology of congestion and progression of HF (adapted with permission from Adamson et al. [7]).

cardiovascular diseases [13]. Machine learning (ML) algorithms can identify and categorize patterns in underlying data in order to classify or predict an individual's health status. AI has the potential to enhance the current clinical decision support systems by predicting the onset of debilitating physiological conditions such as HF.

AI-driven wearable and invasive devices [14–17] have ushered in a new era of medicine, promising equitable access to clinical diagnostics of an ever-increasing HF population. In this chapter, we present an overview of AI based methods for monitoring the cardiovascular state of HF patients. In addition, we provide a comprehensive review of the various invasive and non-invasive modalities employed for the prediction of HF.

12.2 Search Strategy

The Google Scholar database was manually searched without language restriction for articles published in the 5 years from 2017 to 2021. The literature search was primarily focused on invasive and non-invasive devices (telemonitoring) that incorporated AI for HF diagnosis and prediction. The following keywords were used as search criteria: "(machine learning OR deep learning OR artificial intelligence OR telemonitoring OR invasive devices OR non-invasive devices OR commercial devices OR implantable devices) AND heart failure."

12.3 ML Algorithms

ML is considered a subfield of AI, and involves the study of statistical algorithms that can progressively learn from data and achieve a desired performance on a specific task. The rules, findings, and knowledge derived from the data using ML are expected to be non-trivial. Therefore, ML has been used in tasks that require automation, and especially in cases where humans cannot manually develop such a set of complex instructions to automate the desired tasks. Deep learning (DL) is considered a subfield of ML and focuses on learning data representations using algorithms composed of multiple processing layers. In this chapter, the following ML algorithms have been employed:

Random forest (RF): RF is a supervised learning algorithm, consisting of a group of decision trees trained using the bagging method, wherein, a combination of learning models is utilized to increase the accuracy of the overall result. Hence, RF incorporates multiple decision trees merged together to get more accurate and stable predictions [18]. The multiple decision trees incorporated to create an RF classifier, utilize class label attributes from individual decision trees to provide a more comprehensive classification [18–21].

Support vector machine (SVM): Similarly to RF, SVM utilizes logic-based classification techniques wherein the algorithm learns from a predefined set of rules developed based on the training data, and follows a logical decision making approach to classify the test data [22-25]. Contrary to RF, SVMs uses linear or non-linear classification methods to distinguish data based on features by identifying an optimal hyperplane that separates data points from different classes [22, 24, 26-28].

Artificial neural networks (ANNs): DL is an advanced subfield of ML that employs ANNs with multiple layers of abstraction (networks) to extract features from underlying data distributions [24]. ANNs are generally trained on large amounts of data using graphics processing units, making them highly effective in the classification of data. The neural networks (NNs) essentially consist of multiple interconnected processing layers that identify features from the sample data and utilize detection algorithms to classify test data based on the most useful and important features selected.

Bayesian networks: These are graphical models that use probabilistic processing to represent the conditional dependencies between variables (nodes). Since Bayesian networks can aptly predict the causative relationship between an event and its contributing factors, they are ideal for classifying diseases based on clinical symptoms. Bayesian networks can require large amounts of data to accurately establish probabilistic relationships between a complete set of features and predicted outcomes, hence, more simplistic models, such as the Naive Bayes, have been developed. Herein, the features are assumed to be independent and a probabilistic model is created for each feature; classification is performed by assigning each test feature to the class with the highest probability [29, 30].

Convolutional neural networks (CNNs): A feed-forward NN is a commonly used method, wherein each node in one layer is connected to all the nodes of the subsequent layer, thus supporting decision-making in each layer based on feature information from preceding layers [31]. CNNs are a type of feed-forward NN in which nodes from one layer to the next are connected through a fixed weighting pattern or kernels which extract features based on the correlation among neighboring samples [22].

Recurrent neural networks (RNNs): RNNs are another common DL architecture, wherein a feedback loop within the network is created by connecting the output of a node to the input of a node in the previous layer [22]. RNNs offer an effective modality especially for sequential data processing by exploiting the memory effect created by the feedback loops that utilize the stored information from prior inputs.

12.4 ML and DL Algorithms for Prediction of HF

Application of ML on electrocardiographic (ECG) signals to classify disease states has become an extensive field of research, aiming at efficiently identifying and diagnosing changes in ECG test data, based on prior ECG training data knowledge acquired from healthy and diseased states. Various ML algorithms have been developed specifically for the management of HF [22, 32-37; Table 12.1). Supervised ML algorithms encompassing

Table 12.1 Non-exhaustive chronological summary of ML algorithms applied to existing databases for HF classification and prediction, in the 5 years 2017–2021.

Author/ Study	Year	Aim	AI architecture	Features	Prediction Accuracy
Shah et al. [35]	2015	Phenomapping for novel classification of HF with preserved ejection fraction	Unbiased hierarchical cluster analysis	Clinical, laboratory, ECG, and echocardiographic phenotyping	Phenomapping analysis classified patients into three groups that differed markedly in clinical characteristics, cardiac structure/ function, invasive hemodynamics, and outcomes
Chen et al. [128]	2017	Classify HF vs. non HF patients	Sparse auto-encoder-based DL algorithm	Heart rate variability	Accuracy: 72.41%
Mahajan et al. [129]	2017	Classify HF vs. non HF patients	Bagged decision tree	Probabilistic symbolic pattern recognition, RR intervals	Accuracy: 98.1%, SPE: 100%, SENS: 94.7%
Mdhaffar et al. [130]	2017	Classify HF vs. non HF patients	Complex event processing for HF prediction	Heart rate, ECG, weight and blood pressure	Precision: 84.75%
Sudarshan et al. [131]	2017	Classify HF vs. non HF patients	k-NN, decision tree	Dual tree complex wavelet transform	Accuracy: 99.86%, SENS: 99.78%, SPE: 99.94%
Zhang et al. [132]	2017	Classify HF vs. non HF patients	SVM	Urinary proteome	HR: 1.63 (CI, 1.04–2.55; P=0.032) per 1-SD increment, AUC: 0.70 (95% CI, 0.56–0.82); P=0.0047

(Continued)

Table 12.1 (Continued)

Author/ Study	Year	Aim	AI architecture	Features	Prediction Accuracy
Nirschl et al. [51]	2018	Classify HF vs. non HF patients	Convolutional NN	Histopathology	SENS: 99%, SPE: 94%
Rasmy et al. [50]	2018	Classify HF vs. non HF patients	Recurrent NN	Medications, diagnoses, surgical data	AUC: 82%
Sanchez-Martinez et al. [43]	2018	Classify HF vs. non HF patients	Unsupervised ML	Left ventricular long-axis myocardial velocity patterns	72.6%; 95% CI, 58.1–87.0
Wang et al. [52]	2018	Classify HF vs. non HF patients	NN with LSTM	Holter monitor RR intervals	For segment length N=100, Accuracy: 85.13%, SENS: 73.58%, SPE: 91.78%
Blecker et al. [66]	2018	Identification of HF hospitalization	ML with both structured and unstructured data, logistic regression	Demographics, lab results, vital signs, medications	(Developmental set) AUC: 99%, SENS: 98%, PPV: 43%. (Validation SET) AUC: 99%, SENS: 98%, PPV: 34%
Acharya, U.R. et al. [58]	2019	Automated diagnosis of congestive HF	11-layer deep CNN	ECG	Accuracy: 98.97%; SPE: 99.01%; SENS: 98.87%
Tabbasian et al. [44]	2018	Diagnose HFpEF using ML of spatiotemporal variations in left ventricular deformation	Unsupervised statistical method and a supervised classifier	Velocity, strain, and strain rate traces measured from 18 LV segments by echocardiographic myocardial velocity imaging at rest and during semisupine bicycle exercise	Overall accuracy: 57%; Accuracy for patients with HFpEF: 81%; For asymptomatic vs. symptomatic classification – AUC: 0.89, Accuracy: 85%, SENS: 86%, SPE: 82%

(*Continued*)

Table 12.1 (Continued)

Author/ Study	Year	Aim	AI architecture	Features	Prediction Accuracy
Awan et al. [67]	2019	Predict 30-day readmissions or deaths	MLP, logistic regression, RFs, LASSO regression	Demographics, admission charactersitics, medical history	AUC: 0.62, 0.55, 0.53, 0.58, and 0.54 for MLP, weighted RF, weighted decision trees, logistic regression, and weighted SVM models, respectively.
Ali et al. [68]	2019	Predict HF	Feature-driven decision support system: statistical model, forward best first search, Gaussian Naive Bayes classifier		Max accuracy: 93.33%.
Ali et al. [69]	2019	Predict HF	Stacked SVM		Accuracy: 92.22%.
Attia et al [133].	2019	Identify asymptomatic left ventricular dysfunction	Convolutional NN	Paired 12-lead ECG and echocardiogram data, including the left ventricular ejection fraction	AUC: 0.93, SENS: 86.3%, SPE: 85.7%, Accuracy: 85.7%
Segar et al. [134]	2019	Predict incident HF risk among high-risk patients with type 2 diabetes mellitus	Random survival forest	109 predictor variables	C-index = 0.74
Alotaibi [135]	2019	Predict HF	Decision tree, logistic regression, RF, Naive Bayes, SVM	Cleveland heart disease dataset with multiple attributes (14 selected)	Accuracy: 93.19, 87.36, 89.14, 87.27, 92.30 % respectively
Porumb et al. [57]	2020	Detect congestive HF	Convolutional NN	One raw electrocardiogram (ECG) heartbeat	Accuracy: 100%

(Continued)

Table 12.1 (Continued)

Author/ Study	Year	Aim	AI architecture	Features	Prediction Accuracy
Hussain et al. [136]	2020	Detect congestive HF	SVM linear kernel	HRV signals by extracting multimodal features to capture temporal, spectral, and complex dynamics	TA = 93.1%, AUC = 0.97
Gjoreski et al. [137]	2020	Detect chronic HF from heart sounds	ML and end-to-end DL	Heart sounds (phonocardiogram)	HF detection accuracy is 92.9%, differentiates between CHF phases (decompensated phase vs. recompensated phase) accuracy of 93.2%

DL = deep learning, HF = heart failure, NN = neural network, SVM = support vector machine, LSTM = long short-term memory, MLP = multilayer perceptron, LV = left ventricle, SPE = specificity, SENS = sensitivity, ML = machine learning, AUC = area under curve, HFpEF = HF with preserved ejection fraction

linear or logistic regression [38], decision trees [39], RF [40], SVMs [41], or ANNs [42] have been introduced for ECG classification, based on annotated test data sets [24]. While supervised learning techniques can provide a high degree of accuracy, the limited availability of annotated clinical data makes unsupervised [43] ML algorithms a necessity in performing real-time ECG classification based on unlabeled data using characterization methods like clustering or principal component analysis [22, 24, 44]. Also, multiple studies have proposed probabilistic models based on Bayesian networks to classify ECG, with Naive Bayes [45, 46] being one of the most commonly utilized feature assessment techniques [22, 29, 30, 37]. Supervised, instance-based ML algorithms utilizing non-parametric classifiers to compare the test and training data, such as k-nearest neighbors (k-NN), that label the test data based on the k closest training samples in the feature space [22, 23, 47-49], have also been employed by various studies.

Based on the processing algorithms utilized to identify features and perform classification, there have been multiple DL architectures introduced for the prediction of major HF clinical outcomes [22, 42,50-54; Figure 12.1). CNNs have been shown to be highly effective in image classification [55, 56] and have been utilized widely for HF detection and diagnosis [51, 57, 58]. RNNs have shown success in identifying HF patients [50] and predicting the onset of HF [59-61]. A combination of such architectures creating multiple layers of processing can be utilized to improve performance and prediction efficacy, creating a deep neural network (DNN) [55, 62], which has shown promise in HF prediction [58, 63, 64; Figure 12.1).

Importantly, many ML/DL algorithms have shown superior performance in identifying HF patients compared with traditional statistical approaches and conventional physician diagnosis. Nirschl et al. [51] reported a CNN-based DL classifier to detect HF using endomyocardial biopsy images with 99% sensitivity and 94% specificity. The algorithm was highly accurate and shown to outperform two pathology experts by 20%. Another study, investigating the efficacy of an RNN model for prediction of HF onset and risk, reported an area under curve (AUC) of 82% compared to 79% achieved by logistic regression [61]. Additionally, the study demonstrated the successful transferability of the ML model to data across different hospitals with a conservative 3.6% drop in AUC, highlighting the adaptability of the ML algorithm to the variability in data across patient populations and hospitals [61]. Choi et al. demonstrated the utility of AI based clinical decision support systems in diagnosing HF compared to traditional method of diagnosis by HF specialists [65; Figure 12.1). The AI based system showed high accuracy with a concordance rate of 98% between the AI system and HF specialists. Similarly, multiple other groups have shown ML/DL algorithms to outperform conventional analytical methods [66-69].

12.5 Invasive Monitoring Devices for Prediction of HF

Recent studies have suggested that physiological parameters, other than the traditionally utilized markers of weight or intrathoracic impedance, may be needed for timely detection of HF decompensation [70]. In fact, interventions based on pulmonary artery hemodynamic monitoring [71, 72] have shown a significant reduction in rehospitalization rates.

Invasive ambulatory hemodynamic monitors have shown promise as early-warning systems in HF, with multiple devices having been investigated, including right ventricular (COMPASS-HF [9] and REDUCE HF [73]), left atrial (HOMEOSTASIS[74] and LAPTOP-HF [11, 71]), and pulmonary artery (CHAMPION [12]) pressure measurement systems [7, 10–12]. More recently, in the MultiSENSE [75] study, an algorithm based on physiological data from sensors in the implantable cardiac resynchronization therapy (CRT) defibrillators, showed 70% sensitivity in predicting the risk of HF hospitalizations or worsening of HF. Although, in this case, the risk prediction algorithm (HeartLogic [75]) was constructed by combining heart sounds, respiration, thoracic impedance, heart rate, and activity information and did not involve complex ML/DL algorithms, the study highlighted the potential of utilizing physiological information from implanted CRT devices to predict impending HF decompensation.

The utility of applying ML algorithms to data acquired from invasive cardiovascular devices for the management of HF (Table 12.2) was demonstrated by the COMPANION [76] trial. In this study, an RF ML model developed to predict all-cause mortality or HF hospitalization at 12-month post-CRT implantation produced quartiles of patients with an eightfold difference in survival between those with the highest and lowest predicted probability for events [76]. Furthermore, the model also performed better at discriminating the risk of all-cause mortality or HF hospitalization than traditional methods of assessment based on the bundle branch block morphology and QRS duration [76]. While the conventional diagnosis methods failed to significantly differentiate survival outcomes in patients with CRT, the RF ML model successfully predicted clinical outcomes.

Similarly, a study to predict right-ventricular failure (RVF) following left ventricular assist device (LVAD) therapy using a tree-augmented Naive Bayes model, demonstrated an accuracy of up to 97% [77]. Bayesian prognostic models of RVF applied to patient data from the Inter-Agency Registry for Mechanically Assisted Circulatory Support (INTERMACS) who had an implanted LVAD, were shown to be highly accurate in predicting acute, early, as well as late RVF with sensitivity of around 90%, and achieving a maximum specificity of 99% [77]. The Bayesian model was also shown to outperform previous risk scores such as the right ventricular failure risk score [78] (RVFRS) and Drakos [79], obtained by multivariable logistic regression analysis, when applied to the INTERMACS registry (AUC 54.7% and 49.8%, respectively) [77]. Another study by the same group showed that Bayesian prognostic models applied to the INTERMACS registry accurately (76–87%) predicted mortality as well, with an AUC ranging between 0.70–0.71 [80]. Furthermore, they developed a novel Bayesian model for risk stratification and prediction of mortality at different time points, that is 30 days, 90 days, 6 months, 1 year and 2 years, post-LVAD implantation [81]. The AI algorithm exhibited mortality prediction accuracies of 95, 90, 90, 83, and 78%, at each of the five time-points, respectively, with AUCs of 91, 82, 82, 80, and 81%, respectively, performing significantly better than the traditional logistic regression based HeartMate II Risk Score [82] (AUC 57 and 60%, at 90 days and 1 year, respectively) [81].

There are a number of implantable monitoring devices focused on the management of HF, such as CardioMEMs [83, 84], which are implantable impedance monitors [85] to gauge fluid accumulation [86, 87] and dedicated ML approaches to analyze data from CRT devices, LVADs, and implantable cardioverter defibrillator (ICDs) [22, 32, 33, 43, 45, 88]. While devices like CardioMEMS have shown reduction in HF readmissions [12, 72], a major limitation of these devices is that they are invasively implanted, costly upfront, and demand additional personnel and resources to handle the device implantation and data acquisition. In addition, invasive monitoring devices require specialized hardware and data extraction features, often making them cumbersome and impractical for real-time monitoring and assessment of active, ambulatory patients, especially those who live in underserved areas. Furthermore, their cost-effectiveness remains debatable [89–91], highlighting the need for affordable non-invasive approaches for HF monitoring enabled with effective AI based disease prediction strategies.

12.6 Non-Invasive Wearable Monitoring Devices for Prediction of HF

The utility of wearable monitoring devices [92–96] in cardiovascular healthcare and, in particular, in HF management has been well established [16, 97–99]. Ambulatory non-invasive monitoring devices that assess various physiological parameters, including blood pressure [100], photoplethysmograms (PPGs) [101], seismocardiograms [17], ECG [95, 102], electromagnetic energy-based dielectric properties [103], oxygen saturation [104], and fluid status, weight, activity, and bioimpedance [105], have enabled access to large amounts of patient data which are ideally suited for applying AI algorithms and predicting HF onset or deterioration (Table 12.2; 98, 106–110].

Table 12.2 Chronological summary of invasive and non-invasive modalities for HF prediction

Author/Study	Year	Aim	AI architecture	Invasive or Non-Invasive	Prediction Accuracy
MUSIC Trial [105]	2012	Prediction of acute HF decompensation using a multisensor system capable of intermittent transmission of physiologic signals		Non-invasive	(Development cohort) SENS: 65%, SPE: 90%, False positive rate: 0.7 per patient-year (Validation cohort) SENS: 63%, SPE: 92%, False positive rate: 0.9 per patient-year
Loghmanpour et al. [77]	2016	Predict right ventricular failure following left ventricular assist device therapy	Tree-augmented Naive Bayes model	Invasive	Accuracy: 91%– 97% AUC 0.83–0.90, SENS: 90%, SPE: 98–99%
Kanwar et al. [80]	2018	Predict mortality risk retrospectively for various time points (1, 3, and 12 months) after LVAD implantation (INTERMACS Study)	Tree-augmented Naive Bayes model	Invasive	Accuracy: 76–87%, AUC: 0.70–0.71
Inan et al. [17]	2018	Novel wearable seismocardiography and ML algorithms to assess clinical status of HF patients	Graph mining (graph similarity score).	Non-invasive	Graph similarity score metric: 44.4±4.9 (decompensated HF) vs. 35.2±10.5 (compensated HF); 6 decompensated patients' graph similarity score: 44±4.1 (admitted) vs. 35±3.9 (discharged)

(*Continued*)

Table 12.2 (Continued)

Author/Study	Year	Aim	AI architecture	Invasive or Non-Invasive	Prediction Accuracy
COMPANION (Comparison of Medical Therapy, Pacing, and Defibrillation in Trial [76]	2018	Predict all-cause mortality or HF hospitalization 12 months post-CRT	RF model	Invasive	8-fold difference in survival between those with the highest and lowest predicted probability for events (hazard ratio, 7.96; $P<0.0001$); Discriminated the risk of all-cause mortality or HF hospitalization better than bundle branch block morphology and QRS duration.
Al-Makhadmeh et al. [112]	2019	Utilizing IoT based wearable medical device for heart disease prediction	Higher order Boltzmann deep belief neural network	Non-invasive	Accuracy: 99.03%
Green et al. [101]	2019	Detection of obstructive hypertrophic cardiomyopathy using a wearable biosensor (PPG signals)	Multi-instance ML classifier	Non-invasive	C-statistic: 0.99 (95% CI: 0.99–1.0)
LINK HF multicenter study [15]	2020	Detect precursors of hospitalization for HF exacerbation using a multiparameter patch sensor	ML algorithm similarity-based modeling	Non-invasive	SENS: 76–88%, SPE: 85%
Shah et al. [113]	2020	Detecting HF using wearables	SVM	Non-invasive	Max AUC: 0.87, SPE: 72%, SENS: 90%

HF = heart failure, LVAD = left ventricular assist device, SPE = specificity, SENS = sensitivity, ML = machine learning, AUC = area under curve, IoT = internet of things, PPG = photoplethysmogram, ECG = electrocardiogram

Pulse oximetry constitutes a clinically standardized method for non-invasively assessing the pulse oxygen saturation level, SpO_2, in order to evaluate the presence of hypoxemia commonly associated with acute HF. Pulse oximetry has been shown to be useful in diagnosing HF in acute settings such as myocardial infarction [111]. While there are multiple commercially available wearable pulse oximetry devices like the Masimo MightySat, VitalPatch, EQ02 + Lifemonitor, and VinCense WHMS, that offer user-friendly monitoring of the SpO_2, as well as the pulse rate, many of these lack comprehensive cardiac monitoring to detect abnormal rhythms and ischemic events, making them insufficient to assist patients at risk, by detecting early warning signs of adverse cardiopulmonary events. Another convenient wristband-based SpO_2 monitoring device is the Spryhealth Loop, which has been designed specifically for use by seniors and offers easy assessment of SpO_2 levels, as well as HR and respiration. Furthermore, newer devices, like the Everion, which promise a more complete physiological assessment by monitoring 22 vital signs, are being investigated. Similarly, Current Health has designed a mobile monitoring device for continuous SpO_2, temperature, heart rate, respiration, and movement measurements, for detection of warning signs of health deterioration.

A 2019 study applied DL on medical data acquired from an internet of things (IoT) wearable medical device and successfully predicted heart disease with 99.03% accuracy [112]. A higher order Boltzmann deep belief NN was utilized to extract features from patients' physiological data such as ECG, heart rate, blood pressure, peripheral pulse oximetry (SpO_2) level, glucose level, blood fat level, and pulse rate, acquired using the wearable IoT device and stored on cloud servers, to predict heart disease by recognizing abnormal heart patterns in just 8.5 seconds [112]. Another multicenter study, LINK-HF [15], evaluated the accuracy of non-invasive remote monitoring in predicting HF rehospitalization using a wearable multisensor chest patch interconnected with a smartphone to continuously upload data to a cloud analytics platform. A similarity based ML model detected HF exacerbation and provided early detection of impending rehospitalization with a sensitivity ranging between 76% and 88%, and specificity of 85% [15]. This met the sensitivity and specificity thresholds aimed at for reliable prediction of HF hospitalization (≥70% sensitivity and 85% specificity), and was comparable to the predictive ability achieved by implantable devices, such as in the MultiSENSE study (70% sensitivity) [75].

In 2020, a pilot study by Shah et al. [113] aimed to predict HF using PPG and accelerometry data acquired from a wearable wristband; using a combination of demographics, medical history, vital signals, and data from the wearable, an SVM based ML model was able to classify HF with a 0.8 AUC, 72% specificity, and 90% sensitivity [113]. In another study, a novel wearable seismocardiogram and ECG sensing patch was utilized by Inan et al. [17] to assess the clinical status of HF patients; using an ML based graph analytic technique, they generated a graph similarity score that was able to differentiate between decompensated and compensated HF and also track differences in the clinical progress of the decompensated patients from the time of admission to discharge [17]. Similarly, Green et al. [101] demonstrated the application of a multi-instance ML classifier in detecting obstructive hypertrophic cardiomyopathy using a combination of PPG signals acquired from a wearable biosensor and echocardiograms, with a C-statistic of 0.99 (95% CI: 0.99–1.0).

These promising early studies highlight the utility of AI based technologies to detect and assess HF progression using wearable monitoring technologies. However, there remains substantial untapped potential for using novel ML/DL strategies to identify and predict HF risk using non-invasive remote monitoring devices, which warrants further large-scale multicenter trials to evaluate the clinical efficacy of AI enabled wearables for improved HF management (Figure 12.1).

12.7 Future Outlook on the Use of AI

Computational advances have led to the development of numerous AI approaches for clinical data analyses [114] to assist HF diagnosis and prediction (Table 12.1). Multiple ML/DL strategies with an accuracy of over 90% in classifying HF patients and predicting adverse events have been proposed. However, studies comparing the clinical efficacy of AI based HF prediction models with conventional diagnostic methods have shown mixed results. While some newer predictive models have shown improved performance over conventional methods in classifying and identifying HF patients [22], other studies have shown no improvement in predicting HF readmissions using ML compared to traditional statistical approaches [45, 115]. This discrepancy is due to the fact that the accuracy of AI approaches is greatly influenced by the availability of large amounts of data that can enable optimal feature extraction to efficiently identify patterns in underlying data. Indeed, it has been shown that, while AI algorithms provide good discrimination in identifying HF patients based on demographics and medical history, HF classification efficiency can be affected by the subtleties of the disease progression state (e.g. preserved ejection fraction, mid-range ejection fraction, or reduced ejection fraction) and variability in patient characteristics (e.g. age, gender) [22]. Yet, while novel ML/DL approaches continue to be investigated to address these challenges, improved AI strategies have shown promise in outperforming conventional regression models in predicting HF outcomes and have also demonstrated better accuracy in predicting mortality due to acute HF and HF with preserved ejection fraction [22, 116, 117].

In parallel, remote monitoring devices have seen an uptick in the past decade, with the proliferation of low-cost vital sign monitors available for ambulatory real-time assessment of patients' physiological state. From smartwatches, electronic finger-rings, and smart garments to dedicated wearable cardiac and muscle activity sensors, miniaturized medical grade ambulatory monitoring devices are readily available to assist patient care. Yet, there is sparse availability of devices that merge these two technologies and fully utilize the powers of AI and wearable monitors for cardiac disease management, in particular HF prediction.

This technological gap in medical treatment strategies is expected to be bridged by the embedding of AI algorithms in wearable ambulatory devices, a transition that will enable superior classification and prediction capabilities of cardiovascular disease progression, thus accelerating the transition to precision medicine for all population groups. AI is expected to pave the way to precision medicine by providing patients with self-monitoring opportunities using affordable low-cost monitors, hence improving the general quality of life while also reducing the current healthcare burden of HF management [13,

14, 118, 119]. In addition, AI can account for interpatient variability and provide accurate automated diagnosis based on consideration of multiple clinical factors, which is humanly infeasible.

Despite the clear advantages offered by an AI based ambulatory monitoring framework, the utility of novel invasive and non-invasive health monitoring modalities has been met with skepticism due to the lack of a regulatory framework, as well as reliability, accountability, liability, and security concerns. Recognizing and addressing these critical issues is paramount to the successful implementation, transition, and adoption of AI based ambulatory health monitoring systems:

1. **Legislation and liability**: Enabling the universal adaptability of an automated monitoring paradigm, involves participation of developers, researchers, physicians, and legislators alike, to account for the multiple aspects involved in its design, implementation, and end consumer usage. Proper quality checks during development and production, along with thorough assessment ensured by Food and Drug Administration (FDA) approval will reduce the physician's liability in cases of undesired outcomes [120], enabling a constructive framework for the implementation of an AI based medical system.
2. **Data security**: For ambulatory monitoring devices, cybersecurity is a rising concern, as patient data is recorded on cloud servers and transferred between various digital and IoT platforms. Efficient AI based ambulatory systems need to include reliable signal processing algorithms with data security features protecting patient confidentiality. Similar to the need for informed consent prior to any medical procedure, approval needs to be mandated before the implementation of AI systems as well to ensure effective patient involvement and account for data integrity.
3. **Reliability and accountability**: To standardize the accuracy and efficacy requirements of ambulatory monitoring systems, AI devices and algorithms should be FDA approved. In addition, with advancements in real-time signal processing capabilities, AI algorithms need to be consistently refined to keep up with the updated clinical practices. The end performance of the AI based ambulatory healthcare system depends on participation by multiple stakeholders, including developers, physicians, and technicians in charge of data handling, along with willing involvement by patients. Hence, all stakeholders are equally accountable for the quality and performance of the AI device.
4. **Equity**: Disparities in mortality rates between rural and urban communities has been a growing concern in recent years. Inequitable access to healthcare, socioeconomic differences, and geographic variances are significant attributes for the regional disparity in healthcare efficiency [121–127]. AI based ambulatory monitoring systems hold the potential to enable access to precision medicine by providing clinicians with patient custom methodologies for earlier and improved disease diagnosis. ML/DL algorithms can identify patterns from large physiological observations and provide personalized therapeutic approaches by detecting and potentially eliminating bias from underlying data, hence, enabling a more equitable healthcare paradigm.

12.8 Conclusion

Ambulatory, non-invasive, and invasive monitoring devices that employ AI offer novel promising modalities for the prediction and diagnosis of HF. ML/DL strategies can enable real-time quick diagnosis with increased accuracy by providing physicians with tools for improved personalized disease assessment. Thus, AI devices have the potential to bridge the technological vacuum in medical treatment strategies by enabling superior prediction and classification of cardiovascular disease progression, compared with traditional methods. Furthermore, ambulatory remote monitoring devices embedded with AI are likely to enable and facilitate the realization of precision medicine, by offering patients personalized, affordable, low-cost monitors that can improve the overall quality of life. An effective AI enabled medical healthcare system can be fulfilled by the implementation of a comprehensive regulatory framework that successfully addresses, among many, the challenges of reliability, accountability, liability, and data security.

Funding Support

The work was supported by a Grant-in-Aid (#15GRNT23070001) from the American Heart Association (AHA), the Institute of Precision Medicine (17UNPG33840017) from the AHA, the RICBAC Foundation, NIH grants 1 R01 HL135335-01, 1 R21 HL137870-01, 1 R21EB026164-01 and 3R21EB026164-02S1.

References

1 Adamson, P.B. (2009). Pathophysiology of the transition from chronic compensated and acute decompensated heart failure: New insights from continuous monitoring devices. *Current Heart Failure Reports* 6 (4): 287–292.

2 Ponikowski, P., Anker, S.D., AlHabib, K.F., Cowie, M.R., Force, T.L., Hu, S., et al. (2014). Heart failure: Preventing disease and death worldwide. *ESC Heart Failure* 1 (1): 4–25.

3 Savarese, G. and Lund, L.H. (2017). Global public health burden of heart failure. *Cardiac Failure Review* 3 (1): 7.

4 Benjamin, E.J., Blaha, M.J., Chiuve, S.E., Cushman, M., Das, S.R., Deo, R., et al. (2017). Heart disease and stroke statistics—2017 update: A report from the American Heart Association. *Circulation* 135 (10): e146–e603.

5 Lloyd-Jones, D., Adams, R.J., Brown, T.M., Carnethon, M., Dai, S., De Simone, G., et al. (2009). Heart disease and stroke statistics–2010 update: A report from the American Heart Association. *Circulation* Feb. 23 121 (7): e46–e215.

6 Hunt, S.A., Abraham, W.T., Chin, M.H., Feldman, A.M., Francis, G.S., Ganiats, T.G., et al. (2009). 2009 focused update incorporated into the ACC/AHA 2005 Guidelines for the diagnosis and management of heart failure in adults. A Report of the American College of Cardiology Foundation/American Heart Association Task Force on Practice Guidelines, developed in collaboration with the International Society for Heart and

Lung Transplantation. *Journal of the American College of Cardiology* Apr. 14 53 (15): e1–e90.

7 Adamson, P.B., Magalski, A., Braunschweig, F., Bohm, M., Reynolds, D., Steinhaus, D., et al. (2003). Ongoing right ventricular hemodynamics in heart failure: Clinical value of measurements derived from an implantable monitoring system. *Journal of the American College of Cardiology* Feb. 19 41 (4): 565–571.

8 Wang, T.J., Levy, D., Benjamin, E.J., and Vasan, R.S. (2003). The epidemiology of asymptomatic left ventricular systolic dysfunction: Implications for screening. *Annals of Internal Medicine* 138 (11): 907–916.

9 Bourge, R.C., Abraham, W.T., Adamson, P.B., Aaron, M.F., Aranda, J.M., Jr., Magalski, A., et al. (2008). Randomized controlled trial of an implantable continuous hemodynamic monitor in patients with advanced heart failure: The COMPASS-HF study. *Journal of the American College of Cardiology* Mar. 18 51 (11): 1073–1079.

10 Ritzema, J., Troughton, R., Melton, I., Crozier, I., Doughty, R., Krum, H., et al. (2010). Physician-directed patient self-management of left atrial pressure in advanced chronic heart failure. *Circulation* Mar. 9 121 (9): 1086–1095.

11 Maurer, M.S., Adamson, P.B., Costanzo, M.R., Eigler, N., Gilbert, J., Gold, M.R., et al. (2015). Rationale and design of the left atrial pressure monitoring to optimize heart failure therapy study (LAPTOP-HF). *Journal of Cardiac Failure* Jun. 21 (6): 479–488.

12 Givertz, M.M., Stevenson, L.W., Costanzo, M.R., Bourge, R.C., Bauman, J.G., Ginn, G., et al. (2017). Pulmonary artery pressure-guided management of patients with heart failure and reduced ejection fraction. *Journal of the American College of Cardiology* Oct. 10 70 (15): 1875–1886.

13 Krittanawong, C., Zhang, H., Wang, Z., Aydar, M., and Kitai, T. (2017). Artificial intelligence in precision cardiovascular medicine. *Journal of the American College of Cardiology* 69 (21): 2657–2664.

14 Bachtiger, P., Plymen, C.M., Pabari, P.A., Howard, J.P., Whinnett, Z.I., Opoku, F., et al. (2020). Artificial intelligence, data sensors and interconnectivity: Future opportunities for heart failure. *Cardiac Failure Review* 6.

15 Stehlik, J., Schmalfuss, C., Bozkurt, B., Nativi-Nicolau, J., Wohlfahrt, P., Wegerich, S., et al. (2020). Continuous wearable monitoring analytics predict heart failure hospitalization: The LINK-HF multicenter study. *Circulation. Heart Failure* 13 (3): e006513.

16 D'Amario, D., Canonico, F., Rodolico, D., Borovac, J.A., Vergallo, R., Montone, R.A., et al. (2020). Telemedicine, artificial intelligence and humanisation of clinical pathways in heart failure management: Back to the future and beyond. *Cardiac Failure Review* 6.

17 Inan, O.T., Baran Pouyan, M., Javaid, A.Q., Dowling, S., Etemadi, M., Dorier, A., et al. (2018). Novel wearable seismocardiography and machine learning algorithms can assess clinical status of heart failure patients. *Circulation. Heart Failure* 11 (1): e004313.

18 Breiman, L. (2001). Random forests. *Machine Learning* 45 (1): 5–32.

19 Liaw, A. and Wiener, M. (2002). Classification and regression by randomForest. *R News* 2 (3): 18–22.

20 Guidi, G., Pettenati, M.C., Miniati, R., and Iadanza, E. (ed.) (2013). Random forest for automatic assessment of heart failure severity in a telemonitoring scenario. In: *2013 35th Annual International Conference of the IEEE Engineering in Medicine and Biology Society (EMBC)*, IEEE.

21 Masetic, Z. and Subasi, A. (2016). Congestive heart failure detection using random forest classifier. *Computer Methods and Programs in Biomedicine* 130: 54–64.

22 Bazoukis, G., Stavrakis, S., Zhou, J., Bollepalli, S.C., Tse, G., Zhang, Q., et al. (2021). Machine learning versus conventional clinical methods in guiding management of heart failure patients—a systematic review. *Heart Failure Reviews* 26 (1): 23–34.

23 Masetic, Z. and Subasi, A. (2016). Congestive heart failure detection using random forest classifier. *Computer Methods and Programs in Biomedicine* Jul. 130: 54–64.

24 Sevakula, R.K., Au-Yeung, W.T.M., Singh, J.P., Heist, E.K., Isselbacher, E.M., and Armoundas, A.A. (2020). State-of-the-art machine learning techniques aiming to improve patient outcomes pertaining to the cardiovascular system. *Journal of the American Heart Association* 9 (4): e013924.

25 Sahoo, S., Dash, M., Behera, S., and Sabut, S. (2020). Machine Learning Approach to Detect Cardiac Arrhythmias in Ecg Signals: A Survey. IRBM.

26 Cortes, C. and Vapnik, V. (1995). Support-vector networks. *Machine Learning* 20 (3): 273–297.

27 Burges, C.J. (1998). A tutorial on support vector machines for pattern recognition. *Data Mining and Knowledge Discovery* 2 (2): 121–167.

28 Narin, A., Isler, Y., and Ozer, M. (2014). Investigating the performance improvement of HRV Indices in CHF using feature selection methods based on backward elimination and statistical significance. *Computers in Biology and Medicine* Feb. 45: 72–79.

29 Rish, I. (ed). (2001). An Empirical Study of the Naive Bayes Classifier. IJCAI 2001 workshop on empirical methods in artificial intelligence.

30 Duda, R. and Hart, P. 1973. Pattern classification and scene analysis. *A Wiley-Interscience Publication*. Wiley. doi:10.2307/2286028.

31 Haykin, S.S. (2009). Neural Networks and Learning machines. New York: Prentice Hall.

32 Alonso-Betanzos, A., Bolon-Canedo, V., Heyndrickx, G.R., and Kerkhof, P.L. (2015). Exploring guidelines for classification of major heart failure subtypes by using machine learning. *Clinical Medicine Insights. Cardiology* 9 (Suppl. 1): 57–71.

33 Austin, P.C., Tu, J.V., Ho, J.E., Levy, D., and Lee, D.S. (2013). Using methods from the data-mining and machine-learning literature for disease classification and prediction: A case study examining classification of heart failure subtypes. *Journal of Clinical Epidemiology* Apr. 66 (4): 398–407.

34 Isler, Y. (2016). Discrimination of systolic and diastolic dysfunctions using multi-layer perceptron in heart rate variability analysis. *Computers in Biology and Medicine* Sep. 1 (76): 113–119.

35 Shah, S.J., Katz, D.H., Selvaraj, S., Burke, M.A., Yancy, C.W., Gheorghiade, M., et al. (2015). Phenomapping for novel classification of heart failure with preserved ejection fraction. *Circulation* Jan. 20 131 (3): 269–279.

36 Akinyokun, C.O., Obot, O.U., and Uzoka, F.-M.E. eds. Application of neuro-fuzzy technology in medical diagnosis: Case study of heart failure 2009. Berlin, Heidelberg: Springer.

37 Asyali, M.H. (ed). (2003). Discrimination power of long-term heart rate variability measures. *Proceedings of the 25th Annual International Conference of the IEEE Engineering in Medicine and Biology Society (IEEE Cat No03CH37439).* 17–21 Sep.

38 Phillips, K.T. and Street, W.N. (2005). Predicting outcomes of hospitalization for heart failure using logistic regression and knowledge discovery methods. *AMIA Annual Symposium Proceedings AMIA Symposium* 1080.

39 Kang, Y., McHugh, M.D., Chittams, J., and Bowles, K.H. (2016). Utilizing home healthcare electronic health records for telehomecare patients with heart failure: A decision tree approach to detect associations with rehospitalizations. *Computers, Informatics, Nursing: CIN* Apr. 34 (4): 175–182.

40 Guidi, G., Pollonini, L., Dacso, C.C., and Iadanza, E. (2015). A multi-layer monitoring system for clinical management of congestive heart failure. *BMC Medical Informatics and Decision Making* 15 (Suppl. 3): S5.

41 Ramirez, J., Monasterio, V., Minchole, A., Llamedo, M., Lenis, G., Cygankiewicz, I., et al. (2015). Automatic SVM classification of sudden cardiac death and pump failure death from autonomic and repolarization ECG markers. *Journal of Electrocardiology* Jul.–Aug. 48 (4): 551–557.

42 Myers, J., de Souza, C.R., Borghi-Silva, A., Guazzi, M., Chase, P., Bensimhon, D., et al. (2014). A neural network approach to predicting outcomes in heart failure using cardiopulmonary exercise testing. *International Journal of Cardiology* Feb. 1 171 (2): 265–269.

43 Sanchez-Martinez, S., Duchateau, N., Erdei, T., Kunszt, G., Aakhus, S., Degiovanni, A., et al. (2018). Machine learning analysis of left ventricular function to characterize heart failure with preserved ejection fraction. *Circulation. Cardiovascular Imaging* Apr. 11 (4): e007138.

44 Tabassian, M., Sunderji, I., Erdei, T., Sanchez-Martinez, S., Degiovanni, A., Marino, P., et al. (2018). Diagnosis of heart failure with preserved ejection fraction: Machine learning of spatiotemporal variations in left ventricular deformation. *Journal of the American Society of Echocardiography: Official Publication of the American Society of Echocardiography* Dec. 31 (12): 1272–1284 e9.

45 Frizzell, J.D., Liang, L., Schulte, P.J., Yancy, C.W., Heidenreich, P.A., Hernandez, A.F., et al. (2017). Prediction of 30-day all-cause readmissions in patients hospitalized for heart failure: Comparison of machine learning and other statistical approaches. *JAMA Cardiol* Feb. 1 2 (2): 204–209.

46 Koulaouzidis, G., Iakovidis, D.K., and Clark, A.L. (2016). Telemonitoring predicts in advance heart failure admissions. *International Journal of Cardiology* Aug. 1 216: 78–84.

47 Liu, G., Wang, L., Wang, Q., Zhou, G., Wang, Y., and Jiang, Q. (2014). A new approach to detect congestive heart failure using short-term heart rate variability measures. *PLoS One* 9 (4): e93399.

48 Cover, T.M. and Hart, P. (1967). Nearest neighbor pattern classification. *IEEE Transactions on Information Theory* 13 (1): 21–27.

49 Keller, J.M., Gray, M.R., and Givens, J.A. (1985). A fuzzy k-nearest neighbor algorithm. *IEEE Transactions on Systems, Man, and Cybernetics* 4: 580–585.

50 Rasmy, L., Wu, Y., Wang, N., Geng, X., Zheng, W.J., Wang, F., et al. (2018). A study of generalizability of recurrent neural network-based predictive models for heart failure onset risk using a large and heterogeneous EHR data set. *Journal of Biomedical Informatics* Aug. 84: 11–16.

51 Nirschl, J.J., Janowczyk, A., Peyster, E.G., Frank, R., Margulies, K.B., Feldman, M.D., et al. (2018). A deep-learning classifier identifies patients with clinical heart failure using whole-slide images of H&E tissue. *PLoS One* 13 (4): e0192726.

52 Wang, L., Zhou, W., Liu, N., Xing, Y., and Zhou, X. (2018). CHF detection with LSTM neural network. *Conference Proceeding IEEE Engineering in Medicine and Biology Society*. 2018 Jul. 514–517.

53 Golas, S.B., Shibahara, T., Agboola, S., Otaki, H., Sato, J., Nakae, T., et al. (2018). A machine learning model to predict the risk of 30-day readmissions in patients with heart failure: A retrospective analysis of electronic medical records data. *BMC Medical Informatics and Decision Making* Jun. 22 18 (1): 44.

54 Xiao, C., Ma, T., Dieng, A.B., Blei, D.M., and Wang, F. (2018). Readmission prediction via deep contextual embedding of clinical concepts. *PLoS One* 13 (4): e0195024.

55 Krizhevsky, A., Sutskever, I., and Hinton, G.E. (eds.) (2012). Imagenet Classification with Deep Convolutional Neural Networks. Advances in neural information processing systems.

56 LeCun, Y., Bottou, L., Bengio, Y., and Haffner, P. (1998). Gradient-based learning applied to document recognition. *Proceedings of the IEEE* 86 (11): 2278–2324.

57 Porumb, M., Iadanza, E., Massaro, S., and Pecchia, L. (2020). A convolutional neural network approach to detect congestive heart failure. *Biomedical Signal Processing and Control* 55: 101597.

58 Acharya, U.R., Fujita, H., Oh, S.L., Hagiwara, Y., Tan, J.H., Adam, M., et al. (2019). Deep convolutional neural network for the automated diagnosis of congestive heart failure using ECG signals. *Applied Intelligence* 49 (1): 16–27.

59 Chen, R., Stewart, W.F., Sun, J., Ng, K., and Yan, X. (2019). Recurrent neural networks for early detection of heart failure from longitudinal electronic health record data: Implications for temporal modeling with respect to time before diagnosis, data density, data quantity, and data type. *Circulation. Cardiovascular Quality and Outcomes* 12 (10): e005114.

60 Choi, E., Schuetz, A., Stewart, W.F., and Sun, J. (2017). Using recurrent neural network models for early detection of heart failure onset. *Journal of the American Medical Informatics Association* 24 (2): 361–370.

61 Rasmy, L., Wu, Y., Wang, N., Geng, X., Zheng, W.J., Wang, F., et al. (2018). A study of generalizability of recurrent neural network-based predictive models for heart failure onset risk using a large and heterogeneous EHR data set. *Journal of Biomedical Informatics* 84: 11–16.

62 LeCun, Y., Bengio, Y., and Hinton, G. (2015). Deep learning. *Nature* 521 (7553): 436–444.

63 Le, M.T., Vo, M.T., Mai, L., and Dao, S.V. (ed.) (2020). Predicting heart failure using deep neural network. In: *2020 International Conference on Advanced Technologies for Communications (ATC)*, IEEE.

64 Zhang, Y. and Xia, M. (eds.) (2020). Application of deep neural network for congestive heart failure detection using ECG signals. Journal of Physics: Conference Series, Vol.1642, 4th International Conference on Artificial Intelligence Applications and Technologies (AIAAT 2020) 7-9 August 2020, Shenzhen, China.

65 Choi, D.-J., Park, J.J., Ali, T., and Lee, S. (2020). Artificial intelligence for the diagnosis of heart failure. *NPJ Digital Medicine* 3 (1): 1–6.

66 Blecker, S., Sontag, D., Horwitz, L.I., Kuperman, G., Park, H., Reyentovich, A., et al. (2018). Early identification of patients with acute decompensated heart failure. *Journal of Cardiac Failure* Jun. 24 (6): 357–362.

67 Awan, S.E., Bennamoun, M., Sohel, F., Sanfilippo, F.M., and Dwivedi, G. (2019). Machine learning-based prediction of heart failure readmission or death: Implications of choosing the right model and the right metrics. *ESC Heart Failure* 6 (2): 428–435.

68 Ali, L., Khan, S.U., Golilarz, N.A., Yakubu, I., Qasim, I., Noor, A., et al. (2019). A feature-driven decision support system for heart failure prediction based on statistical model and Gaussian naive bayes. *Computational and Mathematical Methods in Medicine*.

69 Ali, L., Niamat, A., Khan, J.A., Golilarz, N.A., Xingzhong, X., Noor, A., et al. (2019). An optimized stacked support vector machines based expert system for the effective prediction of heart failure. *IEEE Access* 7: 54007–54014.

70 Hawkins, N.M., Virani, S.A., Sperrin, M., Buchan, I.E., McMurray, J.J., and Krahn, A.D. (2016). Predicting heart failure decompensation using cardiac implantable electronic devices: A review of practices and challenges. *European Journal of Heart Failure* 18 (8): 977–986.

71 Abraham, W.T., Adamson, P.B., Costanzo, M.R., Eigler, N., Gold, M., Klapholz, M., et al. (2016). Hemodynamic monitoring in advanced heart failure: Results from the LAPTOP-HF trial. *Journal of Cardiac Failure* 22 (11): 940.

72 Abraham, W.T., Adamson, P.B., Bourge, R.C., Aaron, M.F., Costanzo, M.R., Stevenson, L.W., et al. (2011). Wireless pulmonary artery haemodynamic monitoring in chronic heart failure: A randomised controlled trial. *The Lancet* 377 (9766): 658–666.

73 Adamson, P.B., Gold, M.R., Bennett, T., Bourge, R.C., Stevenson, L.W., Trupp, R., et al. (2011). Continuous hemodynamic monitoring in patients with mild to moderate heart failure: Results of the reducing decompensation events utilizing intracardiac pressures in patients with chronic heart failure (REDUCEhf) trial. *Congestive Heart Failure* 17 (5): 248–254.

74 Ritzema, J., Troughton, R., Melton, I., Crozier, I., and Doughty, R. (2010). Hemodynamically guided home self-therapy in severe heart failure patients (HOMEOSTASIS) study group. Physician-directed patient self-management of left atrial pressure in advanced chronic heart failure. *Circulation* 121: 1086–1095.

75 Boehmer, J.P., Hariharan, R., Devecchi, F.G., Smith, A.L., Molon, G., Capucci, A., et al. (2017). A multisensor algorithm predicts heart failure events in patients with implanted devices: Results from the MultiSENSE study. *JACC. Heart Failure* 5 (3): 216–225.

76 Kalscheur, M.M., Kipp, R.T., Tattersall, M.C., Mei, C., Buhr, K.A., DeMets, D.L., et al. (2018). Machine learning algorithm predicts cardiac resynchronization therapy outcomes: Lessons from the COMPANION trial. *Circulation. Arrhythmia and Electrophysiology* 11 (1): e005499.

77 Loghmanpour, N.A., Kormos, R.L., Kanwar, M.K., Teuteberg, J.J., Murali, S., and Antaki, J.F. (2016). A Bayesian model to predict right ventricular failure following left ventricular assist device therapy. *JACC. Heart Failure* 4 (9): 711–721.

78 Matthews, J.C., Koelling, T.M., Pagani, F.D., and Aaronson, K.D. (2008). The right ventricular failure risk score: A pre-operative tool for assessing the risk of right ventricular failure in left ventricular assist device candidates. *Journal of the American College of Cardiology* 51 (22): 2163–2172.

79 Drakos, S.G., Janicki, L., Horne, B.D., Kfoury, A.G., Reid, B.B., Clayson, S., et al. (2010). Risk factors predictive of right ventricular failure after left ventricular assist device implantation. *The American Journal of Cardiology* 105 (7): 1030–1035.

80 Kanwar, M.K., Lohmueller, L.C., Kormos, R.L., Teuteberg, J.J., Rogers, J.G., Lindenfeld, J., et al. (2018). A Bayesian model to predict survival after left ventricular assist device implantation. *JACC. Heart Failure* 6 (9): 771–779.

81 Loghmanpour, N.A., Kanwar, M.K., Druzdzel, M.J., Benza, R.L., Murali, S., and Antaki, J.F. (2015). A new Bayesian network-based risk stratification model for prediction of short-term and long-term LVAD mortality. *ASAIO Journal (American Society for Artificial Internal Organs: 1992)* 61 (3): 313.

82 Cowger, J., Sundareswaran, K., Rogers, J.G., Park, S.J., Pagani, F.D., Bhat, G., et al. (2013). Predicting survival in patients receiving continuous flow left ventricular assist devices: The HeartMate II risk score. *Journal of the American College of Cardiology* 61 (3): 313–321.

83 Ollendorf, D.A., Sandhu, A.T., and Pearson, S.D. (2016). CardioMEMS HF for the management of heart failure—effectiveness and value. *JAMA Internal Medicine* 176 (10): 1551–1552.

84 Volterrani, M., Spoletini, I., Angermann, C., Rosano, G., and Coats, A.J. (2019). Implantable devices for heart failure monitoring: The CardioMEMS™ system. *European Heart Journal Supplements* 21 (Supplement_M): M50–M3.

85 Conraads, V.M., Tavazzi, L., Santini, M., Oliva, F., Gerritse, B., Yu, C.-M., et al. (2011). Sensitivity and positive predictive value of implantable intrathoracic impedance monitoring as a predictor of heart failure hospitalizations: The SENSE-HF trial. *European Heart Journal* 32 (18): 2266–2273.

86 Abraham, W.T., Compton, S., Haas, G., Foreman, B., Canby, R.C., Fishel, R., et al. (2011). Intrathoracic impedance vs daily weight monitoring for predicting worsening heart failure events: Results of the Fluid Accumulation Status Trial (FAST). *Congestive Heart Failure* 17 (2): 51–55.

87 Brachmann, J., Böhm, M., Rybak, K., Klein, G., Butter, C., Klemm, H., et al. (2011). Fluid status monitoring with a wireless network to reduce cardiovascular-related hospitalizations and mortality in heart failure: Rationale and design of the optiLink HF Study (Optimization of Heart Failure Management using optivol fluid status monitoring and care link). *European Journal of Heart Failure* 13 (7): 796–804.

88 Tripoliti, E.E., Papadopoulos, T.G., Karanasiou, G.S., Naka, K.K., and Fotiadis, D.I. (2017). Heart failure: Diagnosis, severity estimation and prediction of adverse events through machine learning techniques. *Computational and Structural Biotechnology Journal* 15: 26–47.

89 Sandhu, A.T., Goldhaber-Fiebert, J.D., Owens, D.K., Turakhia, M.P., Kaiser, D.W., and Heidenreich, P.A. (2016). Cost-effectiveness of implantable pulmonary artery pressure monitoring in chronic heart failure. *JACC. Heart Failure* May 4 (5): 368–375.

90 Sandhu, A.T. and Heidenreich, P.A. (2018). Heart failure management with ambulatory pulmonary artery pressure monitoring. *Trends in Cardiovascular Medicine* Apr. 28 (3): 212–219.

91 Schmier, J.K., Ong, K.L., and Fonarow, G.C. (2017). Cost-effectiveness of remote cardiac monitoring with the CardioMEMS heart failure system. *Clinical Cardiology* Jul. 40 (7): 430–436.

92 Armoundas, A.A., Singh, J.P., Heist, E.K., and Isselbacher, E.M. (2021). State of the art on wearable and implantable devices for cardiac and respiratory monitoring. In: Cardiac Bioelectric Therapy Efimov I.R., Ng F.S., Laughner J.I., 353–362. Springer.

93 Sana, F., Isselbacher, E.M., Singh, J.P., Heist, E.K., Pathik, B., and Armoundas, A.A. (2020). Wearable devices for ambulatory cardiac monitoring: JACC State-of-the-Art review. *Journal of the American College of Cardiology* Apr. 7 75 (13): 1582–1592.

94 Kulkarni, K., Awasthi, N., Roberts, Jr J.D., and Armoundas, A.A. (2021). Utility of a smartphone-based system (cvrPhone) in estimating minute ventilation from electrocardiographic signals. *Telemedicine and e-Health.* doi:10.1089/tmj.2020.0507

95 Sohn, K., Merchant, F.M., Abohashem, S., Kulkarni, K., Singh, J.P., Heist, E.K., et al. (2019). Utility of a smartphone based system (cvrPhone) to accurately determine apneic events from electrocardiographic signals. *PLoS One* 14 (6): e0217217.

96 Sohn, K., Merchant, F.M., Sayadi, O., Puppala, D., Doddamani, R., Sahani, A., et al. (2017). A novel point-of-care smartphone based system for monitoring the cardiac and respiratory systems. *Scientific Reports* Research Support, N.I.H., Extramural Research Support, Non-U.S. Gov't. Mar. 22 7: 44946.

97 Aliverti, A. (2017). Wearable technology: Role in respiratory health and disease. *Breathe* 13 (2): e27–e36.

98 DeVore, A.D., Wosik, J., and Hernandez, A.F. (2019). The future of wearables in heart failure patients. *JACC. Heart Failure* 7 (11): 922–932.

99 Dias, D. (2018). Paulo Silva Cunha J. Wearable health devices—vital sign monitoring, systems and technologies. *Sensors* 18 (8): 2414.

100 Radha, M., de Groot, K., Rajani, N., Wong, C.C., Kobold, N., Vos, V., et al. (2018). Wrist-worn blood pressure tracking in healthy free-living individuals using neural networks. *arXiv Preprint arXiv:180509121.*

101 Green, E.M., van Mourik, R., Wolfus, C., Heitner, S.B., Dur, O., and Semigran, M.J. (2019). Machine learning detection of obstructive hypertrophic cardiomyopathy using a wearable biosensor. *NPJ Digital Medicine* 2 (1): 1–4.

102 Sohn, K.D.S., Merchant, F.M., Kulkarni, K., Sana, F., Abohashem, S., Singh, J.P., Heist, E.K., Owen, C., Isselbacher, E.M., and Armoundas, A.A. (2019). Utility of a smartphone based system (cvrphone) to predict short-term arrhythmia susceptibility. *Scientific Reports* 2019 9: 14497.

103 Amir, O., Rappaport, D., Zafrir, B., and Abraham, W.T. (2013). A novel approach to monitoring pulmonary congestion in heart failure: Initial animal and clinical experiences using remote dielectric sensing technology. *Congestive Heart Failure* 19 (3): 149–155.

104 Zhang, Q., Arney, D., Goldman, J.M., Isselbacher, E.M., and Armoundas, A.A. (2020). Design implementation and evaluation of a mobile continuous blood oxygen saturation monitoring system. *Sensors* 20 (22): 6581.

105 Anand, I.S., Tang, W.W., Greenberg, B.H., Chakravarthy, N., Libbus, I., Katra, R.P., et al. (2012). Design and performance of a multisensor heart failure monitoring algorithm: Results from the multisensor monitoring in congestive heart failure (MUSIC) study. *Journal of Cardiac Failure* 18 (4): 289–295.

106 Maini, E., Venkateswarlu, B., and Gupta, A. (eds). (2018). Applying machine learning algorithms to develop a universal cardiovascular disease prediction system. International Conference on Intelligent Data Communication Technologies and Internet of Things. Springer.

107 Faragli, A., Abawi, D., Quinn, C., Cvetkovic, M., Schlabs, T., Tahirovic, E., et al. (2020). The role of non-invasive devices for the telemonitoring of heart failure patients. *Heart Failure Reviews* 26: 1063–1080.

108 Dovancescu, S., Saczynski, J.S., Darling, C.E., Riistama, J., Kuniyoshi, F.S., Meyer, T., et al. (2015). Detecting heart failure decompensation by measuring transthoracic bioimpedance in the outpatient setting: Rationale and design of the SENTINEL-HF study. *JMIR Research Protocols* 4 (4): e121.

109 Suh, M.-K., Chen, C.-A., Woodbridge, J., Tu, M.K., Kim, J.I., Nahapetian, A., et al. (2011). A remote patient monitoring system for congestive heart failure. *Journal of Medical Systems* 35 (5): 1165–1179.

110 Ahmed, F.Z., Taylor, J.K., Green, C., Moore, L., Goode, A., Black, P., et al. (2020). Triage-HF Plus: A novel device-based remote monitoring pathway to identify worsening heart failure. *ESC Heart Failure* 7 (1): 108–117.

111 Masip, J., Gayà, M., Páez, J., Betbesé, A., Vecilla, F., Manresa, R., et al. (2012). Pulse oximetry in the diagnosis of acute heart failure. *Revista Española de Cardiología (English Edition)* 65 (10): 879–884.

112 Al-Makhadmeh, Z. and Tolba, A. (2019). Utilizing IoT wearable medical device for heart disease prediction using higher order Boltzmann model: A classification approach. *Measurement* 147: 106815.

113 Shah, A.J., Isakadze, N., Levantsevych, O., Vest, A., Clifford, G., and Nemati, S. (2020). Detecting heart failure using wearables: A pilot study. *Physiological Measurement* 41 (4): 044001.

114 Au-Yeung, W.-T.M., Sevakula, R.K., Singh, J.P., Heist, E.K., Isselbacher, E.M., and Armoundas, A.A. (2021). State of the art in artificial intelligence and machine learning techniques for improving patient outcomes pertaining to the cardiovascular and respiratory systems. In: Cardiac Bioelectric Therapy Efimov I.R., Ng F.S., Laughner J.I., 335–352. Springer.

115 Desai, R.J., Wang, S.V., Vaduganathan, M., Evers, T., and Schneeweiss, S. (2020). Comparison of machine learning methods with traditional models for use of administrative claims with electronic medical records to predict heart failure outcomes. *JAMA Netw Open* 3 (1): e1918962–e.

116 Angraal, S., Mortazavi, B.J., Gupta, A., Khera, R., Ahmad, T., Desai, N.R., et al. (2020). Machine learning prediction of mortality and hospitalization in heart failure with preserved ejection fraction. *JACC. Heart Failure* 8 (1): 12–21.

117 Kwon, J.-M., Kim, K.-H., Jeon, K.-H., Lee, S.E., Lee, H.-Y., Cho, H.-J., et al. (2019). Artificial intelligence algorithm for predicting mortality of patients with acute heart failure. *PLoS One* 14 (7): e0219302.

118 Barrett, M., Boyne, J., Brandts, J., Brunner-La Rocca, H.-P., De Maesschalck, L., De Wit, K., et al. (2019). Artificial intelligence supported patient self-care in chronic heart failure: A paradigm shift from reactive to predictive, preventive and personalised care. *Epma Journal* 10 (4): 445–464.

119 Johnson, K.W., Torres Soto, J., Glicksberg, B.S., Shameer, K., Miotto, R., Ali, M., et al. (2018). Artificial intelligence in cardiology. *Journal of the American College of Cardiology* 71 (23): 2668–2679.

120 Price, W.N., II, Gerke, S., and Cohen, I.G. (2019). Potential liability for physicians using artificial intelligence. *JAMA*.322(18): 1765–1766 doi:10.1001/jama.2019.15064

121 Cosby, A.G., McDoom-Echebiri, M.M., James, W., Khandekar, H., Brown, W., and Hanna, H.L. (2019). Growth and persistence of place-based mortality in the United States: The rural mortality penalty. *American Journal of Public Health* 109 (1): 155–162.

122 Jones, I., López-Carr, D., and Dalal, P. (2011). Responding to rural health disparities in the United States: The geography of emergency care and telemedical technology. *Networks and Communication Studies* 25 (3-4): 273–290.

123 Dwyer-Lindgren, L., Bertozzi-Villa, A., Stubbs, R.W., Morozoff, C., Mackenbach, J.P., van Lenthe, F.J., et al. (2017). Inequalities in life expectancy among US counties, 1980 to 2014: Temporal trends and key drivers. *JAMA Internal Medicine* 177 (7): 1003–1011.

124 Marcin, J.P., Shaikh, U., and Steinhorn, R.H. (2016). Addressing health disparities in rural communities using telehealth. *Pediatric Research* 79 (1): 169–176.

125 Eberhardt, M.S. and Pamuk, E.R. (2004). The importance of place of residence: Examining health in rural and nonrural areas. *American Journal of Public Health* 94 (10): 1682–1686.

126 Hartley, D. (2004). Rural health disparities, population health, and rural culture. *American Journal of Public Health* 94 (10): 1675–1678.

127 Merwin, E., Snyder, A., and Katz, E. (2006). Differential access to quality rural healthcare: Professional and policy challenges. *Family & Community Health* 29 (3): 186–194.

128 Chen, W., Liu, G., Su, S., Jiang, Q., and Nguyen, H. (eds). (2017). A CHF detection method based on deep learning with RR intervals. *2017 39th Annual International Conference of the IEEE Engineering in Medicine and Biology Society (EMBC)*. 11–15 July 2017

129 Mahajan, R., Viangteeravat, T., and Akbilgic, O. (2017). Improved detection of congestive heart failure via probabilistic symbolic pattern recognition and heart rate variability metrics. *International Journal of Medical Informatics* Dec. 108: 55–63.

130 Mdhaffar, A., Bouassida Rodriguez, I., Charfi, K., Abid, L., and Freisleben, B. (2017). CEP4HFP: Complex Event Processing for Heart Failure Prediction. *IEEE Transactions on Nanobioscience* Dec. 16 (8): 708–717.

131 Sudarshan, V.K., Acharya, U.R., Oh, S.L., Adam, M., Tan, J.H., Chua, C.K., et al. (2017). Automated diagnosis of congestive heart failure using dual tree complex wavelet transform and statistical features extracted from 2s of ECG signals. *Computers in Biology and Medicine* Apr. 1 83: 48–58.

132 Zhang, Z.Y., Ravassa, S., Nkuipou-Kenfack, E., Yang, W.Y., Kerr, S.M., Koeck, T., et al. (2017). Novel Urinary Peptidomic classifier predicts incident heart failure. *Journal of the American Heart Association* Aug. 7 6 (8).

133 Attia, Z.I., Kapa, S., Lopez-Jimenez, F., McKie, P.M., Ladewig, D.J., Satam, G., et al. (2019). Screening for cardiac contractile dysfunction using an artificial intelligence–enabled electrocardiogram. *Nature Medicine* 25 (1): 70–74.

134 Segar, M.W., Vaduganathan, M., Patel, K.V., McGuire, D.K., Butler, J., Fonarow, G.C., et al. (2019). Machine learning to predict the risk of incident heart failure hospitalization among patients with diabetes: The WATCH-DM risk score. *Diabetes Care* 42 (12): 2298–2306.

135 Alotaibi, F.S. (2019). Implementation of machine learning model to predict heart failure disease. *International Journal of Advanced Computer Science and Applications* 10 (6): 261–268.

136 Hussain, L., Awan, I.A., Aziz, W., Saeed, S., Ali, A., Zeeshan, F., et al. (2020). Detecting congestive heart failure by extracting multimodal features and employing machine learning techniques. *BioMed Research International* 2020 4281243 doi:10.1155/2020/4281243.

137 Gjoreski, M., Gradišek, A., Budna, B., Gams, M., and Poglajen, G. (2020). Machine learning and end-to-end deep learning for the detection of chronic heart failure from heart sounds. *IEEE Access* 8: 20313–20324.

13

Future Techniques and Perspectives on Implanted and Wearable Heart Failure Detection Devices

Muhammad E. H. Chowdhury, Amith Khandaker, Yazan Qiblawey, Fahmida Haque, Maymouna Ezeddin, Tawsifur Rahman, Nabil Ibtehaz, and Khandaker Reajul Islam

13.1 Introduction

Heart failure (HF) affects 1–2% of the population of developed countries [1] and the number of people affected is increasing day by day. More than 30% of the patients visiting clinics require hospitalization within 12 months [2]. The common clinical practice is to make a decision about a patient based on a single short clinical visit or on many short visits, often repeated over several months. However, advancements in implantable and wearable technology and in the machine learning domain have significantly reduced the number of hospital admissions in recent years. Moreover, medical doctors have more patient data from less symptomatic patients compared to more symptomatic patients and the number of self-reported patients has significantly increased over the years [3]. Self-reported patient data, commonly done using a set of questions in a self-report tool, is a common method that is used to collect medical information and can be used to understand the patient's perspective regarding their own health conditions. Most implantable devices are very expensive and only a limited number are approved for clinical applications; on the other hand, the number of users of wearable devices has significantly grown over the years and it has become evident from the outcome of several research studies of large patient cohorts that wearable devices can play a vital role in the disease screening process; this has been particularly evident during the outbreak of the coronavirus pandemic in 2019 (COVID-19) [4–10].

Implantable devices are a common approach that has been used for a long time to monitor and detect HF, beginning in 1960 with the creation of the first implantable pacemaker. Since then, countless lives have been saved [11]. The first implantable pacemaker, a battery-powered pacemaker with a myocardial lead, was developed in a hospital in Buffalo, New York [12]. According to local news, this work helped the first patient to carry on his life for 21 years. With the advances of wearable sensors and the growth of the smartphone market, a change in the healthcare system is possible by introducing personalized healthcare to billions of people. Moreover, these devices are becoming

Predicting Heart Failure: Invasive, Non-Invasive, Machine Learning, and Artificial Intelligence Based Methods, First Edition. Edited by Kishor Kumar Sadasivuni, Hassen M. Ouakad, Somaya Al-Maadeed, Huseyin C. Yalcin, and Issam Bait Bahadur.

increasingly sophisticated and accurate and can be considered biological sensors, which can transform several fields in healthcare including the management of HF, where mobile applications can remotely monitor hundreds of thousands of patients for signs and symptoms and can notify them to change medication or contact their doctors. Management of HF is unique among medical circumstances, in that it requires continuous management of data such as weight, heart rate, blood pressure, and volume status that may require adjusting daily medication.

Wearable health devices are already available in the market, although most of them are for fitness, these devices are creating a unique opportunity to improve HF care. With the advances in technology, some companies have started including biosignal sensors to measure biomedical signals such as heart rate and electrocardiographic information. Several trials [13–15], using commercial devices, have been conducted on using wearable devices for HF management. These studies have confirmed that wearable devices can be used to manage HF patients. However, several problems still exist, such as how to use the devices, data transmission, analyzing the data, and correlating the data with existing records [14, 15]. Advances in machine learning and accessibility to extensive patient information in the electronic medical records play an important role in improving HF management tools. Several studies have shown that machine learning can predict HF diagnosis with reasonable accuracy, classify HF cases, and identify HF a long time before the clinical diagnosis [16]. Studies exist that have used machine learning to create predictive models for HF [16, 17]. The models are trained on different data types, such as ambulatory blood pressure and activity level. The models can either identify the factors that increase the risk of HF, such as diastolic blood pressure, or identify patients at risk, or patients who are at risk of readmission to hospital [18, 19].

This chapter discusses the applications and challenges of implantable devices for HF monitoring, as well as their prospects and limitations, and lists some of the data sets recently collected from wearable devices. Finally, the application of machine learning for detecting HF using wearable devices and its prospects are discussed.

13.2 Applications of Implantable Devices in HF Detection

Implantable devices are extensively used to monitor patients with cardiovascular diseases (CVDs). CVDs contribute to 45% of deaths in Europe and 720,000 people suffer from heart attacks every year in the US [20, 21]. Several studies have confirmed that there is a close relationship between high blood pressure and increased CVD risk in the elderly population. Between 2004 and 2014, there was a significant increase (~34%) in deaths in the world population due to high blood pressure, which was attributed to ever-increasing socioeconomic pressure, as well as to lack of awareness of preventive or monitoring measures, etc [21]. Several implantable devices are clinically being used or are under clinical trial for monitoring HF patients invasively. Among these, low arterial pressure monitors, intrathoracic impedance monitors, and lung fluid monitors are prominent. However, very few remote monitoring systems for HF patients are approved by the US Food and Drug Administration (FDA); the Cardio-Microelectromechanical system (CardioMEMS^{TM}) [22, 23] is one of them. This is a pulmonary artery pressure (PAP) device to directly monitor pressure with the help of implanted sensors, and the data is communicated to the healthcare provider for better patient management (Figure 13.1). Clinical trials have reported that the rate of hospitalization has reduced with the application of the CardioMEMS device [24].

Apart from cardiovascular information, blood pressure provides information about other conditions, such as sleep apnea, dementia, and hypertensive multiple sclerosis complications [25, 26]. Implantable pressure sensors with wireless communication can be effectively used for long-term monitoring. This PAP monitoring has significant research importance. It has been reported that HF can be detected several weeks earlier by monitoring the changes in blood pressure [27]. Non-invasive solutions for real-time arterial blood pressure monitoring can significantly ease the process. One major contribution toward this objective has been reported recently, namely the extraction of arterial blood pressure non-invasively using the photoplethysmogram (PPG) signal [28]. A PPG is an optically obtained plethysmogram that can be used to detect blood volume changes in the microvascular bed of tissue. It is often obtained by using a pulse oximeter which illuminates the skin and measures changes in light absorption. There have been studies conducted by the authors to detect blood pressure using PPG signals using machine learning approaches on already available labeled datasets [28, 29]. These studies reported a deep learning-based approach for predicting the continuous arterial blood pressure (ABP) waveform through a non-invasive approach using PPG signals, an approach that is suitable for wearable devices and remote patient monitoring.

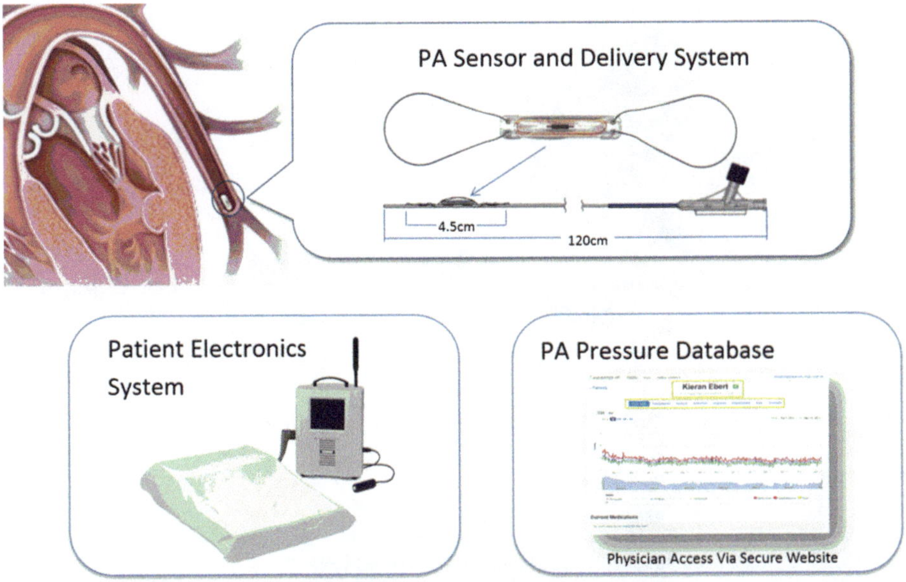

Figure 13.1 The system architecture of the CardioMEMS system [25].

A cardiac pacemaker generates electrical impulses to be delivered to the atria and ventricles to contract and pump blood to the body. By contrast, a cardiac resynchronization therapy defibrillator (CRT-D) is a life-saving device for HF patients who are at high risk of cardiac arrest in that it not only helps to sustain normal heart rhythms like a pacemaker, but also helps to deliver small electrical impulses to both ventricles to contract them simultaneously (Figure 13.2). To monitor the progression of HF, intracellular and extracellular ion concentrations can be monitored and clinical trials with CRT-D and these kinds of sensors can help to save lives by ensuring better patient management. Wireless communication from implantable cardioverter-defibrillators (ICDs) to medical personnel and patients' caregivers has now become a reality [30].

The ICDs continuously monitor the heart signal and, if there are any abnormal heart rhythms detected, it immediately works to correct the rhythms. Moreover, if a cardiac arrest occurs and the heart stops its pumping action, these devices restore heart function by applying an electric shock to revert the situation. These devices are FDA-approved and are quite reliable for critical patient management, although patients have to maintain a very restricted lifestyle.

The rise in left atrial pressure (LAP) usually is gradual and precedes symptom onset. Therefore, accurate monitoring of LAP using an implantable LAP sensing device (as shown in Figure 13.3) could allow earlier identification. A small clinical trial with eight HF patients being monitored with LAP devices twice a day resulted in no deaths, no unplanned HF clinic visits, and no hospital admissions for HF [33].

There is a wide range of cardiac implantable devices available in the market. Figure 13.4 shows some of the implantable devices, with different form factors, from different companies.

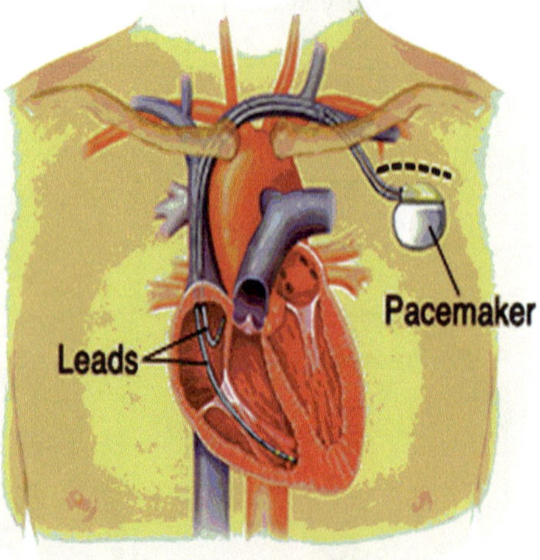

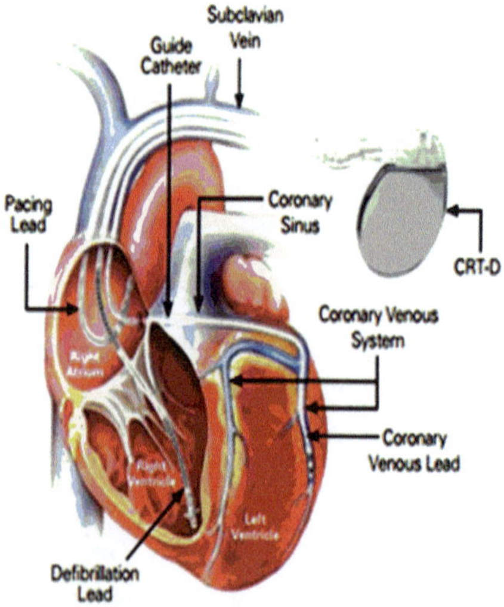

Figure 13.2 Cardiac pacemaker (left) [31] and CRT-D (right) [32].

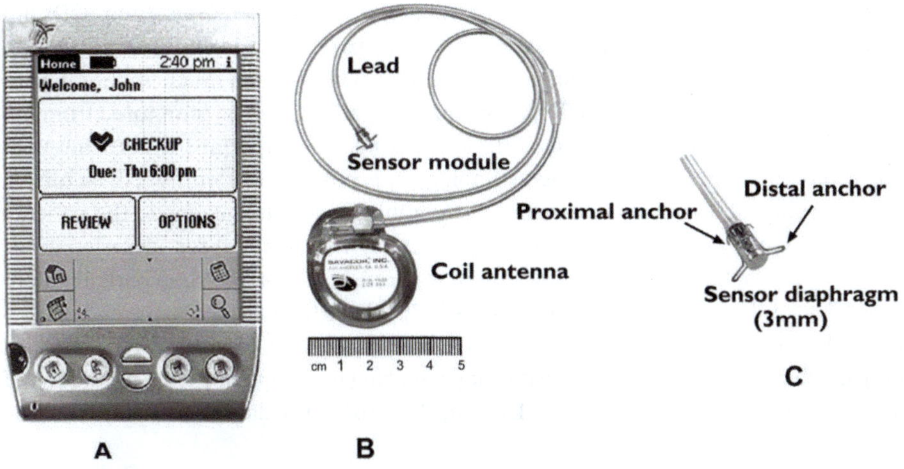

Figure 13.3 Left atrial pressure (LAP) sensing device: Patient advisory module (A), LAP sensing device (B), Sensor tip (C) [33]). With permission from Springer Nature.

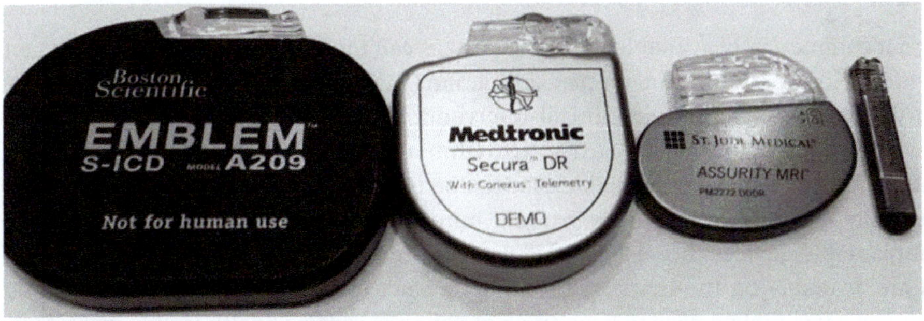

Figure 13.4 Implantable cardiac devices.

13.3 Wearable Devices in HF Detection Application

Consumer health technology has grown to an annual market of billions of dollars and almost 20% of Americans are now using wearable devices for fitness tracking applications [34]. The market of wearable devices is growing very fast and is expected to be more than $27 billion by 2026 [35]. These wearable consumable devices have increasingly become more sophisticated, accurate, and closer to medical-grade devices. They will allow more personalized and precise monitoring of the patients with HF along with more frequent and appropriate adjustment of therapy and care. Moreover, early detection and diagnosis of the disease can help in immediate intervention and save a significant number of lives. At present, patients with a history of HF are monitored within the clinic or hospital and remotely using implantable cardiac devices. Commercial off-the-shelf devices like sphygmomanometers, left ventricular assist devices (LVADs), and ICDs are typically used for HF detection, risk assessment, and patient management [36]. On the other hand, wearable devices can be used in a similar way but on a much wider range of the population, with and without HF history, and the patients can be monitored from the clinic and hospitals when they are in a different setting. It is important to note that with the advancement in machine learning technology, it is possible to identify risk factors by utilizing the clinical data available from the wearable devices to categorize the patients into potentially higher risk groups and to ask them to visit hospital for advanced intervention or even implantable device placement to monitor high-risk group patients more precisely. The authors have done similar work [37], where they ranked features from the collected data using different feature-ranking techniques and then used the best-performing machine learning classifier to develop a scoring technique for early prediction of mortality amongst patients; similar work can be done using the data collected from wearable devices.

13.4 Integrating Wearables Technology into the Healthcare System

Different commercially available wearable devices can monitor steps, heart rate, oxygen saturation, blood pressure, and electrocardiogram (ECG) signals, which can help the clinician in decision-making and clinical intervention. Wearable devices typically, however, focus on predicting HF or cardiac arrhythmia with the help of clinicians. There is a limited number of devices available that can be used to automatically detect a clinical abnormality of the patient reliably without human intervention. Most of such devices are implantable devices; however, these devices are very expensive and only a few of them are available on the market. Therefore, a safe, reliable, and effective automatic system like a wearable device to keep track of patients' cardiac health is very important. Different types of wearable devices in different form factors are shown in Figure 13.5. The name and specifications of the devices from the left to right (top row 1–5; bottom row 6–10) are:

1. Scosche Rhythm +: This is an optical heart band monitor and, thus, is one of the best heart rate monitors for weight lifters.
2. Fitbit Flex 2: This is one of the best heart rate monitors for swimmers who want to use the Fitbit app to track distance and calories burned. The battery life is adequate, and this device will track steps, distance, calories burned, and sleep.
3. Wahoo Tickr X and Polar H7: These are the best heart rate monitors for the money for those who might not want to workout with their phone, a watch, or something on their wrist. They strap comfortably around the chest and record workout data with or without a phone. Anyone can later sync it to their app to maximize the full potential of this device. It will give about 16 hours of workout battery, easily one of the longest on the market. The Polar H7 is both comfortable and light enough to not get in the way of a workout, as well as being relatively cheap.

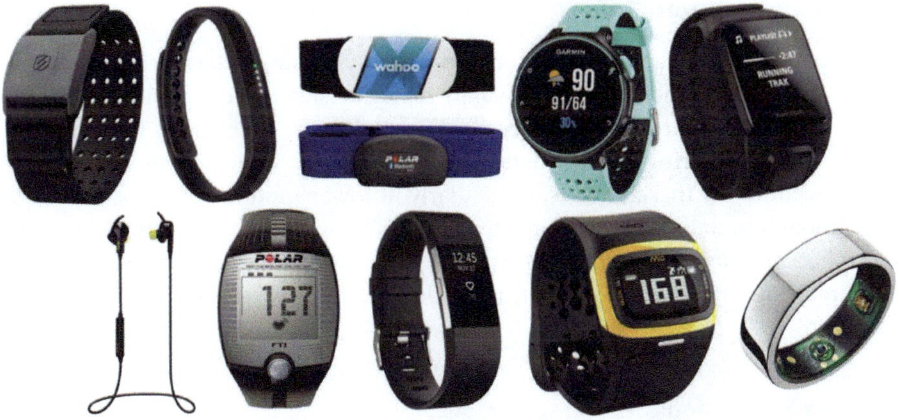

Figure 13.5 Different types of wearable devices in different form factors [38].

4. Garmin Forerunner 235: This is another intelligent heart rate monitor watch that is going to be one of the best heart rate monitors for the professional multitasker interested in a high-end solution.
5. TomTom Spark: The TomTom Spark is one of the best heart rates monitors out there for those wanting a reasonably priced device with some added bells and whistles. It's packed with capabilities that justify its price, including 24/7 activity tracking, GPS, goal-setting applications, sleep tracking, calories burned, and a multisport mode.
6. Jabra Sports Pulse: A unique "heart rate monitor," this is a combined pair of earbud headphones, and a heart rate tracker. It is one of the best dual-functioning heart rate monitors, especially for those who do not want to wear extra equipment while working out.
7. Polar FT1: This is one of the best-priced and budget-friendly heart monitors on the market today. The screen display is also pretty big, making it easy to read anyone's heart rate mid-workout. It comes with a chest strap to ensure that the device is picking up the heart rate.
8. Fitbit Charge 2: This syncs through Bluetooth on a smartphone and records activities through an app associated with the device. The app will track steps, movement, calories, and sleep patterns, and even has a built-in GPS for mapping workouts. It gives a personalized fitness plan and improvement tips, designating a Cardio Fitness Score based on several health factors.
9. Mio Alpha 2: This is one of the best heart rate monitors on the market for swimmers because it can resist 30 feet of water. In addition to being waterproof, the Alpha 2 has a good battery life, lasting between 20 and 24 hours.
10. Ōura ring: The Ōura ring is a discreet, finger-based health tracker that can help keep tabs on activity level, sleep, and general well-being.

13.4.1 Activity Monitors

The most popular form of activity monitoring devices available on the market are a ring, wristband, wristwatch, chest strap, and smart insole or shoe. These devices use three degrees of freedom accelerometers to identify the activity type of the user. They are suitable for activity monitoring and fall detection, but the type of movement significantly affects the accuracy of these devices, particularly at lower motion activities. Wearable devices, although initially designed for activity monitoring, can now be utilized to monitor several other body parameters and every day the list of parameters increases as do their accuracy and reliability. However, these devices are not yet directly used for HF identification.

13.4.2 Heart Rate Monitors

Most of the wearable devices utilize an optical heart rate monitor using the PPG technique, which uses the incident of light of particular wavelengths entering the skin, then measuring the perfusion of blood in the dermis and subcutaneous tissue by capturing the different amounts of light refracted by varying volumes of blood flow occurring due to heart pumps (Figure 13.6). It uses a light-emitting diode (LED) to illuminate a capillary bed and thus monitor pulsatile changes in light absorption by a photodiode, which is similar to a pulse oximeter [13]. It was reported recently that the accuracy of heart rate monitors from wearable PPG devices depends on the type of activity being performed and the heart rate range of the user.

The signal acquired using the PPG techniques can be used to generate metrics about heart rate, blood pressure, breathing rate, and several other usable metrics, as shown in Figure 13.7.

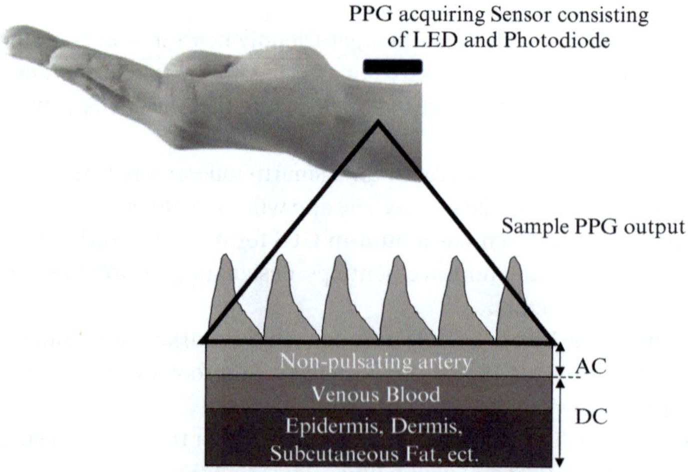

Figure 13.6 Concept of PPG which uses a light-emitting diode and photodiode in the PPG acquiring sensor to measure changing blood volume changes due to the pumping of the heart.

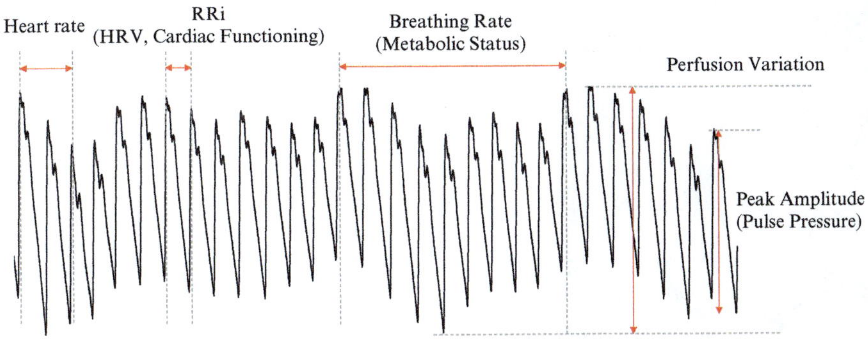

Figure 13.7 Different signal processing and machine learning techniques can be applied to PPG signals to extract useful metrics.

13.4.3 Wearable Devices for HF Prognostic Application

It was reported from a study of 50 patients with HF that the step-counts for two weeks can significantly differentiate New York Heart Association classes [39]. This cohort used accelerometer data to monitor the physical activity during HF as a prognostic measure. Another retrospective study [40] on 189 patients with self-reported HF showed that physical activity has a significant relation with HF-related mortality. This study was also carried out using accelerometer data. A similar prospective study was done on 170 Japanese HF patients, which showed that activity data acquired through the wrist-worn devices were associated with mortality; in both the studies randomized controlled clinical trials and physical activity monitoring using the smartwatches were used for epidemiological investigation (e.g. increased aerobic capacity and better health-related quality of life) [41]. Regular, daily physical activity can lower the risk of heart disease as, primarily, it can help to control weight and reduce the chances of developing other straining heart conditions such as high blood pressure, high cholesterol, and type 2 diabetes [42, 43]. Although it can be summarized from these studies that that wearing devices for HF prognostic application has a strong relationship with reducing HF-related mortality, to the best of our knowledge, there is no clinical HF-related service available yet in the world to routinely use the wearables to assess the patient activity.

13.4.4 Monitoring Blood Pressure

Hypertension is one of the major causes of HF. Clinical therapy has mostly been offered based on a single assessment in the clinic or in home visit by the clinicians. In general, wearable devices still lack reliability in measuring blood pressure; however, the Omron™ HeartGuide (Figure 13.8) has met the American National Standards Institute criteria for measuring blood pressure and such wearable devices can be used to monitor potential HF patients and also the implication of therapeutic treatment on blood pressure.

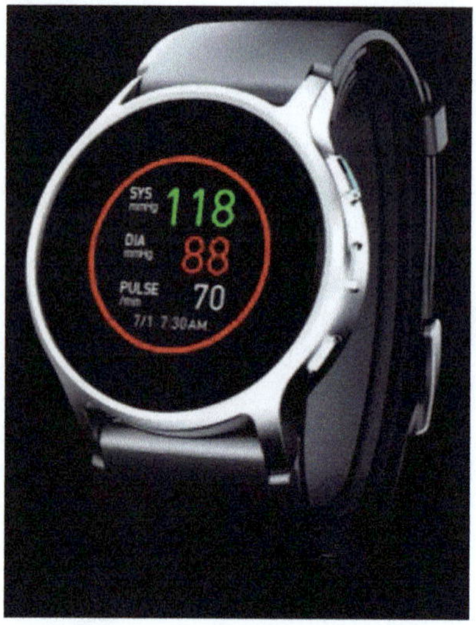

Figure 13.8 Omron HeartGuide [44].

13.4.5 Arrhythmia Detection

Several life-threatening arrhythmias that lead to HF are atrial fibrillation (AF or AFib), ventricular tachycardia (VT or V-tach), and ventricular fibrillation (VF or VFib). However, there are very few wearable solutions available for real-time monitoring and detection of VT and VF. On the other hand, there is a good number of wearable solutions available for AF detection. The main challenges in wearable VT or VF detection are due to the complexity of developing an ECG system in wristwatches and wristbands. Moreover, irregular pulses cannot be easily detected by analyzing the PPG signal without confirming the ECG signals [46]. Ambulatory monitoring of the ECG signals is often done using Holter monitors, but Cardioskin, Carnation™ patch, VivaLNK™, and similar chest patches are becoming popular because they can be used for several days comfortably for ECG monitoring and are more convenient than the Holter devices (Figure 13.9) [47].

The Cardioskin is a wearable, wireless medical device, which allows the acquisition, recording, storage, transmission, and display of a 15-lead ECG to analyze potential cardiac pathological abnormalities. The Carnation Ambulatory Monitor (CAM) – is a lightweight, bandage-size cardiac patch monitor engineered to capture low amplitude, low-frequency electrical signals that form the P-wave. This focus on the P-wave is a major advancement for cardiologists and cardiac rhythm specialists to aid in diagnosing an arrhythmia. The CAM patch is designed to be accurate, promote patient compliance, streamline clinical workflow, and yield clinically actionable data. VivaLNK is stuck to the skin to record ECG waveforms, respiratory rate, heart rate, RR interval, and patient movement, and so has potential to help detect cardiac arrhythmias such as AF. Weighing only 0.26 ounces (7.5 grams), it has all the electronics of a single-lead ECG, an accelerometer, a rechargeable battery, and wireless connectivity. Electrodes can also be woven

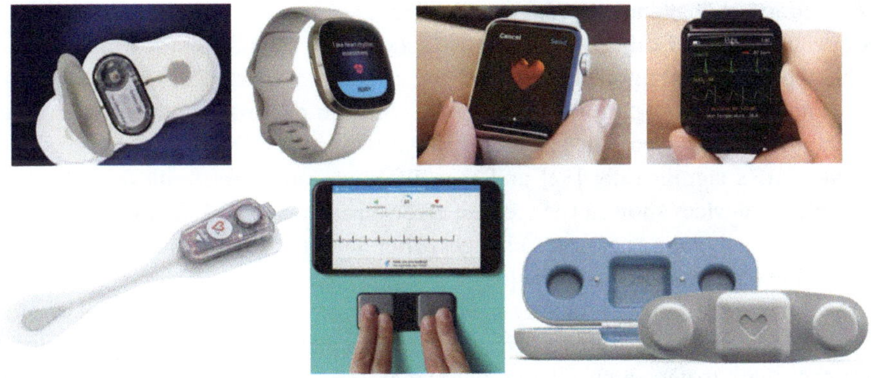

Figure 13.9 Smart wearable devices for arrhythmia detection.

into a "smart textile" vest for prolonged multilead ECG monitoring. ECG monitoring through wearables can therefore be useful for the diagnosis of AF. All three can be worn for several days at a time for continuous ECG monitoring more comfortably and for longer than a standard Holter monitor. The Apple Heart Study has utilized a PPG-based algorithm to identify irregular pulses which can be utilized to screen AF patients without previous history of AF [48]. However, these types of studies should be validated with the concurrent ECG recording in adopting these devices for clinical applications. KardiaMobile, from AliveCor (Mountain View, CA) is typically paired with a smartphone to monitor ECG signals in mobile phones and can be used for AF detection. Philips has released a cardio and motion monitoring module called Philips health watch, which can detect bradycardic and tachycardia with a sensitivity of 85% and 99%, respectively [49]. The E4 wristband from Empatica Inc. (Boston, MA) has a smart application that can discriminate AF from atrial tachycardia and flutter, and premature ventricular contractions with an accuracy of 0.8 using a machine learning algorithm [49]. These devices have received clearance from the US FDA.

A significant increase in the interest in remote monitoring of cardiac and coronavirus disease (COVID-19) patients and their hemodynamic monitoring was reported in patients with implantable sensors and wearable ECG sensors for detecting AF using off-the-shelf solutions HeartLogic™ and CardioMEMS [45].

13.4.6 Technology in Development for Early Detection of HF Decompensation

ZOLL μCor is a patch-based ECG monitor using a radiofrequency sensor and transmitter to measure pulmonary fluid content in the heart and was assessed for predicting HF decompensation in a clinical trial [1]. Several electrodes were embedded in the textile to measure heart rate, heart rate variability, respiration rate, and cardiothoracic impedance with a device-level algorithm using HeartLogic [50]. A smart sock was proposed by [51] to monitor edema and activity using the accelerometer and stretch sensor, which showed high accuracy in measuring ankle circumference and activity for a healthy cohort.

13.4.6.1 Practical Challenges to Wearable Devices

There are hundreds of off-the-shelf smartwatches, smart bands, chest straps/patches available which can monitor physical activity, sleep, and heart rate. However, smartwatches and bands do not perform similarly to a chest strap or patch. It has been reported that even on healthy subjects the performance of different wearable devices in measuring heart rate varies significantly [52] and that although, on a treadmill, there is some agreement, the devices showed the greatest error during cycling [52]. Most of the them fail in measuring dynamic heart rate changes. Therefore, these devices are most suitable for measuring resting-state heart rate [53].

Due to the wide range of variability in activity, subject movements, and form factors of wearable devices (smartwatches, smart band, earbuds, ring, etc.), up to now it has been very difficult to get a high-fidelity PPG signal from them, leading to erroneous calculations of heart rate and other parameters [54]. From its beginnings in watches and wristbands, wearable technology has now moved to being available even in a ring form factor. Ōura [55] is a ring that has infrared LEDs, a temperature sensor, accelerometer, and gyroscope. As described at the beginning of this section, it can capture heart rate, temperature, and body movements and sleep patterns. Moreover, five major challenges can affect the performance of the optical monitoring devices: optical noise, sensor location, skin tone, crossover, and low perfusion [56]. The main technical challenge of processing a PPG signal is the noise, which will escalate in the presence of the motion artifact, thus affecting the analysis, which is mostly dependent on clean PPG signals. There have been studies done by the authors to reduce the motion artifacts from PPG signals using signal processing techniques and machine learning [57]. Only 1% of the incident light reflected the photodetector, 1% of which is modulated by the heart pumping-related blood flow variations. The rest of the incident light is scattered from the skin and body materials and, therefore, time-varying motion noise due to dynamic activities of the user makes it difficult to differentiate from real blood flow-related variations. The ear, lower or upper arm, and wrist are the popular wearable device locations. The earlobe is the best place among them as it can provide the best quality signals with minimum affect from the motion artifacts. However, the wrist should be choice for wearable devices to ensure the acquisition of better quality motion-free signals, while the upper arm or forearm can be the better option, compared to the wrist, for higher signal-to-noise (SNR) PPG signal acquisition as there is a higher density of blood vessels close to the surface of the skin. There is a wide variety of skin tones present among the world population and there are six classes among them according to Fitzpatrick Scale [58]. Skin tone variation changes the pattern of absorption. PPG sensor depends on the skin tone of the user's wearing the sensor. Darker skin will absorb more green light and will make it hard to produce reliable PPG signals and thereby other metrics. One of the major challenges of these wearable devices is observed with periodic activity. Most often periodicity of this activity falls with the range of heartbeats. The process of delivering blood to the capillary bed is called perfusion, which significantly varies among the population particularly with diabetes, heart problem, obesity, and other arterial problems.

13.5 Summary of the Cardiac and Wearable Device Data Sets

There is a large number of data sets publicly available for ECG recording. Recently, several data sets have been released for research and PhysioNet has a large collection of ECG data sets. A team from Chapman University and Shaoxing People's Hospital (Shaoxing Hospital Zhejiang University School of Medicine) has collected and disseminated a novel database that contains 12-lead ECGs of 10,646 patients with a 500 Hz sampling rate that features 11 common rhythms and 67 additional cardiovascular conditions, all labeled by professional experts. The data set consists of 10-second, 12-dimension ECGs and labels for rhythms and other conditions for each subject [59]. Another large recent large ECG data set is the PTB-XL ECG dataset [60] containing 21,837 clinical 12-lead ECGs from 18,885 patients of 10-second length. The raw waveform ECG data was annotated by two cardiologists, who assigned potentially multiple ECG statements in each record.

An ECG image data set was released for CVD and COVID-19 patients with 1937 distinct patient records [61]. The data were collected using the ECG device EDAN SERIES-3 from different healthcare institutes across Pakistan. The data set was manually reviewed by experts to categorize them into five distinct categories (COVID-19, abnormal heartbeat, myocardial infarction (MI), previous history of MI, and normal person). ECG data were collected using a 12-lead ECG device which can be used for machine learning-based model development for CVD detection among COVID and other CVD patients.

Bogu et al. [5] reported heart rate and steps data from 106 individuals using wearable devices. There were 25 COVID-19 +, 11 non-COVID-19 illnesses with self-reported symptoms, and 70 healthy individuals with no symptoms or illness during the COVID-19 period (February 2020 to June 2020) were reported in this data set. Resting heart rate was computed by selecting the heart rate intervals where steps were zero for 12 minutes ahead of an interrogated time point.

Similarly, Mishra et al. [10] used the data from consumer smartwatches for the presymptomatic detection of COVID-19. Using retrospective smartwatch data, they showed that 63% of the COVID-19 cases could have been detected before symptom onset in real-time via a two-tiered warning system based on the occurrence of extreme elevations in the resting heart rate relative to the individual baseline. The investigation was carried out on nearly 5300 participants; however, 32 patients infected with COVID-19 were identified from the cohort, and the rest weree in the control group.

The MyHeart Counts study [62] used an iOS app among 110,056 users from March 9, 2015, to October 28, 2015. The study cohort described here is composed of contributions from study participants who designated broad sharing of their data (n = 34,189). Among consenting participants, 4900 (10.2%) completed a 6-minute walk test at the end of day 7 in the study. The 6-minute walk test activity not only collects distance traveled but also accelerometry during the walk. Additionally, MyHeart Counts users were able to upload data from wearable devices compatible with HealthKit. Table 13.1 summarizes some recent cardiac and wearable device data sets.

Table 13.1 Summary of different wearable device studies' data sets on heart disease.

Study	Device Design	Number of Patients with HF	Primary Outcome	Main Findings
Hershman et al. [62]	MyHeart Counts Study	50,000	Physical activity, sleep, and cardiovascular health data	Importance of physical activity and fitness for long-term cardiovascular health
Bogu et al. [5]	Fitbit-One (San Francisco, CA)	106	Heart rate and steps	An abnormal resting heart rate during the period of viral infection (7 days before the symptom onset and 21 days after) in 92%
Mishra et al. [10]	Fitbit-One (San Francisco, CA), smartwatch, Apple watches, and Garmin device	5262	Disease dates, as well as symptom dates, diagnosis dates, heart rate, and steps	Physiological and activity data from 32 individuals infected with COVID-19, identified from a cohort of nearly 5300 participants, and found that 26 of them (81%) had alterations in their heart rate, number of daily steps, or time asleep
Wagner et al. [60]	12-lead ECG system	18,885	Four class ECG data	Data set released for investigation
Zheng et al. [59]	GE MUSE ECG system	10,646 patients including 5956 males and 4690 females	11 common rhythms and 67 additional cardiovascular conditions	Data set released for investigation
Cook et al. [63]	Fitbit-One (San Francisco, CA)	22	Steps/day, length of stay, discharge disposition	Wireless monitoring of mobility after major surgery was feasible and practical
Thorup et al. [64]	Fitbit-One (San Francisco, CA)	13	Pedometer	Cardiac telerehabilitation at a call center can support walking activity using commercial pedometers
Redfield et al. [65]	Kersh activity monitor (Richardson, TX) Kionix Accelerometer (Ithaca, NY, subsidiary of ROHM, Inc. Japan)	110	Daily activity level	During all dosage regimens, activity in the isosorbide mononitrate group was lower than that in the placebo group

(Continued)

Table 13.1 (Continued)

Study	Device Design	Number of Patients with HF	Primary Outcome	Main Findings
Dontje et al. [66]	Sense Wear Pro3 armband (BodyMedia, Inc., Pittsburgh, PA)	68	Steps/day; METs	The variance in daily physical activity in patients with HF is considerable; approximately half of the patients had a sedentary lifestyle
Athilingam et al. [15]	Zephyr BioHarness and/or BioPatch (Medtronic, Dublin, Ireland)	25	Confidence in the use of a device	Patients reported moderate self-confidence in using HeartMapp, a mobile health application for the management of chronic HF
Chan et al. [67]	AliveCor, (San Francisco, CA)	97	AF detection	Community screening for AF with smartphone-based wireless single-lead ECG was feasible and it identified a significant proportion of citizens with newly diagnosed AF
Amir et al. [68]	ReDS	50	HF readmission	HF readmissions at 3 months were reduced by 87%
Bensimhon et al. [69]	Seismocardiography	110	Blood flow through the arteries accompanying each heartbeat	Hospital discharge with the vest and found 32% of patients had significant residual lung congestion
Inan et al. [70]	Ballistocardiogram and seismocardiogram device	45	6-minute walk test	Seismocardiogram signal analysis from a wearable can assess compensated and decompensated HF states
Elian et al. [71]	Textile sensors	161	Weight accuracy	Weight measurements from shoe integrated pressure sensors are inaccurate

13.6 Machine Learning for Improving Cardiac Health of HF Patients

The advances in machine learning for biomedical applications have stimulated the use of wearables for continuous monitoring and abnormality detection [35]. The authors have worked on solutions to detect heart attacks amongst drivers using models trained on public databases (MIT-BIH ST Change Database) and a conventional machine learning model (support vector machine algorithm), showing an accuracy of about 97.4 % and 96.3 % in detecting ST-elevation myocardial infarction (STEMI) and non-ST-elevation MI (NSTEMI), respectively [72].

The authors have also worked on another solution to continuously monitor the heart sound and use it to train the machine learning model on the 2016 PhysioNet Challenge database, consisting of different classes of heart sounds, to detect abnormal heart sounds with an accuracy of 97% [73]. There have been studies to use machine learning techniques to classify HF patients using the eight strongest derived predictors (age, creatinine, hemoglobin, weight, heart rate, systolic blood pressure, mean arterial pressure, and income) of mortality, these have shown much more promising classification of HF patients than conventional methods, in terms of prognostication and response to medications [74]. In the future, the life-saving LVAD for HF patients can be further improved in HF prediction, using machine learning techniques with the help of a miniature high-configuration low-power-consuming microcontroller (Figure 13.10).

Machine learning techniques can be useful even in the management aspects of HF patients, e.g. identification of patients who might adhere to the prescribed medications or might need additional measures for treatment adherence. Machine learning approaches can also be utilized to identify HF patients at high risk for additional comorbidities (such as depression) or in remote HF monitoring systems to improve HF clinical outcomes. To protect implantable devices from cybersecurity assaults, effective machine learning algorithms have been used. When compared with traditional methodologies, machine learning approaches have been successful in developing score models with improved measure estimates regarding the prediction of cardiac resynchronization therapy (CRT) responders.

ECG-based wearables, such as the Apple Watch (Apple, Cupertino, CA), mobile ECG equipment, and temporary patches are all helping to advance ambulatory heart rhythm assessment (e.g. Zio patch from iRhythm Technologies, San Francisco, CA). Wearables can generate a multiple-lead ECG with a single touch, allowing patients to self-screen in the event of any symptomatic episode. As mentioned in section 13.4.5, machine learning models are used with AliveCor's KardiaMobile, which combines cellphones as a mobile ECG monitor. In the iTransmit13 and iREAD14 tests, these wireless devices had 100% percent and 96.6% sensitivity and 97% and 94.1% specificity for AF detection, respectively, using machine learning models. Tison et al. in [76] trained a deep neural network using PPG heart rate recordings exhibited a sensitivity of 98.0% and specificity of 90.2% in detecting AF, compared to a 12-lead ECG-based analysis. The sensitivity and specificity

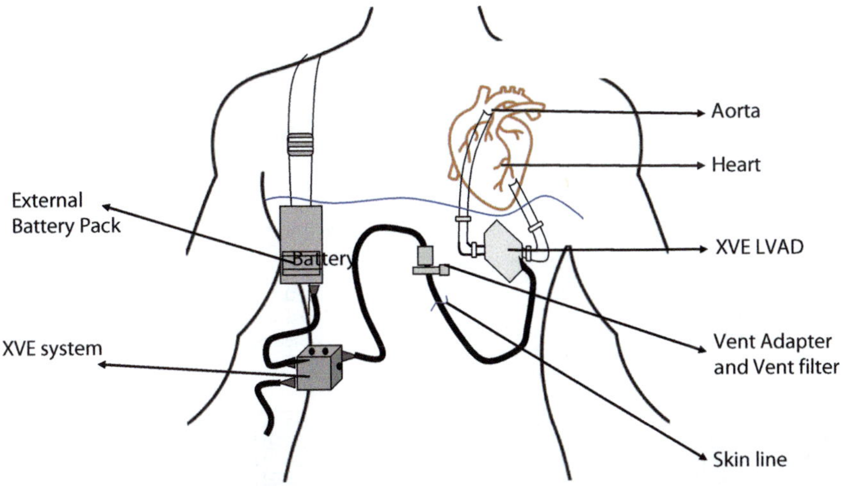

Figure 13.10 Using machine learning algorithms in LVAD to take actions when symptoms of HF are detected.

of smart bands were found to be in a range of 75.4–97.0% and 94–100%, respectively, while smartwatches showed a sensitivity of 67.7–100% and a specificity of 67.6–98%.

There have been studies that proposed the use of selfies and machine learning models to detect heart abnormalities such as coronary artery diseases (CADs). Facial appearance has long been identified as a marker of cardiovascular risk, with features such as male pattern baldness, earlobe crease, xanthelasmata, and skin wrinkling being the most common predictors. Information extracted from the analysis of an individual's facial photo utilizing the proposed technology can unquestionably benefit the individual, the attending physician, and the healthcare system altogether. Early detection of individuals at risk for CAD can initiate lifestyle and other personal mitigation approaches, guide medication treatment, and inspire a novel approach in diagnostic testing and screening algorithms for the general population. Despite these challenges, the full potential of such novel and out-of-the-box diagnostics lies ahead to the research community. The framework proposed in [77] suggested the use of facial images and deep learning techniques for early detection of patients with risk of CAD (Figure 13.11).

Lin et al. [78] evaluated this framework, where they conducted a multicenter cross-sectional study of patients undergoing coronary angiography or computed tomography angiography at nine Chinese sites to train and validate a deep convolutional neural network for the detection of CAD (at least one > 50% stenosis) from patient facial photos. The performance was compared with radiologist diagnosis. Results concluded that a deep learning algorithm based on facial photos could assist in CAD detection in the Chinese cohort. This technique holds promise for pre-test CAD probability assessment in outpatient clinics or CAD screening in the community. Table 13.2 summarizes the findings of different studies.

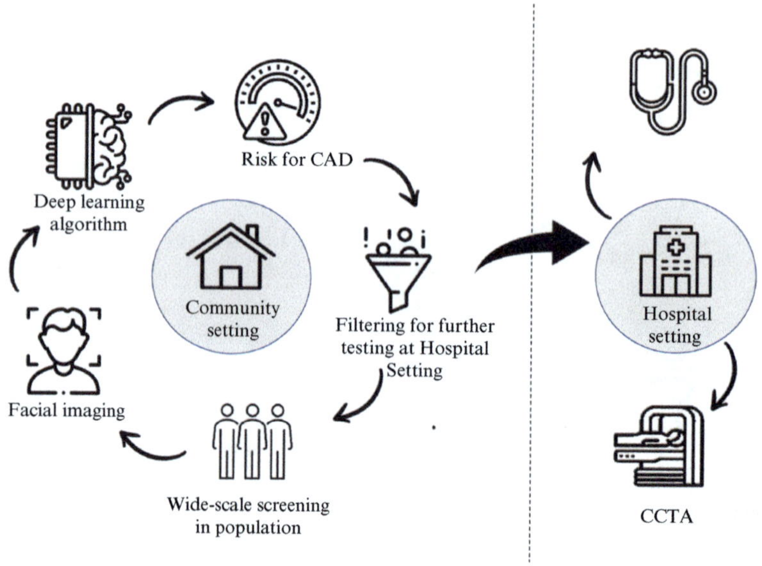

Figure 13.11 Proposed framework to use selfies to screen patients with CAD.

Table 13.2 Summary of researches to improve cardiac health of HF patients.

Study	Description	Key Findings
Chowdhury et al. [72]	Heart attack amongst drivers using machine learning models on MIT-BIH ST Change Database	ST-elevation and non-elevation myocardial infarction detection accuracies are 97.4% and 96.3%, respectively.
Chowdhury et al. [73]	Abnormal heart condition detection using heart sounds from 2016 PhysioNet Challenge Database	Heart abnormality detection accuracy of 97%
Bazoukis et al. [74]	Classify HF patients' mortality using the eight predictors (age, creatinine, hemoglobin, weight, heart rate, systolic blood pressure, mean arterial pressure, and income)	Better classification of HF patients than conventional methods, in terms of prognostication and response to medications
Eisen [75]	Life-saving LVAD for HF patients for HF prediction using machine learning techniques	LVADs may be alternatives to cardiac transplantation in selected patients
Ip et al. [48]	Apple Heart Study has utilized a PPG-based algorithm to identify the irregular pulses	Better screening AF patients without previous history of AF
Dagher et al. [49]	KardiaMobile (AliveCor) can be used for AF detection while Philips health watch can detect bradycardic and tachycardia.	Philips health watch has a sensitivity of 85% and 99%, respectively.

(Continued)

Table 13.2 (Continued)

Study	Description	Key Findings
Dagher et al. [49]	E4 wristbands discriminate AF from atrial tachycardia and flutter, and premature ventricular contractions using machine learning algorithm	E4 wristband has an AUC of 0.8
Miller et al. [45]	HeartLogic and CardioMEMS can be used for AF detection	Implantable sensors and wearable ECG sensors were used for detecting AF
Singhal et al. [1]	ZOLL μCor ECG monitor using a radiofrequency sensor and transmitter to measure pulmonary fluid content in the heart to assess HF decompensation	Successfully used for clinical trial
Tison et al. [76]	A deep neural network was trained using PPG heart rate recordings in detecting AF	This exhibited a sensitivity of 98.0% and specificity of 90.2%
Kotanidis et al. [77]	A framework to use the facial images and deep learning techniques for early detection of patients with risk of CAD	It shows a potential use of facial images using mobile phone to detect risk of CAD disease
Lin et al. [78]	A multicenter cross-sectional study of patients undergoing coronary angiography or computed tomography angiography at nine Chinese sites was conducted to train and validate a deep convolutional neural network for the detection of CAD	This technique hold promise for pre-test CAD probability assessment in outpatient clinics or CAD screening

13.7 Future Directions of Wearables for Early Prediction of HF

It is well known that an ECG of healthy individuals can have morphological variabilities/abnormalities at the baseline with variable prevalence. Similarly, patients following cardiac abnormalities can develop persistent abnormal ECG changes, which can be detected early if they are continuously monitored. This is where machine learning can play a really important role. Machine learning models can be used to detect heart abnormalities at an early stage, but the models should be made aware of how abnormalities might look and that they might be different for different patients. The authors are working on such a machine learning paradigm that can detect cardiac abnormalities for a specific patient early and can instruct the patient, along with their doctor and caregiver, to take precautionary actions (Figure 13.12).

Such a system would adhere to the following framework: (i) continuously record the ECG signals of a patient using a chest strap or patch, (ii) the existing benchmark database will be used to develop a machine learning model to classify the abnormal heart condition, (iii) the existing data set of HF patients will always have healthy and unhealthy ECG signals; healthy ECG signals of a person will be used to generate unhealthy signals of that patient and will be validated with the existing database, (iv) real-time acquired

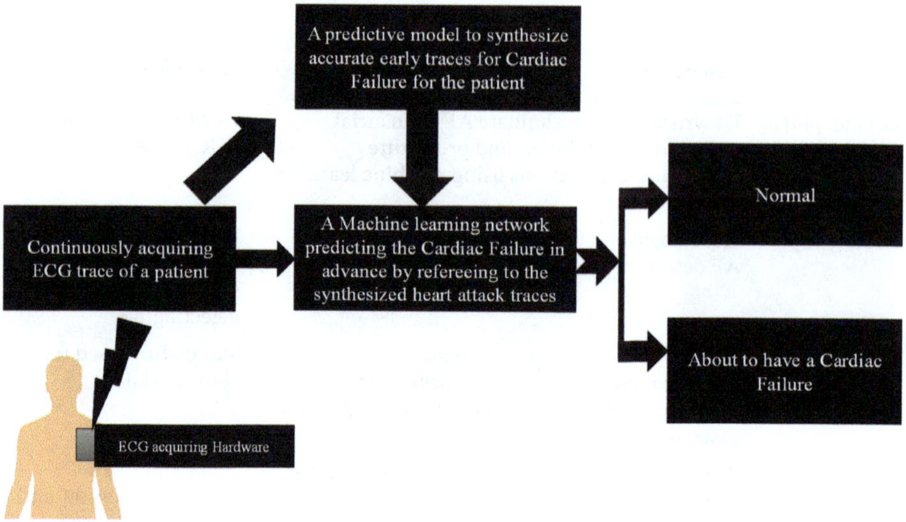

Figure 13.12 Concept of machine learning in automatically detecting a cardiac failure.

ECG signals will be used to continuously monitor the HF patient's heart condition to immediately identify if there is an abnormal heartbeat being produced, and (v) abnormal beats will be recorded and notified to the user, doctor, and caregiver, significantly helping inpatient management.

Acknowledgment

This work was made possible by NPRP12S-0227-190164 and NPRP11S-0108-180228 from the Qatar National Research Fund, a member of the Qatar Foundation, Doha, Qatar. The statements made herein are solely the responsibility of the authors.

References

1 Singhal, A. and Cowie, M.R. (2020). The role of wearables in heart failure. *Current Heart Failure Reports* 17: 125–132.
2 Maggioni, A.P., Dahlström, U., Filippatos, G., Chioncel, O., Leiro, M.C., Drozdz, J., et al. (2013). EURObservational Research Programme: Regional differences and 1-year follow-up results of the Heart Failure Pilot Survey (ESC-HF Pilot). *European Journal of Heart Failure* 15 (7): 808–817.
3 Ioana Dumitru, M.M.B. (2021). *Heart Failure Treatment & Management* [Online]. Available https://emedicine.medscape.com/article/163062-treatment. [February 20, 2020].
4 Drew, D.A., Nguyen, L.H., Steves, C.J., Menni, C., Freydin, M., Varsavsky, T., et al. (2020). Rapid implementation of mobile technology for real-time epidemiology of COVID-19. *Science* 368 (6497): 1362–1367.

5 Bogu, G.K. and Snyder, M.P. (2021). Deep learning-based detection of COVID-19 using wearables data. *medRxiv*.

6 Seshadri, D.R., Davies, E.V., Harlow, E.R., Hsu, J.J., Knighton, S.C., Walker, T.A., et al. (2020). Wearable sensors for COVID-19: A call to action to harness our digital infrastructure for remote patient monitoring and virtual assessments. *Frontiers in Digital Health* 2: 8.

7 Khan, H., Kushwah, K., Singh, S., Urkude, H., Maurya, M.R., and Sadasivuni, K.K. (2021). Smart technologies driven approaches to tackle COVID-19 pandemic: A review. *3 Biotech* 11 (2): 1–22.

8 Radin, J.M., Wineinger, N.E., Topol, E.J., and Steinhubl, S.R. (2020). Harnessing wearable device data to improve state-level real-time surveillance of influenza-like illness in the USA: A population-based study. *The Lancet Digital Health* 2 (2): e85–e93.

9 Whitelaw, S., Mamas, M.A., Topol, E., and Van Spall, H.G. (2020). Applications of digital technology in COVID-19 pandemic planning and response. *The Lancet Digital Health*.

10 Mishra, T., Wang, M., Metwally, A.A., Bogu, G.K., Brooks, A.W., Bahmani, A., et al. (2020). Pre-symptomatic detection of COVID-19 from smartwatch data. *Nature Biomedical Engineering* 4 (12): 1208–1220.

11 Shah, M., Zimmer, R., Kollefrath, M., and Khandwalla, R. (2020). Digital technologies in heart failure management. *Current Cardiovascular Risk Reports* 14 (8): 9.

12 Jeffrey, K. and Parsonnet, V. (1998). Cardiac pacing, 1960–1985: A quarter century of medical and industrial innovation. *Circulation* 97 (19): 1978–1991.

13 Thorup, C., Hansen, J., Grønkjær, M., Andreasen, J.J., Nielsen, G., Sørensen, E.E., et al. (2016). Cardiac patients' walking activity determined by a step counter in cardiac telerehabilitation: Data from the intervention arm of a randomized controlled trial. *Journal of Medical Internet Research* 18 (4): e69–e69.

14 DeVore, A.D., Wosik, J., and Hernandez, A.F. (2019). The future of wearables in heart failure patients. *JACC. Heart Failure* 7 (11): 922–932. 2019/11/01/.

15 Athilingam, P., Labrador, M.A., Remo, E.F.J., Mack, L., San Juan, A.B., and Elliott, A.F. (2016). Features and usability assessment of a patient-centered mobile application (HeartMapp) for self-management of heart failure. *Applied Nursing Research* 32: 156–163.

16 Wu, J., Roy, J., and Stewart, W.F. (2010). Prediction modeling using EHR data: Challenges, strategies, and a comparison of machine learning approaches. *Medical Care* 48 (6).

17 Awan, S., Sohel, F., Sanfilippo, F., Bennamoun, M., and Dwivedi, G. (2017). Machine learning in heart failure: Ready for prime time. *Current Opinion in Cardiology* 33: 1. 11/01.

18 Austin, P.C., Tu, J.V., Ho, J.E., Levy, D., and Lee, D.S. (2013). Using methods from the data-mining and machine-learning literature for disease classification and prediction: A case study examining classification of heart failure subtypes. *Journal of Clinical Epidemiology* 66 (4): 398–407.

19 Kang, Y., McHugh, M.D., Chittams, J., and Bowles, K.H. (2016). Utilizing home healthcare electronic health records for telehomecare patients with heart failure: A decision tree approach to detect associations with rehospitalizations. *Computers, Informatics, Nursing: CIN* 34 (4): 175–182.

20 Wilkins, E., Wilson, L., Wickramasinghe, K., Bhatnagar, P., Leal, J., Luengo-Fernandez, R., et al. (2017). European cardiovascular disease statistics 2017. Brussels: European Heart Network. https://ehnheart.org/images/CVD-statistics-report-August-2017.pdf

21 Benjamin, E.J., Blaha, M.J., Chiuve, S.E., Cushman, M., Das, S.R., Deo, R., *et al.* (2017). Heart disease and stroke statistics—2017 update: A report from the American Heart Association. *Circulation* 135 (10): e146–e603.

22 Volterrani, M., Spoletini, I., Angermann, C., Rosano, G., and Coats, A.J. (2019). Implantable devices for heart failure monitoring: The CardioMEMS™ system. *European Heart Journal Supplements* 21 (Suppl. M): M50–M53.

23 Iellamo, F., Sposato, B., and Volterrani, M. (2020). Telemonitoring for the management of patients with heart failure. *Cardiac Failure Review* 6.

24 Shah, M., Zimmer, R., Kollefrath, M., and Khandwalla, R. (2020). Digital technologies in heart failure management. *Current Cardiovascular Risk Reports* 14 (8): 1–8.

25 (2021). *Cardiomems Implantation* [Online]. Available https://www.azheartarrhythmia.com/contents/ep-procedures/cardiomems-implantation. [February 15, 2020].

26 Nelson, B.D., Karipott, S.S., Wang, Y., and Ong, K.G. (2020). Wireless technologies for implantable devices. *Sensors* 20 (16): 4604.

27 Ristow, B., Ali, S., Ren, X., Whooley, M.A., and Schiller, N.B. (2007). Elevated pulmonary artery pressure by Doppler echocardiography predicts hospitalization for heart failure and mortality in ambulatory stable coronary artery disease: The Heart and Soul Study. *Journal of the American College of Cardiology* 49 (1): 43–49.

28 Ibtehaz, N. and Rahman, M.S. (2020). PPG2ABP: Translating photoplethysmogram (ppg) signals to arterial blood pressure (ABP) waveforms using fully convolutional neural networks. *arXiv Preprint arXiv:2005.01669.*

29 Chowdhury, M.H., Shuzan, M.N.I., Chowdhury, M.E., Mahbub, Z.B., Uddin, M.M., Khandakar, A., et al. (2020). Estimating blood pressure from the photoplethysmogram signal and demographic features using machine learning techniques. *Sensors* 20 (11): 3127.

30 Kadish, A. and Mehra, M. (2005). Heart failure devices: Implantable cardioverter-defibrillators and biventricular pacing therapy. *Circulation* 111 (24): 3327–3335.

31 (2021). *Pacemaker Insertion* [Online]. Available https://www.spectrumhealthlakeland.org/population-health/health-library/Content/92/P07980. [Accessed on: 05th May].

32 Lal, D.B. (2016). *Pacemaker, ICD & CRT Implantation* [Online]. Available https://www.drlaldaga.com/Pacemaker.html. [February 23, 2020].

33 Troughton, R.W., Ritzema, J., Eigler, N.L., Melton, I.C., Krum, H., Adamson, P.B., et al. (2011). Direct left atrial pressure monitoring in severe heart failure: Long-term sensor performance. *Journal of Cardiovascular Translational Research* 4 (1): 3–13.

34 Mccarthy, J. (2019). *One in Five* U.S. *Adults Use Health* Apps, *Wearable Trackers* [Online]. Available https://news.gallup.com/poll/269096/one-five-adults-health-apps-wearable-trackers.aspx. [February 18, 2020]

35 Chowdhury, M.E., Khandakar, A., Qiblawey, Y., Reaz, M.B.I., Islam, M.T., and Touati, F. (2020). Machine learning in wearable biomedical systems. In: *Sports Science and Human Health-Different Approaches*, IntechOpen Book Series doi: 10.5772/intechopen.93228.

36 DeVore, A.D., Wosik, J., and Hernandez, A.F. (2019). The future of wearables in heart failure patients. *JACC. Heart Failure* 7 (11): 922–932.

37 Chowdhury, M.E., Rahman, T., Khandakar, A., Al-Madeed, S., Zughaier, S.M., Doi, S.A., et al. (2021). An early warning tool for predicting mortality risk of COVID-19 patients using machine learning. *Cognitive Computation* Apr 1–16 doi: 10.1007/s12559-020-09812-7.

38 Sean. (2018). *The Top 10 Best Heart Rate Monitors in the Market.* The Wire Realm. [Online]. Available https://www.wirerealm.com/guides/top-10-best-heart-rate-monitors. [February 20, 2020]

39 Baril, J.-F., Bromberg, S., Moayedi, Y., Taati, B., Manlhiot, C., Ross, H.J., et al. (2019). Use of free-living step count monitoring for heart failure functional classification: Validation study. *JMIR Cardio* 3 (1): e12122.

40 Loprinzi, P.D. (2016). The effects of free-living physical activity on mortality after congestive heart failure diagnosis. *International Journal of Cardiology* 203: 598–599.

41 Izawa, K.P., Watanabe, S., Oka, K., Hiraki, K., Morio, Y., Kasahara, Y., et al. (2013). Usefulness of step counts to predict mortality in Japanese patients with heart failure. *The American Journal of Cardiology* 111 (12): 1767–1771.

42 Kannel, W., Wilson, P., and Blair, S. (1985). Epidemiological assessment of the role of physical activity and fitness in development of cardiovascular disease. *American Heart Journal* 109 (4): 876–885.

43 King, A.C., Jeffery, R.W., Fridinger, F., Dusenbury, L., Provence, S., Hedlund, S.A., et al. (1995). Environmental and policy approaches to cardiovascular disease prevention through physical activity: Issues and opportunities. *Health Education Quarterly* 22 (4): 499–511.

44 (2020). *Blood Pressure Anytime, Anywhere* [Online]. Available https://omronhealthcare.com/products/heartguide-wearable-blood-pressure-monitor-bp8000m. [accessed on: May 5, 2020].

45 Miller, J.C., Skoll, D., and Saxon, L.A. (2021). Home monitoring of cardiac devices in the era of COVID-19. *Current Cardiology Reports* 23 (1): 1–9.

46 Chan, P.H., Wong, C.K., Poh, Y.C., Pun, L., Leung, W.W.C., Wong, Y.F., et al. (2016). Diagnostic performance of a smartphone-based photoplethysmographic application for atrial fibrillation screening in a primary care setting. *Journal of the American Heart Association* 5 (7): e003428.

47 Vardas, P., Cowie, M., Dagres, N., Asvestas, D., Tzeis, S., Vardas, E.P., et al. (2020). The electrocardiogram endeavour: From the Holter single-lead recordings to multilead wearable devices supported by computational machine learning algorithms. *EP Europace* 22 (1): 19–23.

48 Ip, J.E. (2019). Wearable devices for cardiac rhythm diagnosis and management. *JAMA* 321 (4): 337–338.

49 Dagher, L., Shi, H., Zhao, Y., and Marrouche, N.F. (2020). Wearables in cardiology: Here to stay. *Heart Rhythm: The Official Journal of the Heart Rhythm Society* 17 (5): 889–895.

50 Boehmer, J.P., Hariharan, R., Devecchi, F.G., Smith, A.L., Molon, G., Capucci, A., et al. (2017). A multisensor algorithm predicts heart failure events in patients with implanted devices: Results from the MultiSENSE study. *JACC. Heart Failure* 5 (3): 216–225.

51 Fallahzadeh, R., Pedram, M., and Ghasemzadeh, H. (2016). SmartSock: A wearable platform for context-aware assessment of ankle edema. In: *2016 38th Annual International Conference of the IEEE Engineering in Medicine and Biology Society (EMBC)*. 6302–6306.

52 Cadmus-Bertram, L., Gangnon, R., Wirkus, E.J., Thraen-Borowski, K.M., and Gorzelitz-Liebhauser, J. (2017). Accuracy of heart rate monitoring by some wrist-worn activity trackers. *Annals of Internal Medicine* 167 (8): 607–608.

53 Moayedi, Y., Abdulmajeed, R., Posada, J.D., Foroutan, F., Alba, A.C., Cafazzo, J., et al. (2017). Assessing the use of wrist-worn devices in patients with heart failure: Feasibility study. *JMIR Cardio* 1 (2): e8.

54 Bayoumy, K., Gaber, M., Elshafeey, A., Mhaimeed, O., Dineen, E.H., Marvel, F.A., et al. (2021). Smart wearable devices in cardiovascular care: Where we are and how to move forward. *Nature Reviews: Cardiology* 18, 581–599.

55 (2021). *Know why you feel how you feel* [Online]. Available https://ouraring.com. [February 20, 2020]

56 LeBoeuf, S. (2016). *Five challenges of optical heart rate monitoring*. Available: https://www.fierceelectronics.com/components/five-challenges-optical-heart-rate-monitoring. [February 18, 2020].

57 Shuzan, M.N.I., Chowdhury, M.H., Chowdhury, M.E., Uddin, M.M., Khandakar, A., Mahbub, Z.B., et al. (2021). A novel non-invasive estimation of respiration rate from photoplethysmograph signal using machine learning model. *arXiv Preprint arXiv:2102.09483.*

58 Makrides, G., Zinsser, B., Phinikarides, A., Schubert, M., and Georghiou, G.E. (2012). Temperature and thermal annealing effects on different photovoltaic technologies. *Renewable Energy* 43: 407–417.

59 Zheng, J., Zhang, J., Danioko, S., Yao, H., Guo, H., and Rakovski, C. (2020). A 12-lead electrocardiogram database for arrhythmia research covering more than 10,000 patients. *Scientific Data* 7 (1): 1–8.

60 Wagner, P., Strodthoff, N., Bousseljot, R.-D., Kreiseler, D., Lunze, F.I., Samek, W., et al. (2020). PTB-XL, a large publicly available electrocardiography dataset. *Scientific Data* 7 (1): 1–15.

61 Khan, A.H., Hussain, M., and Malik, M.K. (2021). ECG images dataset of cardiac and COVID-19 patients. *Data in Brief* 34: 106762.

62 Hershman, S.G., Bot, B.M., Shcherbina, A., Doerr, M., Moayedi, Y., Pavlovic, A., et al. (2019). Physical activity, sleep and cardiovascular health data for 50,000 individuals from the MyHeart counts study. *Scientific Data* 6 (1): 1–10.

63 Cook, D.J., Thompson, J.E., Prinsen, S.K., Dearani, J.A., and Deschamps, C. (2013). Functional recovery in the elderly after major surgery: Assessment of mobility recovery using wireless technology. *The Annals of Thoracic Surgery* 96 (3): 1057–1061.

64 Thorup, C., Hansen, J., Grønkjær, M., Andreasen, J.J., Nielsen, G., Sørensen, E.E., et al. (2016). Cardiac patients' walking activity determined by a step counter in cardiac telerehabilitation: Data from the intervention arm of a randomized controlled trial. *Journal of Medical Internet Research* 18 (4): e69.

65 Redfield, M.M., Anstrom, K.J., Levine, J.A., Koepp, G.A., Borlaug, B.A., Chen, H.H., et al. (2015). Isosorbide mononitrate in heart failure with preserved ejection fraction. *New England Journal of Medicine* 373 (24): 2314–2324.

66 Dontje, M.L., van der Wal, M.H., Stolk, R.P., Brügemann, J., Jaarsma, T., Wijtvliet, P.E., et al. (2014). Daily physical activity in stable heart failure patients. *Journal of Cardiovascular Nursing* 29 (3): 218–226.

67 Chan, N.-Y. and Choy, C.-C. (2017). Screening for atrial fibrillation in 13 122 Hong Kong citizens with smartphone electrocardiogram. *Heart* 103 (1): 24–31.

68 Amir, O., Ben-Gal, T., Weinstein, J.M., Schliamser, J., Burkhoff, D., Abbo, A., et al. (2017). Evaluation of remote dielectric sensing (ReDS) technology-guided therapy for decreasing heart failure re-hospitalizations. *International Journal of Cardiology* 240: 279–284.

69 Bensimhon, D., McLean, D., Chase, P., Wood, D., Garman, V., and Curran, L. (2017). Readiness for discharge of heart failure patients based on ReDS lung fluid measurement. *Journal of Cardiac Failure* 23 (8): S66.

70 Inan, O.T., Baran Pouyan, M., Javaid, A.Q., Dowling, S., Etemadi, M., Dorier, A., et al. (2018). Novel wearable seismocardiography and machine learning algorithms can assess clinical status of heart failure patients. *Circulation: Heart Failure* 11 (1): e004313.

71 Elian, A., Sada, N., Elfadel, I., Saeed, M., and Shabra, A. (2016). A preliminary evaluation of continuous, shoe-integrated weight measurements for heart failure patients. In: *2016 38th Annual International Conference of the IEEE Engineering in Medicine and Biology Society (EMBC)*. 4768–4771.

72 Chowdhury, M.E., Alzoubi, K., Khandakar, A., Khallifa, R., Abouhasera, R., Koubaa, S., et al. (2019). Wearable real-time heart attack detection and warning system to reduce road accidents. *Sensors* 19 (12): 2780.

73 Chowdhury, M.E., Khandakar, A., Alzoubi, K., Mansoor, S., Tahir, A.M., Reaz, M.B.I., et al. (2019). Real-time smart-digital stethoscope system for heart diseases monitoring. *Sensors* 19 (12): 2781.

74 Bazoukis, G., Stavrakis, S., Zhou, J., Bollepalli, S.C., Tse, G., Zhang, Q., et al. (2021). Machine learning versus conventional clinical methods in guiding management of heart failure patients—a systematic review. *Heart Failure Reviews* 26 (1): 23–34.

75 Eisen, H.J. (2019). Left ventricular assist devices (LVADS): History, clinical application and complications. *Korean Circulation Journal* 49 (7): 568.

76 Tison, G.H., Sanchez, J.M., Ballinger, B., Singh, A., Olgin, J.E., Pletcher, M.J., et al. (2018). Passive detection of atrial fibrillation using a commercially available smartwatch. *JAMA Cardiology* 3 (5): 409–416.

77 Kotanidis, C.P. and Antoniades, C. (2020). Selfies in cardiovascular medicine: Welcome to a new era of medical diagnostics. *European Heart Journal* 41(46): 4412–4414.

78 Lin, S., Li, Z., Fu, B., Chen, S., Li, X., Wang, Y., et al. (2020). Feasibility of using deep learning to detect coronary artery disease based on facial photo. *European Heart Journal* 41 (46): 4400–4411.

Index

Predicting Heart Failure: Invasive, Non-Invasive, Machine Learning, and Artificial Intelligence Based Methods, First Edition. Edited by Kishor Kumar Sadasivuni, Hassen M. Ouakad, Somaya Al-Maadeed, Huseyin C. Yalcin, and Issam Bait Bahadur.

X

Printed in the USA/Agawam, MA
September 16, 2026

910661.049